RENEWALS 458-4574

DATE DUE

GAYLORD			PRINTED IN U.S.A.

IMPROVING HEALTHCARE TEAM COMMUNICATION

For those who serve in healthcare

Improving Healthcare Team Communication
Building on Lessons from Aviation and Aerospace

Edited by

CHRISTOPHER P. NEMETH
The University of Chicago, USA

ASHGATE

Published by
Ashgate Publishing Limited
Gower House
Croft Road
Aldershot
Hampshire GU11 3HR
England

Ashgate Publishing Company
Suite 420
101 Cherry Street
Burlington, VT 05401-4405
USA

Ashgate website: http://www.ashgate.com

British Library Cataloguing in Publication Data
Improving healthcare team communication : building on
    lessons from aviation and aerospace
    1. Health care teams 2. Communication in medicine
    I. Nemeth, Christopher P.
    362.1'068

Library of Congress Cataloging-in-Publication Data
Improving healthcare team communication : building on lessons from aviation and aerospace
/ [edited] by Christopher P. Nemeth.
    p. cm.
    Includes bibliographical references and index.
    ISBN 978-0-7546-7025-4 (hardback : alk. paper)
    1. Health care teams. 2. Communication in medicine. I. Nemeth, Christopher P.
[DNLM: 1. Communication. 2. Patient Care Team. 3. Group Processes. 4. Interprofessional
Relations. 5. Risk Management. W 84.8 I34 2008]

    R729.5.H4I47 2008
    362.1--dc22

2007046577

ISBN 978-0-7546-7025-4

Printed and bound in Great Britain by TJ International Ltd, Padstow, Cornwall.

Contents

PART 3: HEALTHCARE TEAM COMMUNICATION IN THE FIELD

PART 4: FUTURE TRENDS

List of Figures

List of Tables

Notes on Contributors

Charles E. Billings is affiliated with the Cognitive Systems Engineering Laboratory at the Ohio State University. He is a Clinical Professor Emeritus in Preventive Medicine at the Ohio State University and a Fellow of the Aerospace Medical Association and the Royal Aeronautical Society. Prior to returning to the University, he was chief scientist at the NASA Ames Research Center, where in 1975 he and his colleagues developed and implemented the NASA Aviation Safety Reporting System (ASRS).

Adelaïde Blavier has a PhD in psychology and works as a senior researcher thanks to a grant of the Belgian National Fund of Scientific Research at the Department of Cognitive Ergonomics (Prof. AS Nyssen) of the University of Liège, Belgium. With a background in neuropsychology and cognitive psychology, her domain of research concerns the visual perception and more specifically, the depth perception, visual attention and eye movements, in relation to human errors in complex systems.

Marianne J. Brandwijk, MD practices Pediatric Critical Care Medicine. While performing her fellowship in pediatric critical care at The University of Chicago Medical Center, Dr. Brandwijk studied how clinicians perform cognitive work in the Pediatric Intensive Care Unit (PICU) with particular attention to technical work issues.

Jeffrey P. Brown, MEd, is engaged in patient safety research and improvement initiatives concerned with interdisciplinary decision making and teamwork. In 2002, he joined a cardiac surgery care team in receiving a John M. Eisenberg Patient Safety Award for System Innovation from the Joint Commission and the National Quality Forum. He served as advisor and consultant in the development of an interdisciplinary decision-making methodology that significantly improved the safety and quality of care for post-operative open heart surgery patients. His affiliations include Klein Associates Division of Applied Research Associates and the University System of New Hampshire, USA. Prior to 1996, he served as a faculty member and department chair for university aviation programs. He has authored and co-authored a number of articles and book chapters on patient safety. Brown earned his MEd and BS degrees from the University of Maine.

Richard I. Cook, MD is a physician, educator, and researcher at the University of Chicago. His current research interests include the study of human error, the role of technology in human expert performance, and patient safety. He is internationally recognized as a leading expert on medical accidents, complex system failures, and human performance at the sharp end of these systems. Dr. Cook's most often cited publications are 'Gaps in the continuity of patient care and progress in patient safety', 'Operating at the Sharp End: The complexity of human error', 'Adapting to New Technology in the Operating Room', and the report 'A Tale of Two Stories:

Contrasting Views of Patient Safety.' Dr. Cook regularly practices clinical procedures at various sites in the University of Chicago Medical Center. Home page : <http://www.ctlab.org/Cook.cfm>

Brian Cuthbertson (MD, FRCA) is a Senior Lecturer in Anaesthesia and Intensive Care at the University of Aberdeen. His research interests include the improvement of patient outcomes from critical illness, with investigations focusing upon patient safety, teamwork, the early recognition of critical illness, and quality of life after ICU care.

Eric M. Eisenberg, PhD, is Professor of Communication at the University of South Florida. He received his doctorate from Michigan State University in 1982. Dr Eisenberg twice received the National Communication Association Award for the outstanding research publication in organizational communication, as well as the Burlington Foundation award for excellence in teaching. He is also the recipient of the Ohio University Elizabeth Andersch Award for significant contributions to the field of communication. Dr Eisenberg is the author of over 75 articles, chapters, and books on the subjects of organizational communication, health communication, and communication theory. His best-selling textbook *Organizational Communication: Balancing Creativity and Constraint* (currently in its fifth edition) received the Academic Textbook Author's "Texty" award for the best textbook of the year. He is an internationally recognized researcher, teacher, and consultant specializing in the strategic use of communication to promote positive organizational change. Home page: <http://www.cas.usf.edu/communication/eisenberg/index.html>.

Rod Elford, BPE, MD, CCFP, MSc, is the first Canadian physician to complete formal training in telehealth, specifically a two-year international clinical research fellowship in telemedicine and a master's degree in child telepsychiatry. He is a founding member of the Canadian Society of Telehealth and the International Society for Telemedicine. Dr Elford is the co-founder and director of Digital Telehealth Incorporated and has worked as a telemedicine consultant for many organizations, including the Canadian Space Agency. He is a Clinical Assistant Professor at the University of Calgary, associated with the Centre for Health Information Technology Innovation. Currently, Dr Elford is the Medical Director for Health Link Alberta, a province-wide health call center. He continues to practice as an urgent care physician.

Mica R. Endsley, PhD, is recognized as a world leader in the study and application of situation awareness in advanced systems. Dr Endsley has authored over 200 scientific articles and reports on situation awareness and is often cited in professional journals. Dr Endsley has a PhD in Industrial and Systems Engineering from the University of Southern California. As founder and president of SA Technologies, Dr Endsley leads a team of researchers, designers and engineers in situation awareness research, advanced system design, and professional writing and seminars.

Rhona Flin (Bsc, PhD Psychology) is Professor of Applied Psychology in the School of Psychology at the University of Aberdeen, UK. She directs a team of psychologists working with high risk industries and health care on research and consultancy projects concerned with the management of safety. The group focuses on topics such as human error, decision-making, situation awareness, teamwork, leadership, safety climate and risk perception.

Ute Fischer is a research scientist in the School of Literature, Communication and Culture at the Georgia Institute of Technology. After receiving her PhD in Cognitive Psychology from Princeton University, she was a post-doctoral fellow and then a senior research scientist at the NASA Ames Research Center. Her current projects concern the effects of team composition and team training approaches on the interaction and decision strategies of small teams, such as flight crews and mission specialists.

Leila Johannesen, PhD, is a user experience engineer with IBM, focusing on database information management tools. Her areas of speciality are: usable graphical user interfaces, usability testing, accessibility for persons with disabilities, autonomic systems, and human error. She received her PhD from Ohio State University's Cognitive Systems Engineering program in 1994.

Madelyn Kahana, MD is the Associate Chair of Pediatrics for Education and the Program Director for the Pediatric Residency Program at The University of Chicago Medical Center. She is Section Chief of Pediatric Critical Care and a Professor of Anesthesia and Pediatrics. She is board certified in pediatrics, anesthesiology and critical care medicine. Dr. Kahana has specific interest and expertise in the perioperative care of the child with congenital heart disease and pediatric sedation and pain management. She has a national reputation for excellence in clinical care and teaching and regularly attends in the pediatric intensive care unit and on the pediatric sedation service.

P. Allan Klock, MD, is a board certified anesthesiologist, and an Associate Professor and Vice Chair for Clinical Affairs in the Department of Anesthesia and Critical Care at the University of Chicago. He has an undergraduate degree in Biomedical Engineering and specializes in anesthesia for urologic surgery and difficult airway management. His research interests include difficult airway management, patient outcomes and administrative and economic issues.

Julie Kowalsky, MD recently completed studies for her medical degree at The University of Chicago and is scheduled to begin her residency in radiation oncology. While in the Summer Research Program in 2004, Dr. Kowalsky performed research on the technical work of critical care medicine with particular attention to the analysis of between shift hand-offs.

David M. Musson, MD, PhD, is a physician and social psychologist whose work focuses on the human performance under stress and in safety critical settings. He completed his MD at the University of Western Ontario in 1988, and a rotating internship at the University of Toronto in 1990. He served as a flight surgeon in the Canadian Forces for five years where he was involved in flight safety and fighter aircrew support. He received a PhD in Social and Personality Psychology in 2003 at the University of Texas at Austin under the supervision of Robert Helmreich. Dr

Musson is currently the Academic Director of the Centre for Clinical Simulation at McMaster University, and an Associate Professor in the Department of Anesthesia. His recent research has examined the role of personality testing in astronaut selection, the nature of professional cultures, and the translation of error reduction strategies, such as Crew Resource Management, from aviation to medicine.

Christopher P. Nemeth, PhD, studies human performance in complex high hazard environments as a Research Associate (Assistant Professor) at the Cognitive Technologies Laboratory at the University of Chicago. Recent research interests include technical work in complex high stakes settings, research methods in individual and distributed cognition, and understanding how information technology erodes or enhances system resilience. His design and human factors consulting practice and his corporate career have encompassed a variety of application areas from healthcare to transportation and manufacturing. His consulting practice has included human factors analysis, expert witness, and product development services. His academic career has included adjunct positions with Northwestern University's McCormick College of Engineering and Applied Sciences (Associate Professor), and Illinois Institute of Technology. He retired from the Navy in 2001 at the rank of Captain after a 30-year active duty and reserve career. His book on human factors research methods, *Human Factors Methods for Design*, is now available from Taylor and Francis/CRC Press. Home page: <http://www.ctlab.org/Nemeth.cfm>.

Mark Nunnally, MD is a physician, educator and researcher at the University of Chicago. As a clinician, Dr. Nunnally performs surgical procedure anesthesia in the operating room. He also performs critical care medicine as an attending intensivist in the Surgical, Cardiothoracic and Burn Intensive Care Units (ICUs). Dr. Nunnally's research interests concern the role of technology in patient safety. His work explores a technology fallacy: that technology, instead of consistently improving patient safety, often contributes to failure in novel, unexpected ways. His work to date has focused on infusion devices, delivery systems and incident reporting.

Anne-Sophie Nyssen is Doctor of Work Psychology and Professor of Cognitive Ergonomics at the University of Liege, Belgium. Her main interest is in the study of human error in cognitive complex systems. Her PhD research on Human Error in Anaesthesia identified the role of contextual, cognitive, and organizational variables on performance. Progressively, the research extended in scope to assess the impact of technology changes on cognition. For the last ten years, she has contributed to the development and use of simulations for training and research on medical expertise. In 1999, she received a grant from NATO to do post-PhD research at Stanford University with Professor David Gaba. In the same year, her research project to develop a system-wide health care critical incident reporting system in Belgium was approved for funding by the Office of the Prime Minister of Belgium. Central to her lab is the use of multiple techniques to collect data in order to understand the complexity of work systems: *in situ* observation, questionnaire, interview, observation of performance in simulated situations and spartan lab settings.

Michael F. O'Connor, MD is a physician, educator and researcher at the University of Chicago. His clinical work is a combination of critical care medicine (where he attends in the Medical, Surgical, Cardiothoracic and Burn ICUs), and operating room anesthesia, where his activity has been centered on anesthesia for liver transplantation. His educational activity is centered around his clinical activity. Dr. O'Connor is also Director of the Senior Medical Student Selective 'Vignettes in Physiology'. His clinical research has included new drug development (atracurium, sevoflurane, propofol, etomidate, methylnaltrexone, antithrombin, activated recombinant protein C, linezolid, and several blood substitutes), clinical research in critical care (bedside assessment of autoPEEP, use of propofol as a sedative, management of sedation in critically ill patients), and now patient safety. He has lectured about the social science of accidents in a variety of settings.

Judith Orasanu, PhD, is a Principal Investigator at the NASA Ames Research Center where she studies team communication, distributed team decision making, and crew performance in aviation and space environments. Her research on shared mental models, decision strategies, risk assessment, and error detection and correction has been adopted in the aviation, medical, nuclear power, military, offshore oil and other high-risk industries. Dr Orasanu's current research is concerned with developing tools and technologies to support space flight crews for NASA exploration missions to the Moon. Her contribution to the nascent field of naturalistic decision making resulted in the first book in the field, *Decision Making in Action: Models and Methods* (edited by G. Klein, J. Orasanu, R. Calderwood, and C. Zsambok, Ablex Publishers, 1993).

Emily S. Patterson, PhD, conducts human factors research to improve joint cognitive system performance in complex, socio-technical settings, including healthcare, military, intelligence analysis, space shuttle mission control, emergency response, and emergency call centers. She is a Research Scientist at the VA Getting at Patient Safety (GAPS) Center and the Institute for Ergonomics at the Ohio State University. Her current lines of research include medical informatics to improve patient safety, handover communications to transfer authority, making systems resilient to human error, and rigor in information analysis. She has published extensively in diverse academic outlets, including 26 journal articles and eight book chapters. She serves as a Centers Communication Advisory Group Member for the Joint Commission International Center for Patient Safety, Advisory Board Member for ECRI's Health Technology Forecast, and Editorial Board Member for *Human Factors*.

Tom Reader, MA, PhD Psychology, is a research psychologist within the Industrial Psychology Research Centre at the University of Aberdeen. His primary research interests include patient safety, teamwork and situation awareness in intensive care and other acute medical environments. Further research interests include safety climate, risk perception, and worker health and well-being in sectors such as oil and gas, aviation, and air traffic control. Prior to his academic career, Tom worked in the UK offshore oil and gas industry. Home page: <http://www.abdn.ac.uk/~psy409/dept/>

Philip J. Smith is affiliated with the Cognitive Systems Engineering Laboratory at the Ohio State University. He is a Professor in the Industrial and Systems Engineering program, with extensive experience in the design of distributed work systems and decision support tools, including the design of the Post-Operations Evaluation Tool, an analysis system used by the FAA and the airlines to evaluate performance in the US airspace system.

Amy L. Spencer is affiliated with the Cognitive Systems Engineering Laboratory at the Ohio State University. She is a doctoral student in the Industrial and Systems Engineering program, and also has considerable previous work experience in the design of cognitive tools to support collaborative decision making in the airspace system.

Jennifer Watts-Perotti, Ph.D., is a Cognitive Engineer in the Work Practices team, in the Xerox Innovation Group. She has conducted ethnographic studies at Microsoft, Apple, NASA, Kodak, and Xerox. She is currently studying human interaction with production printing systems. Prior to her current position, she worked as an interface designer, ethnographer, and user experience researcher at Kodak. She received her Masters and Ph.D. from Ohio State University, where the research presented in her chapter was conducted.

Robert L. Wears, MD, MS is an emergency physician and holds an advanced degree in computer science. He is currently Professor in the Department of Emergency Medicine at the University of Florida, and Visiting Professor with the Clinical Safety Research Unit at Imperial. Dr Wears has been an active writer and researcher with interests in technical work studies, joint cognitive systems, and particularly the impact of information technology on safety and resilient performance. His work has been funded by the Agency for Healthcare Research and Quality, the National Patient Safety Foundation, the Emergency Medicine Foundation, the Society for Academic Emergency Medicine, the Army Research Laboratory, and the Florida Agency for Health Care Administration. Dr. Wears performs regular shifts as an active member of the emergency department clinical staff at his medical center.

David D. Woods, PhD, is affiliated with the Cognitive Systems Engineering Laboratory at the Ohio State University. He is a Professor in the Industrial and Systems Engineering program, with extensive experience with research in resilience engineering, first in nuclear power (Nuclear Regulatory Commission), later in aviation (Federal Aviation Administration), in healthcare (as Associate Director of the first VA Midwest Patient Safety Center of Inquiry from 1999-2003) and most recently at NASA as part of the Columbia Investigation Accident Board (CAIB).

Melanie C. Wright, PhD, is an Assistant Professor in the Department of Anesthesiology at the Duke University Medical Center. She completed her PhD in Industrial Engineering at North Carolina State University. She has 15 years' experience in engineering and research in the areas of human performance, usability analysis, and human-machine system design. Dr Wright is currently active in research related to information management in the peri-operative environment, and the training and assessment of team coordination skills in dynamic environments.

Foreword

Significant questions about healthcare safety demand substantive answers. What needs to be changed in order to improve healthcare work efficiency, reliability, and safety? What changes will actually make a difference? Without an adequate basis in research, notions about how to improve healthcare safety amount to only a collective guess.

Current ideas about how to improve healthcare safety have the nature of folk remedies that are passed along without understanding whether or how they actually work. Many are imported from other sectors such as manufacturing with no proof that they actually create an improvement or, if they do, whether they are suited to healthcare. This is not new. Observers within healthcare have noted this lack of insight for decades (see Cook, Woods and McDonald 1989). Clinicians' conventional views on what is admissible as scientific activity have prevented them from understanding this (Auerbach, Landefeld and Shojania 2007) and from relying on other professionals from outside healthcare. As a result, healthcare has few skills or resources to genuinely study safety at the systems level when compared with other high hazard sectors such as nuclear power generation, the military, and aviation. This shortfall makes it difficult to know what does and does not matter in the clinical setting, much less what to do about it.

While interventions suggest progress, interventions with no basis in science do more damage than good. They make systems more brittle (Sarter, Woods and Billings 1997): unable to change in response to circumstances. They induce unforeseen outcomes, waste time and resources that could be spent more productively, and delay progress toward genuine improvement. Efforts to improve healthcare safety must start with understanding it as a system (Woods and Cook 2002). This begins with understanding its *technical work*, which is the planning and management that is intimately bound up with medical care (Cook, Woods and Miller 1998). Surveys and statistical analyses have attempted to describe what occurs at the sharp (operator) end of healthcare, but these are one or more steps removed from what actually happens in the real world. Rather than illuminate the complexity of clinical work, they obscure it by averaging out complex internal details (Cilliers 1998). By contrast, the authors in this book have immersed themselves in healthcare's messy, confusing, and challenging details in order to discover how clinicians develop their own strategies to confront and surmount daily challenges (Nemeth, Cook and Woods 2004). Insights from such studies reveal how gaps can occur in care continuity (Cook, Render and Woods 2002), how systems change to fit demand, and how people anticipate and respond with gap-filling adaptations to delay or prepare for upcoming events (Woods and Hollnagel 2006). Knowing the actual nature of real work leads to the creation of more resilient systems that are able to anticipate and respond to inevitable change (Hollnagel, Woods and Leveson 2006).

These chapters are the start of a core of knowledge about the healthcare technical work that is based in well-considered, scientific, methodical research. Using this approach makes it evident how work is actually done. This is altogether different from the way that work is imagined by those who do not understand it. The difference matters, because notions about how to improve the work of healthcare and get traction in the real world must start with the deep understanding that this text describes.

David Woods
Institute for Ergonomics
The Ohio State University

References

Auerbach, A.D., Landefeld, C.S. and Shojania, K.G. (2007), 'The Tension between Needing to Improve Care and Knowing How to Do It', *New England Journal of Medicine* 357:6, 608–13.

Cilliers, P. (1998), *Complexity and Postmodernism: Understanding Complex Systems* (London, UK: Routledge).

Cook, R., Render, M. and Woods, D. (2000), 'Gaps in the Continuity of Care and Progress on Patient Safety', *British Medical Journal* 320, 791–4.

Cook, R., Woods, D. and McDonald, J.S. (1989), 'On Attributing Critical Incidents to Factors in the Environment', *Anesthesiology* 71:5, 808.

Cook, R., Woods, D. and Miller, C. (1998), *A Tale of Two Stories: Contrasting Views of Patient Safety* (Chicago: National Health Care Safety Council of the National Patient Safety Foundation, American Medical Association). <http://www.npsf. org>, accessed June 8, 2002.

Hollnagel, E., Woods, D. and Leveson, N. (2006), *Resilience Engineering: Concepts and Precepts* (Aldershot, UK: Ashgate Publishing).

Nemeth, C., Cook, R. and Woods, D. (2004), 'The Messy Details: Insights from Technical Work in Healthcare', in C. Nemeth, R. Cook and D. Woods (eds), Special Issue on Studies in Healthcare Technical Work, *IEEE Transactions on Systems, Man and Cybernetics-Part A* 34:6, 689–92.

Sarter, N., Woods, D. and Billings, C. (1997), 'Automation Surprises', in G. Salvendy (ed.), *Handbook of Human Factors and Ergonomics* (New York: John Wiley and Son) 1926–43.

Woods, D. and Cook, R.I. (2002), 'Nine Steps to Move Forward from Error', *Cognition, Technology and Work* 4:2, 137–44.

Woods, D. and Hollnagel, E. (2006), *Joint Cognitive Systems: Patterns in Cognitive Systems Engineering* (Boca Raton, FL: Taylor and Francis; CRC Press).

Preface

Among 24 gaps in patient safety research, Cooper (2000: 5, 69) identified four that bear directly on human factors, and "research about communication and information sharing among healthcare providers" was ranked third. This book strives to fill that gap.

As a service sector, healthcare relies heavily on the availability, quality, accuracy, and timing of information. Sharing problem detection and problem solving among members of a team broadens expertise and the range of attention, it avoids fixation, and it makes it easier to work in parallel and reorganize (Klein 2006). Communication is the vehicle for the information that is crucial to effective teamwork, as tasks and roles are broken into manageable parts, performed, and reassembled into a whole. The chapters in this book show how research reveals the ways in which clinicians capture, modify, use, and share information that changes continuously in response to the large and small challenges and opportunities of daily work.

This text deals primarily with communication among clinicians as a verbal experience at the task level. Certainly, there are other approaches to communication that can shed light on the topic such as theoretical models, social network theory, non-verbal communication, social psychology, and large scale coordination of cognitive work. Also, recent work (Xiao et al. 2001; Wears et al. 2003; Nemeth et al. 2006) has described how clinicians develop and use cognitive artifacts to maintain a distributed cognition. Inter-personal communication among clinicians and with patients is often cited as a problem that healthcare organizations need to improve (Meryn 1998). In fact, some consider clinician–patient communication to be the main ingredient in medical care. Because that topic has been well covered elsewhere (Ong et al. 1995), the goal of this book is to explore communications between and among health professionals, which is substantial enough to fill an entire volume.

This text takes a pragmatic approach in order to "cut to the chase" by addressing real issues that clinicians need to grasp and apply directly to their work. I invite your interest in, and comments on, the chapters that follow.

Christopher P. Nemeth
Cognitive Technologies Laboratory
The University of Chicago

References

Cooper, J.B. (2000), *Current Research in Patient Safety in the US* (Chicago: National Patient Safety Foundation).

Klein, G. (2006), 'The Strengths and Limitations of Teams for Detecting Problems', *Cognition, Technology and Work* 8:4, 227–36.

Meryn, S. (1998), 'Improving Doctor Patient Communication: Not an Option, But a Necessity', *British Medical Journal* 316:7149, 1922–30.

Nemeth, C., O'Connor, M., Klock, P.A. and Cook, R.I. (2006), 'Discovering Healthcare Cognition: The Use of Cognitive Artifacts to Reveal Cognitive Work', in Special Issue on Naturalistic Decision Making, R. Lipshitz (ed.), *Organization Studies* 27:7, 1011–35.

Ong, L.M., deHaes, J.C., Hoos, A.M. and Lammes, F.B. (1995), 'Doctor-Patient Communication: A Review of the Literature', *Social Science and Medicine* 40:7, 903–18.

Wears, R.L., Perry, S.J., Shapiro, M., Beach, C., Croskerry, P. and Behara, R. (2003), 'A Comparison of Manual and Electronic Status Boards in the Emergency Department: What's Gained and What's Lost?', *Proceedings of the Human Factors and Ergonomics Society 47th Annual Meeting* (Santa Monica, CA: HFES).

Xiao, Y., Lasome, C., Moss, J., Mackenzie, C.F. and Faraj, S. (2001), 'Cognitive Properties of a Whiteboard: A Case Study in a Trauma Centre', *Proceedings of the Seventh European Conference on Computer-Supported Cooperative Work* (Norwell, MA: Kluwer Academic Publishers) 259–78.

Acknowledgements

The editor thanks Robert Wears, MD, for his gracious service and insightful comments as reviewer for each chapter in this text.

Thanks to David Woods and Ashgate Publishing editor Guy Loft for the opportunity to edit this volume. Thanks also to Michael F. O'Connor who offered insightful comments on drafts of Chapter 1.

The authors who have contributed to this text have been generous with their time and thoughts. Those who are the subjects of study, from many walks of life and kinds of work, have made this publication possible. I offer my thanks and appreciation to all.

Dr Nemeth's research is funded by support from the Agency for Healthcare Research and Quality, and the US Food and Drug Administration.

Chapter 1

The Context for Improving Healthcare Team Communication

Christopher P. Nemeth

It is not unusual to find communication failure cited as a "root cause" of healthcare accidents. Single factor solutions, such as standards for how to conduct hand-offs, are recommended in reaction to such conclusions. James Reason's (1997) description of the factors that contribute to adverse events makes it clear that changing a single factor such as communication cannot overcome the multiple threats to safety in complex systems. This text, then, is not about whether improvement to communications between and among clinicians and patients can solve issues related to healthcare safety. It is: "How can healthcare information be shared better?" and "What can we expect from its improvement, and how do we get there?"

Erik Hollnagel (2004) suggests in Figure 1.1 how understanding adverse events and their causes evolves through time as we develop and use established ways of thinking about how an accident happens. Among technology and equipment, organizations, and human performance, attributions to the latter have peaked over the past 40 years. By implication, attributions to the organization are on the upswing. Among sequential, epidemiologic, and systemic accident models, the systemic model suggests that adverse as well as positive results emerge from daily operations. The research in this text largely follows the systemic model to account for the interactions of clinicians with technology and equipment as well as organizations. The traits of healthcare systems mold the properties, needs, and strategies that require team communication.

Like its high hazard sector counterparts such as aviation, nuclear power generation, ground transportation, and the military, healthcare is typically risky, complex, uncertain, and time-pressured. Staff resources are constrained in a number of ways including availability, qualifications, shift, and rank. Decisions can, and do, have severe consequences. However, healthcare has additional characteristics that make it unique from other high hazard sectors. Guidelines for clinical practice are not consistent and in some instances actually conflict with each other. Demands for care are uncertain, vary widely, and are in a continual state of change. Work is performed on compromised systems (patients) whose affliction and response to treatment is not predictable, can be difficult to assess, and may vary widely. Patients may, or may not, comply with therapeutic regimens. Patient condition, diagnoses, and the procedures to treat them are highly context-specific and individualized. In order to meet these characteristics of the demand for care, equipment and supplies are configured ad hoc—assembled and adapted to fit the individual patient and specific procedure. Decisions on the acquisition of highly sophisticated clinical equipment are routinely made by staff members who have no clinical experience and are advised by clinicians who have no experience in the technical evaluation of complex products or systems.

% Attributed cause

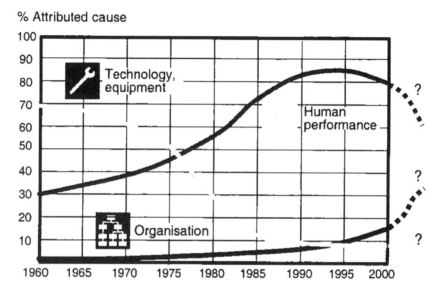

Figure 1.1 Trends in causes attributed to "accidents"
Source: Hollnagel 2004: 46.

Medical care for patients requires substantial cognitive work. *Technical work* (Cook, Woods and Miller 1998), which is the many practical and essential activities that are needed to perform medical care, also requires cognitive work. This is because what is needed for an individual patient depends on the timely synchronization of people, equipment, tools, and facilities. The planning and management of procedures for an entire suite of operating rooms (ORs) or an intensive care unit (ICU) require a similar kind of coordination. Both the individual level and the collective unit level require the performance of cognitive tasks that include the assessment of resource availability, resource allocation, the anticipation and prediction of future events, speculation about the best courses of action, negotiation to develop consensus, and trade-off decisions.

Characteristics of work in an organization can be compared to a wedge that has both sharp and blunt ends. At the sharp end, practitioners perform work applying expertise and actions using the resources at hand to generate results. Care providers work in various kinds of groups than can be ill-defined, fluid, and may overlap. They must negotiate multiple constraints in their work domains as they perform complex activities that routinely have significant consequences. The blunt (management) end develops policies, procedures, resources, and constraints that support and shape work at the sharp end (Cook, Woods and Miller 1998: 13, 36). While blunt end cognitive work is more evident, cognition is more difficult to discern the closer one gets to the sharp end. This is because sharp end knowledge is dense, complex, changes rapidly, and is embedded in a complex social setting that resists exposure to those who are considered to be "outsiders." Clinicians deliberately set the thresholds for access to this setting higher in order to thwart scrutiny and each facility imposes additional controls to protect patient privacy.

Why This Text Matters

One of the reasons behind the popularity of "fixing" healthcare communications is that it is an available target. After all, facilities are costly to build and take a long time. Equipment is complex and requires specialized knowledge to develop and manufacture. Arduous certification procedures take time, money, and effort. People, though, are available and adaptable. The presumption is that if clinicians can be made to behave differently, the difficulties that are brought on by all manner of contributing factors might be eliminated or at least reduced. This view flows from the notion of iatrogenic medical malpractice, which is based on a traditional model that emphasizes individual practitioner agency and accountability. It also stems from hindsight bias (Agans and Shaffer 1994), which leads those who know what happened after the fact to consistently overestimate what others who lacked that knowledge could have known. In reality, practitioners act in concert, collectively coping with system defects that were "created by poor design, incorrect installation, faulty maintenance and bad management decisions" (Reason 1990: 173). Multiple causes of an adverse outcome are usually present in a system as a characteristic of its routine operation. It is poor system design, poor job design, and failed systems that "contribute significantly to harmful error by providing the conditions under which error will thrive" (Sharpe and Faden 1998: 61–77, 138, 234). If failure occurs, it is a "consequence and not a cause" because failures are "shaped and provoked by upstream, workplace and organizational factors" (Reason 1997: 126) such as limited or declining resources.

Healthcare communication must necessarily be as complex as the domain that it is intended to control (Ashby 1956; Conant and Ashby 1970). Contributions by Jens Rasmussen, James Reason, Erik Hollnagel, David Woods, Richard Cook, Yan Xiao and others have demonstrated how healthcare is a variable high stakes sector that is molded by a complex array of factors. "Team" encompasses more than a few individuals, from shifts, clinics, and departments, to clinicians, managers, technicians, suppliers, patients, consultants, and other transferring or receiving care organizations. Healthcare teams can also be fluid, shifting, can overlap, and include strangers as well as colleagues. "Communication" encompasses verbal exchange, but also includes other means to transfer information that include physical artifacts (for example, lists, status boards, schedules, orders, records, and notes), electronic systems (for example, databases, software programs, equipment displays, and controls), as well as phones, pagers, and personal digital assistants.

Views of the way that work is performed also shape notions of the tools that are intended to support it. Recent research into cognition at large scale (Nemeth 2007) in healthcare demonstrates the scope and level of effort that is necessary to understand it. Such studies rely on cognitive systems engineering (CSE) methods (Hollnagel and Woods 1983; 2005) to elicit information about work domains and to derive criteria for the development of information and communications technology (ICT) tools that are intended to aid such work. The insights that the chapters in this text contain can be used to guide the development of ICT that is intended to support healthcare cognitive work. Without the scientific analysis of such complex work, healthcare ICT systems will certainly remain clumsy (Weiner 1985), brittle (Sarter, Woods and Billings 1997), and fail to be a useful team player (Christoffersen and Woods 2002).

Team communications as it is performed in aviation is often proposed as a model for healthcare to adopt. That assumption's pristine simplicity belies the reality of healthcare's messy details (Nemeth, Cook and Woods 2004). A number of authors including Helmreich (2000), Helmreich, Musson and Sexton (2001), and Powell, Haskins and Sanders (2005) have encouraged the healthcare community to emulate the models of communications that have been developed in aviation research. Research in aviation team communication cannot be imported in its entirety to healthcare. As the introduction to this chapter explained, the domains are too different for such a simple solution to succeed. Instead, aviation should be understood in terms of what lessons will benefit healthcare communications. Rather than an ending point, research into communication in aviation provides a starting point. This text draws the connection between the lessons that have been learned through cognitive research in aviation and aerospace to cognitive research that is underway in healthcare.

How This Text is Organized

Five sections address improvement to healthcare team communications. Guest author Eric Eisenberg applies his considerable experience in team communications to describe issues that apply across high hazard sectors and to healthcare in particular. This is a valuable contemporary view of organizational communication, with a vocabulary and a framework that we can use to address the very real challenges that face healthcare systems.

Part 1 surveys the origins of research in aviation team communications as a starting point to improve communications in healthcare. Few authors have published on aviation safety as extensively as Judith Orasanu and Ute Fischer. They account for key findings in the aviation literature on aircrew effectiveness, efficiency, breakdown, interrelationships, and error mitigation, then point to lessons from that foundation which can be applied to healthcare. David Musson dispels widely held myths about crew resource management (CRM), which is one of the most popular aspects of aviation communication. Rather than leap into CRM programs, Musson cautions clinicians to better understand the presumed benefits of CRM before adopting them for use.

Part 2 covers recent work in aviation and aerospace that are less well known than flightdeck group studies and CRM, yet provide compelling lessons for healthcare. Asynchrony (conveying healthcare information across time and locations) is growing as the number of participants, and pace and complexity of the care process grows. The potential for gaps in care continuity (Cook, Render and Woods 2000) grows along with it. Two of the chapters in this section share valuable insights into effective ways to deal with asynchrony. Charles Billings, Philip Smith, and Amy Spencer leverage Dr Billings' seminal work on the Aviation Safety Reporting System to explain the implications for reporting adverse events in healthcare. Emily Patterson describes the National Aeronautic and Space Administration (NASA) use of voice loops that enables staff members to communicate asynchronously and efficiently. Melanie Wright and Mica Endsley explain the close link between healthcare communication and situation awareness—the understanding of dynamic information that is critical for task performance.

In Part 3, recent research in acute healthcare provides a well-grounded understanding of cognitive work and communication among teams. Tom Reader, Rhona Flin, and Brian Cuthbertson describe how variations in care provider perceptions influence ICU team communication. Nemeth et al. describe how clinicians create their own highly plastic forms of hand-offs between shifts in a pediatric ICU as a way to minimize gaps in the continuity of care. Jeff Brown reveals how clinicians collaboratively cross-check each other by detecting, verbalizing, and correcting work in order to sustain safety. Leila Johannesen employs an analytic approach to show how teams maintain a common ground of understanding during complex and extended surgical procedures in the OR.

Part 4 looks to the future of team communications in healthcare, taking particular note of the role that technology will play in both public and professional settings. Anne-Sophie Nyssen and Adélaïde Blavier examine how the addition of a major player – a robotic surgery unit – affects team communication in the OR. Rod Elford shares his insights into telehealth, noting how the ways that remote populations currently rely on Internet resources for healthcare information suggest future aspects of communication among patients and clinicians. Finally, Nemeth and Robert Wears offer thoughts on the future of healthcare team communication and what it will take for further research in this arena to get traction in the real world of clinical practice.

Conclusion

The chapters amply draw the connection from one high hazard sector to another, demonstrating that lessons from aviation and aerospace do inform team communication in healthcare. Their value lies not in the wholesale adoption of procedures, though, but rather in the insights that come from intense study of complex sharp end activities. More than anything, aviation and aerospace research points out *how to learn* about team communication. The text's value is not to provide definitive conclusions, but rather to signal a research approach and agenda that will make it possible to better understand and improve team communications in healthcare.

References

Agans, R.P. and Shaffer, L.S. (1994), 'The Hindsight Bias: The Role of the Availability Heuristic and Perceived Risk', *Basic and Applied Social Psychology* 15:4, 439–49.

Ashby, W.R. (1956), *An Introduction to Cybernetics* (London: Chapman and Hall).

Christoffersen, K. and Woods, D. (2002), 'How to Make Automated Systems Team Players', in E. Salas (ed.), *Advances in Human Performance and Cognitive Engineering Research* 2, 1–12.

Conant, R.C. and Ashby, W.R. (1970), 'Every Good Regulator of a System Must Be a Model of That System', *International Journal of Systems Science* 1:2, 89–97.

Cook, R., Render, M. and Woods, D. (2000), 'Gaps in the Continuity of Care and Progress on Patient Safety', *British Medical Journal* 320:7237, 791–4.

Cook, R.I., Woods, D.D. and Miller, C. (1998), *A Tale of Two Stories: Contrasting Views of Patient Safety* (Chicago: National Health Care Safety Council of the National Patient Safety Foundation, American Medical Association). <http://www.npsf.org>, accessed June 8, 2002.

Helmreich, R. (2000), 'On Error Management: Lessons from Aviation', *British Medical Journal* 320:7327, 781–5.

Helmreich, R., Musson, D. and Sexton, J.B. (2001), 'Applying Aviation Safety Initiatives to Medicine', *Focus on Patient Safety: A Newsletter from the National Patient Safety Foundation* 4:1, 1–2.

Hollnagel, E. (2004), *Barrier Analysis and Accident Prevention* (Aldershot, UK: Ashgate Publishing).

Hollnagel, E. and Woods, D. (1983), 'Cognitive Systems Engineering: New Wine in New Bottles', *International Journal of Man Machine Studies* 18:6, 583–600.

Hollnagel, E. and Woods, D.D. (2005), *Joint Cognitive Systems: Foundations of Cognitive Systems Engineering* (New York: CRC Press).

Nemeth, C. (ed.) (2007), 'Special Issue on Large Scale Coordination: The Study of Groups at Work in Healthcare', *Cognition, Technology and Work* 9:3, 127–76.

Nemeth, C., Cook, R. and Woods, D. (2004), 'The Messy Details: Insights from Technical Work in Healthcare', in C. Nemeth, R. Cook and D. Woods (eds), Special Issue on Studies in Healthcare Technical Work, *IEEE Transactions on Systems, Man and Cybernetics-Part A* 34:6, 689–92.

Powell, S.M., Haskins, R.M. and Sanders, W. (2005), 'Improving Patient Safety and Quality of Care Using CRM', *Patient Safety and Quality Care*, July/August, <http://www.psqh.com/julaug05/delivering.html>, accessed September 26, 2006.

Reason, J. (1990), *Human Error* (New York: Cambridge University Press).

Reason, J. (1997), *Managing the Risks of Organizational Accidents* (Brookfield, VT: Ashgate Publishing).

Sarter, N., Woods, D. and Billings, C. (1997), 'Automation Surprises', in G. Salvendy (ed.), *Handbook of Human Factors and Ergonomics* (New York: John Wiley and Son) 1926–43.

Sharpe, V. and Faden, A. (1998), *Medical Harm* (Cambridge, UK: Cambridge University Press).

Weiner, E. (1985), 'Beyond the Sterile Cockpit', *Human Factors* 27:1, 75–90.

Chapter 2

The Social Construction of Healthcare Teams

Eric M. Eisenberg

Human nature is essentially collaborative. Beginning with the earliest societies, people have joined forces to pursue what they need, creating in the process a myriad of informal groups and formal institutions aimed at accomplishing various goals. Humans are social animals situated at the intersection of multiple social institutions and relationships (Eisenberg, Goodall and Tretheway 2007). Human survival literally depends on the ability to effectively form and navigate collaborative relationships.

There are, of course, many levels and kinds of collaboration. The challenge of collaboration varies in complexity depending upon the characteristics of the people and the situation at hand. A small, culturally homogenous, like-minded group of co-located people will likely find collaboration easier than a large, diverse, and geographically dispersed group. While effective communication is critical to both groups' success, what constitutes effectiveness in each case can be very different.

This chapter explores what might be meant by effective communication in the context of healthcare teams. Unlike other chapters in this book, which offer useful examples of collaborative techniques, this chapter takes a step back to consider our assumptions about communication. From this vantage point, we can better see how these assumptions affect both our understanding of and ability to engage in successful collaboration.

In the first part of the chapter, I present two contrasting models of communication as transmission and communication as social construction, and explore the criteria for effectiveness associated with each. I then provide an overview of leading social theories that present a unified view of social life by taking into account both communication models.

In the second part of the chapter, I describe the current healthcare environment, focusing on those factors that influence the effectiveness of communication and collaboration. In so doing, I compare the organizing challenges in healthcare to those faced by social institutions more generally, namely of coordinating across diverse, distributed individuals in an equivocal, shifting environment.

In the third part, I identify practical techniques for supporting coordinated action, followed by a discussion of likely impediments and obstacles to collaboration and how they might be overcome. I close with recommendations for researchers and practitioners as they seek to improve healthcare team communication.

Defining Communication and Collaboration

The first challenge facing anyone with an interest in healthcare teams is defining what is meant by effective teamwork, which in turn rests on implicit definitions of communication and collaboration. Too often, researchers and practitioners are satisfied to adopt the lay understanding of communication as linear *transmission* of messages through a conduit (Axley 1984). According to this "information engineering" approach, effective communication is the faithful and uninterrupted transmission of information that results in understanding (Feldman and March 1981; Stohl and Redding 1987). Seen this way, the main obstacle to effectiveness is physical and psychological noise in the system that can cause communication to "break down." Readers are familiar with this approach, since JCAHO's efforts to reduce medication errors and improve patient hand-offs have employed this information engineering approach almost exclusively. Callbacks, improved dispensing technology, and written orders are all laudable attempts to improve the fidelity of information transfer.

While this definition of communication as information transfer—and the practical improvements that derive from it—is useful, it does not tell the whole story. The conduit model treats communication as a defined process that occurs *within* an already established social context, and in so doing limits our ability to appreciate other, potentially more powerful, social dynamics. In contrast, *the social construction* approach focuses on the ways in which team communication creates the very context in which people work (see Leeds-Hurwitz and Galanes (forthcoming) for a recent review). This perspective maintains that "communication, rather than merely a neutral conduit for transmitting independently existing information, is the primary social process through which our meaningful common world is constructed" (Craig 2007: 127).

From a social construction perspective, efforts to improve information transmission are inherently limited because they fail to address how enduring patterns of communication both create and sustain a team's definition of itself and its situation. Seen this way, team communication is both about transmission *and* the social construction of reality, of the spoken and unspoken frameworks the team develops regarding appropriate goals, roles, and behavior. Focusing directly on the social construction of healthcare teams opens the possibility for deeper, second-order change that can be achieved through alterations in the social context. Pearce (2006: 3) underscores this optimistic stance in his characterization of social construction thinking:

> This fashion of thinking treats the events and objects of the social world—such things as beliefs, personalities, attitudes, power relationships, and social and economic structures— as *made*, not *found* (Pearce 1989, 3–31). Taking a communication perspective, the most useful questions are not "can you hear me?" or even "do you understand me?" They are "what are we making together?" or, referring to specific events or objects such as a person, an organization, or a culture, "how is it being made in the process of interaction?" or, "how can we make better social worlds?"

An illustration of the difference between the two approaches is in order. One of the most vexing problems in health communication is facilitating effective transitions of care. While mechanisms to promote effective hand-offs do exist (white boards, electronic charts, and rounding at the beginning and ends of shifts) they rarely work as well as one might hope. A commonly identified obstacle to effective communication in this context is level of acoustical noise on the unit, and many facilities have made great strides in creating a quieter environment for patients and staff. Based in a transmission model of communication, physical noise reduction makes sense as one effective tactic for improving quality of care.

The social construction approach poses a different kind of question: Not "how can the noise level be reduced?" but rather "what are the social forces that make and sustain the unit as a loud environment?" These forces include how employees are socialized and oriented to the institution and the unit; professional expectations established in school for acceptable noise levels; architectural and technological choices that promote or discourage particular interaction patterns; and so on. The social construction perspective, then, both exposes and complicates what we take for granted about communication situations by interrogating why things are as they are and proposing alternatives.

To date, most work on healthcare teams has focused squarely on information transmission, despite more than two decades of work in the field of communication developing the idea of social construction. Taking seriously the social construction of healthcare teams requires us to look more closely at what these teams are making together when they communicate, as well as how they might choose to make something different. The next section provides some theoretical and historical context for approaching communication in this way.

Communication in Social Theory

The philosopher Immanuel Kant imagined the goal of human society to be "maximum individuality within maximum community" (cf., Eisenberg 1984). This dialectical relationship between self and society has been called the central problem in social theory, reflecting humans' dual desires for agency and belonging. Moreover, this tension between individual agency and social constraint characterizes each and every social interaction, from physician rounds to faculty meetings to baseball fields to political debate. But how is this dialectical balancing act accomplished?

We create connections between self and other through communication, defined as "the moment to moment working out of the tension between individual creativity and organizational constraint" (Eisenberg, Goodall and Tretheway 2007: 36). This perspective seeks a middle ground between those who imagine human potential as largely unconstrained and those who see it as largely determined by social and economic factors (cf., Wentworth 1980). This reconciliation is achieved by recognizing how constraints develop over time, and specifically through a unique focus on the *emergent qualities of structure*.

While it is tempting to regard the social structures that constrain our activities as fixed, the social construction view argues that they are anything but. For example, health professionals are socialized to think about *time* as a scarce resource, and this way of thinking permeates every team meeting. Similarly, social forces conspire to perpetuate a status hierarchy in healthcare, which may affect how people communicate and collaborate with one another. Certain patterns of behavior get repeated over time and may eventually become reified, meaning that participants no longer see them as human creations but rather as unquestionable "reality" (Berger and Luckmann 1967).

What is needed is a more provisional concept of social structures that includes an emphasis on how they are made and reinforced over time. One proponent of such an approach is sociologist Anthony Giddens (1984), who seeks to bring a different kind of order to the long-standing micro/macro debate. Specifically, Giddens speaks of "the duality of structure," referring both to how constraints emerge from human agency and gain power over future actions. Similarly, Taylor and Van Every (2000) view human organizing as the continual interplay between texts (established rules and structures) and conversations (use of these rules and structures in daily life). In each of these perspectives, what one might call "context" is not a static container for communication, but rather a dynamic, living picture of social reality that is continually created through communication. As we look closer at healthcare teams, we should examine both their immediate patterns of communication within the present social context and the ways in which their communication over time has served to create, reinforce, or modify that context. We have a responsibility to examine the effectiveness of information transmission within social contexts *as well as* the process by which these social contexts are created.

Organizing Challenges to Healthcare Teams

A number of factors are changing the nature of work today, putting pressure on existing processes and structures. Probably the most significant change has to do with the *urgency* that healthcare institutions feel to respond to increasing demands for their services in a way that both conserves limited resources and ensures quality and safety. This sense of urgency derives in part from rising expectations for services of all kinds, and in part from increasing competition for customers.

A second trend that affects all healthcare organizations—and by implication all healthcare teams—is the rising *complexity* of their work. While a few hospitals and clinics have managed to narrowly define their mission and patient population, most continue to respond to a broad range of increasingly specialized and complex conditions. Add to this picture the uncertainty associated with the possibility of a catastrophic public health event, and the knowledge needs of the system become almost unbearable.

Moreover, the healthcare system in the United States does not have to look far to see the costs of fragmentation and complexity. Institutional responses to the terrorist attacks of 9-11 provide ample evidence of what can happen when a myriad of well-intentioned agencies fail to sufficiently coordinate their actions. Moreover, analysis of the 9-11 Commission transcripts reveal an unhelpful preoccupation with seeking to assign blame to one agency or another when there was more than enough to go around (Cooper 2007). What has become clear is that traditional models of organizing, based on armies and factories and the assumption of a placid environment, do not work in our current situation. But what might work better?

Throughout this book, you will encounter examples of institutions that are experimenting with alternatives to hierarchical organization. The most promising way of dealing with the urgency and complexity of the current environment is to design more distributed systems, with less centralized control and the capacity to act quickly to address urgent, emerging issues. This is easier said than done, as evidenced by the 9-11 report, which demonstrates the persistence of hierarchical thinking in contemporary organizational life. At the same time, there is also an indication of the power of distributed systems in the wake of 9-11, as evidenced by the superiority of ad hoc clean-up efforts over a more bureaucratic approach (Langewiesche 2003).

The kinds of communication that are effective in a distributed system are different from those found in a team existing within a traditional hierarchy. This hierarchical bias and focus on status relationships characterizes the culture of medicine and presents a significant obstacle to change. New technology and new patterns of communication to promote shared awareness can be tried in these teams, but will be limited in their effects to the extent that the overall team reality is constrained by formal rules and roles. Our challenge is to attend simultaneously to the new forms of communication we wish to advance within teams and to the communication that sustains (or could potentially transform) the social structures surrounding these new forms.

The driving force behind the formation of healthcare teams is the desire to combat fragmentation by engaging multiple perspectives on complex problems (Ellingson 2004). There exists broad consensus that to succeed in healthcare today, we must treat the whole person, and the systems perspective permeates both organizational life and everyday lived experience. No one likes fragmentation, and we like the results of it even less; hence we are responsible for collecting as much context as possible in making sense of any patient's condition. Interdisciplinarity is the spoken but rarely achieved mantra of complex organizations.

One useful way to think about the perils of fragmentation and the need for context is Browning's (1992) theory of organizational "lists and stories" that my colleagues and I have applied to emergency medicine (Eisenberg et al. 2005). We studied the difference between technical rationality—*lists* of symptoms and potential diagnoses—and narrative rationality, the patient's *story* of what was happening to them. We found patients repeatedly telling their story throughout their hospital stay to be a way of ensuring sufficient context for health team decision making. All the while, the physician's desire for certainty and the urgency of the emergency environment put constant pressure on the team to go with their lists and forgo the story.

From a social construction perspective, we can acknowledge that healthcare teams today are formed to combat fragmentation, to both encourage the flow of information and to better cope with the complexity of the environment. They succeed when they make the time to work together (no small feat), encourage individual initiative, eschew centralized control, suspend assumptions about how things are "supposed to work," and take an experimental attitude with new approaches to care and communication. But simply *calling* a group of people a healthcare team means little—the real challenge is in how that team is able to define itself in new and productive ways, along with the repertoire of practices it develops to sustain that definition. I turn next to a more detailed consideration of these practices.

Collaboration and Communication in Action

From a communication perspective, meaning only exists in context. So-called "raw data" means dramatically different things depending upon contextual information. To use a simple example from daily life, when we come across a friend who is crying, we do not immediately know what to say or do—we must first look to the context to form our interpretation (Happy or sad? Dust storm? Torn contact lens?) The same is true in healthcare teams, but the stakes are significantly higher. Still the questions are the same: "What's going on here?" and "What should we do?"

It is helpful to think of the health team context as a dynamic construction that reflects the experience of team members and updates with each new action. The implication is that teams must remain *ambivalent* toward their experience, recognizing simultaneously the value of past lessons and the possibility that the next situation may require an entirely new approach. In healthcare, there is a strong bias toward certainty, for finding the "good story" amidst a complex and often conflicted mass of information. While we must apply the lessons of experience, an over-reliance on these lessons is at the root of most incorrect action; we get into trouble when we become too attached to any particular interpretive frame or course of action and consequently lose our ability to think and act in new ways (Eisenberg et al. 2005).

The other characteristic of context in healthcare teams is that it is undeniably plural. While we may believe that teams operate with common assumptions, the reality is much more diverse. Individual sense-making is based upon personal and professional life experiences. When a team is formed, the members initially trust their judgment over that of the team. In research on group dynamics, the first stage of team development is called "storming," because the initial encounter between team members' world views is predictably conflicted. Over time, members can construct a common perspective and gain appreciation for how the varied world views represented on the team can in fact lead to better decisions than one might make individually.

The main challenge of healthcare teams, then, is to continually provide the *centripetal force* to draw members together. This is needed to build some shared view of the situation, and to engage in communication practices that encourage the airing of multiple perspectives, which may in turn cause the team to either reinforce or elaborate upon their present understanding. All the while, a host of *centrifugal forces* threaten to tear the team apart, in accord with their personal practices, professions, and commitments.

Nonetheless, it is possible to exert this centripetal force in healthcare teams, and there are numerous examples of how it can work. The rest of this chapter is organized around three aims of health team communication that together can create this centripetal force. They are:

1. Building shared situational awareness of the context. Team members engage in dialogue that promotes both diverse points of view and contributes to the development of shared mental models or world views (Senge 1990).
2. Refreshing and updating the team's understanding of the (changing) context with new information. Team members systematically scan the environment for new developments that must be taken into account in their ongoing practice.
3. Deepening each team member's capacity for heedful interrelating, that is, for acting with each other's (and the team's) perspective in mind (Weick and Sutcliffe 2001). Team members adopt a notion of team accountability and clearly connect their work to the success of the team.

Building Shared Situational Awareness

Students of organizational communication believe that an organization's effectiveness—both in terms of productivity and quality of life for employees—is determined largely by the quality of conversations that can occur there. The worst institutional environments are those where fear and politics constrain both the quantity and quality of discourse. But the best environments approximate something akin to real dialogue, the critical but supportive exchange of multiple perspectives on an issue. My colleagues and I have identified three levels of dialogue that may occur in organizations, and they are applicable to healthcare teams (Eisenberg, Goodall and Tretheway 2007). The first, dialogue as equitable transaction, occurs when "all participants have the ability to voice their opinion and perspectives" (p. 48). While straightforward, even this level of dialogue can be challenging in organizations. For example: Who gets invited to be on the team? Are there others with valuable perspectives that have been excluded because of their status or professional training? Also, when the team assembles, does the leader or facilitator create an environment where everyone feels it is safe to speak, or do the rules of the culture silence certain individuals or groups?

The second, deeper level of discourse is dialogue as empathic conversation. In this kind of communication, team members develop the ability to imagine the world as others on the team see it. This revelation, while still uncommon in healthcare, is critical to organizational effectiveness in a complex, interdependent environment. Manufacturing organizations, for example, learned decades ago that they could not provide quality products or services so long as various departments—sales, engineering, manufacturing—believed that they were the "center of the universe" without which the organization would fail. Their recognition that *everyone is* critical to the success of the whole resulted in the practice of concurrent engineering, wherein all stakeholders work side-by-side in the design process. Unfortunately, there are still many groups and individuals in healthcare who have not yet had this insight, and the teams on which they serve are the worse for it. Empathic conversation requires humility and an awareness that learning can come from anywhere, from housekeeping to administration to social work.

The third, deepest form of dialogue is real meeting, wherein each team member recognizes the common humanity of all of the team members. Put more concretely, this means refusing to treat anyone on the team as a "role," but instead as a whole individual like oneself. In some respects, real meeting is an extension of empathic conversation; it also points toward the idea of heedful interrelating, which I discuss below. Treating others as subjects (like yourself) rather than objects creates an openness to subtle cues and potentially important information that may otherwise be missed.

When team members converse, the quality of their conversation determines the degree of shared situational awareness that develops. Shared situational awareness is a critical competency for healthcare teams because it is the only way to ensure that diffuse decisions made by team members away from their meetings will be consistent. Diagnoses, prognoses, and treatment plans are all part of shared situational awareness, but so too are patient and family stories. While complete shared situational awareness is impossible, the proof is in the pudding—shared situational awareness guides effective coordination of action.

There are already in existence techniques whose main purpose is to create this kind of awareness. Certain shared artifacts—patient charts, orders, whiteboards—are all meant to provide a common point of reference and enhance group cognition. The very existence of multidisciplinary care teams is an acknowledgment of the importance of considering multiple perspectives. But these teams will not create shared situational awareness if they operate in a culture of status or fear. The use of overlapping shifts in the emergency department is another example that originated in aerospace; just as incoming air traffic controllers overlap with outgoing ones and spend that time to develop a feel for the room before they sit down at the console, so do incoming ER doctors use that overlapping time to hear the outgoing doctors and nurses' take on things, and walk the unit to get their own sense of what is happening. Patient rounds in general are designed to promote shared situational awareness, but they are too often fraught with distractions and tremendous time pressures.

Finally, shared situational awareness is not always built through synchronous communication. In a classic study of NASA and the space program, Tompkins (2006) describes in detail lab director Wernher von Braun's use of "Monday Notes" as a prompt for coordinated action. These were weekly assignments for team members to update the director on what was happening in their area, which he read, commented upon (he wrote on the notes) and distributed to the entire team. Reflecting on this process, team members recalled that the decidedly low-tech Monday Notes were one of the main ways that the scientists (especially those that were physically distant) remained on the same page. Work suffered when subsequent leaders abandoned them.

Refreshing and Updating the Context

The complexity of the healthcare environment requires individuals and teams to develop cognitive short cuts for sense-making. The unending flow of needy patients, and the ever-increasing pressure from government and insurance to cut costs, encourage a brutal cognitive environment. In this context, people rely on shorthand scripts and recipes and have little time for idiosyncratic detail.

Fortunately, these recipes work much of the time, and when they do not work, the consequences are usually minor. In a substantial minority of these cases, however, a more deliberate conversation about diagnosis and treatment would have helped tremendously. But who has the power and the will to break the rhythm of routine and call for a deliberate pause? Who has the time and inclination to treat patients whose diagnoses are unclear and hence do not have "a good story?" (Eisenberg et al. 2005).

Effective teams in all industries develop ways to "stop the assembly line" when things are beginning to spin out of control. This is critical because nearly all incorrect action in healthcare settings is caused by a series of contributing factors that unfold over time, none of which alone can account for the outcome. Responding to anomalies in real time, however, is exceedingly difficult for most people. We are inclined to see only those things that are consistent with our beliefs, and to ignore or explain away the rest. Moreover, status hierarchy discourages some members of the team from "pulling the cord" and stopping the action. Even once an adverse event has occurred, it is difficult to step back and understand fully what went wrong. Fortunately, the tradition of M & M conferences encourages at least some reflection (however formulaic), and recent advances in the reporting of "near misses" provide critical data for process improvement.

Obviously, however, the best time to improve sense-making is in the course of action, not after the fact. Teams have a distinct need to update their guiding assumptions, their shared understanding of the situation, in real time. Unfortunately, as I have outlined, there are many disincentives and not many formal opportunities to do so. The updating of context in healthcare teams is typically catch-as-catch-can, inconsistent, and on the fly. New information becomes available daily about the efficacy of medications and procedures, but very few nurses would challenge a physician with this information (nor do many physicians challenge one another). Even when new research information is brought up on health teams, status hierarchy and a general concern with saving face seriously limit the quality of dialogue and hence of decision making.

While I have explored in depth the communication challenges associated with patient hand-offs (Eisenberg et al. 2005), one must also appreciate the value of shift changes for refreshing and updating the context. Shift changes are one occasion where it is acceptable to review and potentially alter the shared understanding of, for example, a patient's situation. Could other opportunities be created for what Argyris and Schön (1978) called "double-loop learning," where team members could take a step back and question the validity of their assumptions and approach to a case? Moreover, what would have to change in the professional training of team members and in the design of facilities to make these "deliberate pauses" possible or even likely?

Promoting Heedful Interrelating

Effectiveness in complex situations requires deliberate efforts by team members to continually (re-)consider the effects of their actions in relation to the goals and actions of others. This process is called "heedful interrelating," and has been described in the context of high reliability organizations like aviation and nuclear power production (Weick and Sutcliffe 2001). The idea is that traditional hierarchies and divisions of labor diffuse responsibility and create a "not my job" attitude. The traditional solution to this state of affairs is greater oversight and centralized controls to ensure that different departments play well together. The problem with this approach is that management can never anticipate every situation where a more holistic approach would be called for; moreover, forcing collaboration through supervision only results in a half-hearted version, which is quick to dissolve when the supervisor looks the other way.

A more robust way of encouraging heedful interrelating is to communicate the big picture to all team members, and to develop practices that, when repeated, create a culture of engagement. Regarding the big picture, team leaders must never assume that members know how the system works, or their precise role in its operation. Very often, simply making the system more visible to employees goes a long way toward building heedful interrelating, in that now people understand how others use and rely upon their work. Reward systems can send a powerful message about the extent to which the organization truly values shared goals and objectives that transcend the work of any single individual or department. It is folly to wish for greater collaboration while only rewarding individual performance. Similarly, information systems can do a great deal to allow and reinforce heedful interrelating; it is easier for one to understand and support the things that one can see.

Returning to the NASA example, Tompkins (2006) celebrates an aspect of the culture that existed at the start but faded over time—automatic responsibility. At NASA, this meant that every scientist assumed responsibility for any problem he saw as within his area of competence, regardless of where it was "assigned" in the broader organization. Considered more generally, automatic responsibility is the willingness on the part of team members to maintain two identities, as a member of their department and of the organization, with critical responsibilities associated with both. We have all experienced examples of this concept in the service industry, where entry-level employees may take it upon themselves to go beyond their area to help a customer solve a problem; there are in fact many hospitals that encourage all their employees to pitch in to solve patient problems wherever they encounter them. Effective healthcare teams are those that feel some sense of shared accountability to the team as a whole, if not the organization, and are willing to act on information that falls outside of their normal job duties.

In fact, careful compliance with job duties can at times be the antithesis of shared situational awareness and heedful interrelating. A review of the 9-11 Commission transcripts (Cooper 2007) reveals few heroic characters. But one who is singled out for almost universal praise is the security screener whose broader sense of the context (and willingness to act on this sense) caused him to bend the rules and stop the last hijacker from boarding a plane that day. Lines were long and he could have easily let the individual pass. What Congress found impressive in his actions that day was his willingness to respond to a broader understanding of the situation, despite specific rules, norms, and pressures to the contrary.

Summary and Recommendations

Effective healthcare team communication is more than the accurate transmission of information. Healthcare teams are socially constructed groups situated at the intersection of multiple institutional and professional cultures. Consequently, very powerful social forces constrain how these teams can work together. In particular, socially accepted constructions of a rigid status hierarchy and a pervasive lack of time to work deliberately are just the two most apparent ones. In examining communication in healthcare teams, we must be sure to look both at the communication and the evolving context.

This book is timely because it begins with the recognition that other industries are ahead of healthcare in thinking about ways to combat fragmentation and promote systems thinking. It is clear that traditional hierarchy and division of labor are ineffective in the current environment. Healthcare teams should be at the forefront in experimenting with alternatives to hierarchy that both promote shared situational awareness and support distributed action.

To be effective, these new approaches to organizing must be aligned with other aspects of the organization, including reporting structure, technology, communication, and rewards. Teams should promote a federalist identity for their members through which they feel equally committed and accountable to their department and the team as a whole. Team leaders and members should practice dialogue skills to promote equitable participation and empathic conversation. Over time, teams should strive to deepen their understanding of one another as individuals and practice heedful interrelating.

At the same time, teams should consider changes to their processes that work in deliberate moments of reflection, opportunities to "check in" about what we know about a case so far and to change direction if necessary. Healthcare teams should take responsibility for creating an environment for their own communication that supports effective collaboration and cognition. Any team that takes on this challenge will surely have the benefit of both the transmissional and constructionist perspectives on communication.

References

Argyris, C. and Schön, D. (1978), *Organisational Learning: A Theory of Action Perspective* (Reading, MA: Addison Wesley).

Axley, S. (1984), 'Managerial and Organizational Communication in Terms of the Conduit Metaphor', *The Academy of Management Review* 9:3, 428–37.

Berger, P. and Luckmann, T. (1967), *The Social Construction of Reality* (New York: Penguin).

Browning, L.D. (1992), 'Lists and Stories as Organizational Communication', *Communication Theory* 2:4, 281–302.

Cooper, S. (2007), *Making Sense of 9-11*, unpublished doctoral dissertation (Department of Communication, University of South Florida).

Craig, R. (2007), 'Pragmatism in the Field of Communication Theory', *Communication Theory* 17:2, 125–45.

Eisenberg, E. (1984), 'Ambiguity as Strategy in Organizational Communication', *Communication Monographs* 51:3, 227–42.

Eisenberg, E., Goodall Jr., H.L. and Tretheway, A. (2007), *Organizational Communication: Balancing Creativity and Constraint*, 5th edition (New York: St. Martin's Press).

Eisenberg, E., Murphy, A., Sutcliffe, K., Wears, R., Schenkel, S., Perry, S. and Vanderhoef, M. (2005), 'Communication in Emergency Medicine: Implications for Patient Safety', *Communication Monographs* 72:4, 390–413.

Ellingson, L. (2004), *Communicating in the Clinic* (New York: Hampton Press).

Feldman, M. and March, J. (1981), 'Information as Signal and Symbol', *Administrative Science Quarterly* 26:2, 171–86.

Giddens, A. (1984), *The Constitution of Society* (Berkeley: University of California Press).

Langewiesche, W. (2003), *American Ground: Unbuilding the World Trade Center* (New York: North Point Press).

Leeds-Hurwitz, W. and Galanes, G. (eds) (forthcoming), *Socially Constructing Communication* (Cresskill, NJ: Hampton Press).

Pearce, B. (2006), 'Toward Communicative Virtuosity', presented at the seminar 'Modernity as a Communication Process (Is Modernity "On Time?")' (Moscow, Russia, April 15).

Pearce, W.B. (1989), *Communication and the Human Condition* (Carbondale, IL: Southern Illinois University Press).

Senge, P. (1990), *The Fifth Discipline* (New York: Free Press).

Stohl, C. and Redding, W.C. (1987), 'Messages and Message Exchange Processes', in F. Jablin, L. Putnam, K. Roberts and L. Porter (eds), *The Handbook of Organizational Communication* (Beverly Hills, CA: Sage) 451–502.

Taylor, J. and Van Every, E. (2000), *The Emergent Organization* (Mahwah, NJ: Lawrence Erlbaum Associates).

Tompkins, P. (2006), *Apollo, Challenger, Columbia: The Decline of the Space Program* (Los Angeles: Roxbury).

Weick, K. and Sutcliffe, K. (2001), *Managing the Unexpected* (San Francisco: Jossey-Bass).

Wentworth, W. (1980), *Context and Understanding* (New York: Elsevier Press).

PART 1
Sources of Team Communication

Chapter 3

Improving Healthcare Communication: Lessons from the Flightdeck

Judith Orasanu and Ute Fischer

Ever since observers first recognized the critical role of flight crew behavior in aviation accidents, crew communication has been in the spotlight (Helmreich and Foushee 1993; Lautman and Gallimore 1987). Several accidents occurred in the 1970s and 1980s that were caused at least in part by crew communication problems. Many of these involved what has come to be known as "monitoring and challenging" errors (NTSB 1994), a form of crew communication with special relevance to healthcare communication. In addition, vague hints at problems, ambiguous terminology, and unwillingness of more senior crew members to attend to concerns of junior crew members have all contributed to accidents. Consider a few examples:

- In 1971 a Convair 340/440 crashed during approach to the New Haven Airport under adverse weather conditions and low visibility. The captain disregarded the first officer's repeated advisories that minimum descent altitude had been reached. The airplane continued to descend without the crew being able to see the runway environment (NTSB 1972).
- In 1978 a DC-8 crashed near Portland, OR, due to fuel exhaustion. It had circled the airport for nearly an hour while the crew tried to resolve a landing gear problem, despite repeated attempts by the flight engineer to call attention to the dwindling fuel situation. When the captain said he needed 15 minutes more, the second officer replied, "Not enough. Fifteen minutes is gonna' really run us low on fuel here." (Kayten 1993; NTSB 1979).
- In a third case, while preparing to take off from Washington National Airport in a snowstorm, the first officer of a B-737 noticed that engine indicators were not quite right. "God, look at that thing, ... That don't seem right, does it? ... Ah, that's not right." The captain replied, "Yes it is, there's eighty," but the first officer persisted, "Naw, I don't think that's right." During the 35-second take-off roll the crew did not discuss the meaning of the abnormal engine behavior or check other indicators that would have told them that their power settings were below normal for take-off (NTSB 1982).

Each of these accidents involved "monitoring and challenging" errors, or the inability of one crew member, usually a junior one, to get the attention of the senior crew member concerning some matter of immense safety importance and change the course of action. The National Transportation Safety Board (NTSB) considers these secondary errors, because they represent failure to correct a primary error such as not monitoring the altitude while descending for landing, the remaining fuel level, or the engine settings on take-off, as well as many other problems (NTSB 1994). Likewise, aviation incident reports, which number in the hundreds of thousands, reflect what Billings and Cheaney (1981) labeled "information transfer" problems. Based on 28,000 reports submitted to the Aviation Safety Reporting System (ASRS) from 1976 to 1981, the authors noted that about 70 per cent reported failed information transfer because (a) the person who had the information did not think it necessary to transfer it, or (b) information was transmitted, but incorrectly.

Each of the above examples illustrates the intimate connection between communication, team cognition, and the safety of operations. These accidents—and many more like them—created the impetus for airlines around the world to launch cockpit resource management (CRM) training programs beginning in the 1970s (Cooper, White and Lauber 1980; Kayten 1993; Lauber 1993). Crew communication was a central component of all of these programs.

Also during the 1970s a research program on "human factors in aviation safety" was initiated at the NASA Ames Research Center at Moffett Field, CA (Cooper, White and Lauber 1980). It included development of a conceptual framework for CRM by a group of industry leaders and the first CRM-related simulation study by Ruffell Smith (Kayten 1993; Ruffell Smith 1979). Since that groundbreaking work, NASA, the FAA, and the military have supported numerous studies of crew behavior under challenging operational conditions. What has been learned from those studies concerning aviation communication and its contributions to flight safety—or lack thereof—is the core of this chapter.

The Relevance of Lessons Learned from Aviation for the Healthcare Industry

One may challenge the relevance of studies of aviation communication to medical environments on the grounds that flying an airplane is nothing like managing patient care in an emergency facility, operating room or hospital. But surely effective and efficient communication is central to successful performance in both domains. Communication difficulties have been identified as a major contributor to adverse outcomes in medical environments as well as in aviation (Donchin et al. 1995; Kohn, Corrigan and Donaldson 2000; Leape et al. 1995; Wilson et al. 1995). Wilson and his colleagues determined that "communication errors were the leading cause and were associated with twice as many deaths as clinical inadequacy" in an Australian study (Wilson et al. 1995). In New Zealand, communication errors were found to be the second most common source of error in recovery room incidents (Kluger and Bullock 2002).

But critics would be correct in pointing out the differences between the two domains. Flying a plane primarily involves two or three people who are similarly trained, which allows first officers to act as "pilot in command" at the discretion of the captain.[1] Despite the captain's ultimate responsibility for the safety of the flight and typical differences in years of experience, the operational differences between the two pilots are more functional: one is the "pilot flying" and the other is the "pilot monitoring," roles that may be alternated during legs of a flight. They have access to identical controls and information. In contrast, medical teams typically are larger (sometimes five to fifteen in a complex surgical environment), and composed of team members who have different skill sets, different responsibilities, and different actions that they are allowed to take or comment on. However, this difference in size and specialization is somewhat misleading because recent definitions of aviation "teams"[2] have been expanded to include flight attendants, gate agents, dispatchers, maintenance, and air traffic control (ATC). As in healthcare environments, each of these specialties has specific training and roles, but frequently contributes at different times. For example, dispatchers plan the flight route and fuel load pre-flight but may become involved during flight when deviations are required from the planned route. Mechanics work on the plane pre-flight, but may become involved if a system fails during flight. Air traffic controllers interact with the flight crew throughout the flight, from taxi out to taxi in. Unlike most medical environments, aviation team members typically are spatially distributed in the air and on the ground at numerous sites. Thus, most of their communication is mediated by radio or some type of automation, except of course within the aircraft.

Perhaps a more significant difference between the two domains is the discrete nature of a flight versus the ongoing nature of many healthcare activities. A flight has a beginning, middle and end. It begins with the crew picking up the flight plan and paperwork at the airport, going through routine pre-flight checks, boarding, and taking off. Phases of flight are totally predictable, from cruise through landing, taxiing to the gate, and post-flight paperwork. Flights typically follow standard routes, and have standardized procedures for abnormal or emergency events. While this discrete event model may be similar to that of a scheduled operation, it is quite different from activities in emergency rooms and intensive care units, which function continuously, with team members coming on shift and going off shift. Moreover, one medical procedure can change into a significantly different one as a result of patient response to treatment, anatomy or newly discovered pathology. This latter type of medical event highlights the need for procedures to support shift-handovers and team flexibility, and for communication strategies for transmission of critical information to personnel coming on duty, thus assuring situation awareness and continuity of care. This type of activity is different from typical aviation operations, except perhaps for extra-long haul flights of 12–14 hours that include one or two extra pilots who take shifts on flying duties.

---

1 The third member of the flight crew, a flight engineer or second officer, is not necessarily trained as a pilot.

2 The terms "team" and "crew" are used interchangeably here. They are distinguished from "groups" in that the former are composed of interdependent individuals with specialized knowledge who have designated roles with respect to a common goal. Groups typically are undifferentiated collections of people who may have transient common interests (Dyer 1984; Orasanu and Sallas 1993; Sundstrom, De Muse and Futrell 1990).

The relatively predictable nature of aviation operations further distinguishes the two domains. Aviation is highly proceduralized and includes standard checklists, procedures for normal, abnormal, and emergency operations, and standard communications. Besides spoken checklists, there are standard call-outs for speed and altitude at specific points in the flight, along with notification of location with respect to navigational points of reference. Part of training as a pilot is learning the required and appropriate verbalizations. This proceduralized aspect of communication does not appear to have a parallel in medical environments, at least not to the degree that it dominates routine talk in aviation. In fact, Xiao et al. (1996) have advocated the development of work procedures in trauma teams that make certain verbalizations mandatory (Fletcher et al. 2002).

A final domain difference is that pilots play a dual role: in addition to being the managers of the flight, in crises they also may be its victims. It has been said, "The pilot is the first at the scene of the accident." Communication norms, procedures, and checklists are designed to minimize pilots' effort and provide them with maximum support to manage dangerous and difficult situations. If pilots make an error they may be injured or die. This is not generally the case with medical personnel (although there certainly are cases in which the health and well-being of medical personnel are threatened by puncture wounds or by contagion from a deadly disease). Different types of stressors may influence medical and aviation teams: losing a patient certainly takes a toll on clinicians just as injury to a passenger has an impact on pilots. Commercial pilots involved in serious incidents or accidents appear to have greater support from their organizations in dealing with the consequences, including critical incident stress management programs, in part demanded by the pilots' unions.

Organizational and regulatory contexts are quite different for the medical and aviation domains. While airlines are highly regulated, with close oversight and established safety standards, the same does not appear to be true for healthcare. Aviation also has substantial support for investigating causes of adverse events. Accidents are investigated by the NTSB, which yields public reports. For the past 30 years, aviation personnel have been able to submit incident reports to the ASRS, yielding broad information on conditions that compromise safety. In contrast, until recently healthcare has been an accumulation of cottage industries with little support for investigations that could make it possible to learn from adverse events. The recently introduced Patient Safety Reporting System (<http://www.psrs.arc. nasa.gov/flashsite/index.html>), modeled on the ASRS, is certainly a step toward accumulating such information. Recent observational research on medical practice has grown significantly in the past two decades, prompting policy and practice changes to enhance patient safety and practitioner well-being (Bogner 1994; Fletcher et al. 2002; Gaba and Howard 2002; Grote and Zala-Mezo 2004; Helmreich and Merritt 1998; Helmreich and Sexton 2004; Kohn, Corridan and Donaldson 2000; Landrigan et al. 2006; Landrigan et al. 2004).

Despite these differences between cockpit crews and medical teams, many similarities exist between the two domains that support the relevance of lessons learned from aviation communication. Both rely on teams of highly trained professionals who perform very complex tasks. Both environments are dynamic, requiring frequent updates of situation or patient models. Conditions may be ambiguous and outcomes highly uncertain. Little time may be available for making diagnostic decisions and taking action. Workload, stress, and interpersonal conflicts may complicate team functioning. And finally, the consequences of human error can be catastrophic in both domains. Because of these similarities, the Department of Defense recently commissioned an evaluation of three different medical team training programs that are grounded in military aviation CRM training (Baker, Beaubien and Holtzman 2006). The general principles were found to be relevant across the domains, despite some differences and problems with implementation.

Lessons Learned from Aviation Communication

In the next section we review some of the major findings from aviation concerning communication practices and strategies that are associated with effective crew performance. These lessons are drawn primarily from research conducted in full-mission simulation environments, but also from other rich sources such as recordings of crew communication from accident investigations, incident reports, and laboratory studies. The section includes four components: a review of various functions of communication on the flightdeck; a description of the data sources used to study aviation communication both by our team at NASA and by others; and lessons learned about both problematic and effective communication practices in aviation.

Functions of Communication

As linguists and social scientists have pointed out, human communication serves two essential functions: it transfers information and it carries relational meaning (Bales 1976; Watzlawick, Beavin and Jackson 1967). Within aviation, communication serves several purposes beyond these two functions that contribute to safe flight operations. Kanki and Palmer (1993) pointed out that communication on the flightdeck helps to establish predictable behavior patterns, to maintain attention to critical events and information, and to manage the flow of cognitive work. For example, procedure-related talk is essential for supporting predictability, which in turn reduces cognitive workload. Orasanu (1990) called this "SOP talk" (for Standard Operating Procedures). It involves the routine management of normal operations, the call-outs and checklists that are associated with the normal flow of the flight. In their analysis of crew performance in a full-mission simulation, Foushee and Manos (1981) found greater uncertainty in low-performing crews because their behavior was less predictable: they did not follow the norms of SOP talk.

In addition to SOP talk, crews engage in "problem-solving talk" or non-standard talk that emerges in response to off-nominal conditions, when the crew must develop new plans to deal with them (Orasanu 1990). It is highly variable and not required by standard flight procedures, but constitutes good practice. Maintaining attention to events and conditions in dynamic conditions is essential for updating situational models. Managing task assignments, plans, and strategies is essential to crew coordination in a busy cockpit, especially during off-nominal conditions. More will be said about non-SOP communication in the next section because it clearly distinguishes more from less effective crews.

While team communication research has identified linguistic markers of task-oriented team cognition in complex work domains, it has largely ignored the social dimension of team interactions (Keyton 1999). The social function comes into play even in the context of professional team interactions (Lauche, Ehbets-Müller and Mbiti 2001), including aviation and medicine. As team members communicate to achieve their task objectives, they also define (or re-affirm) the nature of their relationship, thus creating a social context that may support or impede their joint task work (Keyton 1999). One social aspect that has received some attention in the crew communication literature is the role of status on pilot interactions (c.f., Fischer 1999; Linde 1988; Orasanu and Fischer 1992). More will be said about this topic in later sections on explicitness and monitoring and challenging.

Data Sources

Crew communication research has relied primarily on four data sources: cockpit voice recorders, field studies, flight simulation studies, and experimental research.

Cockpit Voice Recorders (CVRs) CVRs, those black boxes in the cockpit that record flight crew communication, provided initial insights into the critical role of crew communication when accidents occurred in the early 1970s (Helmreich and Foushee 1993). CVRs record on tape loops the last 30 minutes of conversation, usually enough to capture the reactions to (and sometimes the origins of) problems on the flight deck. In conjunction with the flight data recorders (FDRs), which record numerous channels of data from aircraft systems, and audiotapes maintained by ATC of their communication with the crew, these tools provide investigators with the means to reconstruct accident scenarios (Kayten 1993).

Field Studies Field studies are often undertaken to address a particular type of crew behavior. Observers may ride in the "jump seat" (the extra seat in the flight deck used by check airmen, FAA officials or others). Line Operational Safety Audits conducted by Helmreich and his team (Helmreich 2005; Klinect, Wilhelm and Helmreich 1999) found that over half of the 4,500 observed flights involved a communication problem associated with an ATC clearance.

An important field study was conducted by Ginnett (1993), who observed flight crews during their orientation sessions prior to flight. His study illustrated the importance of pre-flight briefings to subsequent crew performance in flight, a topic to which we will return later.

Full-mission Simulation Studies One technique for examining crew performance in nearly realistic conditions is to have crews fly full missions, from pre-flight preparation to landing, in a flight simulator. Standard scenarios can be presented to numerous crews to assess differences associated with, for example, experience levels, prior flight backgrounds, personality, procedures or training protocols. Scenarios can be structured to include challenging and high-risk features that would not be reasonable to introduce in actual flight. High-fidelity simulation combines the control of the laboratory with the realism of the flightdeck to yield useful information, especially given the high levels of motivation that characterize most professional pilots. Crew communication and performance are audiotaped and videotaped for post-mission analysis. The simulator itself collects data on pilot actions and flight parameters. Findings from several full-mission simulation studies will be discussed in the next section.

Laboratory Studies Hypotheses about causal factors in crew behavior may be best studied in the laboratory, which is certainly less expensive than a simulator and involves less effort. Provided that the materials are realistic, laboratory studies can contribute to theory building and examine combinations of factors that may affect communication and practical outcomes. We conducted a series of related studies to address the issue of monitoring and challenging introduced at the beginning of this chapter. The studies included both pencil and paper tasks and a full-mission simulation study involving a retired pilot who served as a research confederate, scripted to commit errors to determine how the other pilot would respond (Fischer and Orasanu 2000; Orasanu and McDonnell 1999).

Problems in Crew Communication

Accident analyses, simulation studies, and laboratory research have revealed several recurring problems in crew communication which are apparent at three levels: the transmission of a message, its content, and the communicative intent. Transmission problems in pilot–pilot communications are frequently the result of distractions. Consequently, pilots do not hear what has been said because some ongoing task demands their attention. This problem has also been recognized in healthcare environments (Coiera et al. 2002; Parker and Coiera 2000). One safeguard against transmission problems is the requirement that pilots acknowledge and read back critical information. Adherence to communication standards characterizes the behavior of high-performing crews.

Misunderstandings are a second type of communication problem. Pilots may fail to establish a common understanding of the problem they face, their goals, plans, or individual responsibilities. Misunderstandings frequently arise because pilots use ambiguous references (Cushing 1997), provide insufficient information, or fail to address critical task components. Crew communication during simulated flight showed significant differences between high-performing and lower-performing crews in the frequency and explicitness of task-related communication (Orasanu and Fischer 1992). Xiao et al. (1996) also found communication breakdowns in trauma care associated with lack of explicit communication, non-routine task demands, and diffuse responsibility.

The final type of communication problem is failure to convey one's intentions. Communication is not just a matter of transmitting information. Speakers use language to induce people to act in particular ways (Austin 1962). However, speakers may fail to realize their intentions because they communicate too indirectly and their addressee does not grasp what they really want. Alternatively, they may be too imposing, thereby alienating their addressee who then refuses to cooperate. First officers have been found to adopt indirect communication strategies, especially in situations in which they intend to disagree with or criticize the captain's actions. In so doing they run the risk of not being heard, at times with tragic consequences, as revealed by accident analyses (Cushing 1997; Fischer and Orasanu 2000; Kayten 1993; Linde 1988). In contrast, captains have been found to favor very direct communication strategies, which first officers considered not very effective in eliciting their cooperation (Fischer and Orasanu 1999; Fischer and Orasanu 2000).

Features of Effective Crew Communication

Simulation, laboratory, and field studies have all provided a basis for observing flight crews performing effectively. On the basis of numerous studies, we have identified five communication strategies that are associated with effective aviation crew performance:

1. Build shared situation models
2. Address plans and decision alternatives to cope with emergent problems
3. Establish a positive crew climate through briefings to support open communication
4. Monitor and manage problems and errors
5. Use explicit, efficient communication

Studies by a number of investigators at NASA Ames Research Center provide most of the findings we report here, supplemented by the work of investigators in other labs who have led complementary efforts. While the number of relevant studies is not sufficiently large to support a meta-analysis, the communication features we describe below have been confirmed in several studies, often with crews of various sizes flying different types of aircraft simulators, both civilian and military, with different types of problems embedded in the flight scenarios. Hence, we have confidence in the robustness of the findings.

To move beyond abstract description, we first provide an example of one simulation study we used to analyze flight crew communication. Professional B-737 pilots flew a simulated flight during which their communication and behaviors were audio- and videotaped. All flew the same scenario: a "missed approach" at their original destination airport due to bad weather, followed by a hydraulic system failure during climb-out which complicated their decision about where to land; a second approach at the original destination or diversion to an alternate airport with better weather. "Check pilots" who routinely assess pilots' skill both in simulators and in flight evaluated crew performance in these challenging situations. The evaluators noted the type and severity of errors, yielding a total performance score for each crew. We compared the highest performing five crews and the lowest performing five crews (out of 22 crews) for analysis.

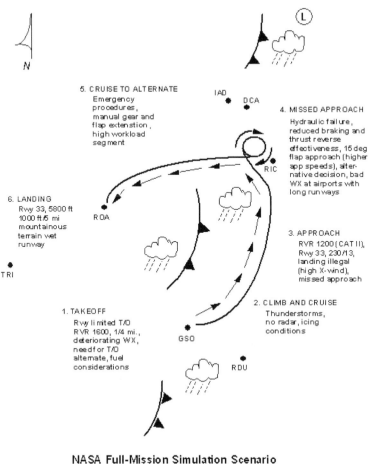

NASA Full-Mission Simulation Scenario
(originally from Foushee, Lauber, Baetge, & Acomb, 1986)
(WX = Weather, X-wind = cross-wind)

Figure 3.1 NASA full-mission simulation scenario
Source: Foushee, Lauber, Baetge and Acomb 1986.

Details of the scenario from Foushee et al. (1986) are presented in Figure 3.1. Departing in bad weather, the flight from Greensboro, NC, to Richmond, VA, was scheduled to take approximately 25 minutes. En route the crew encountered turbulence and icing conditions. The landing at Richmond had to be aborted due to high crosswinds. During climb-out, hydraulic system A failed. These conditions necessitated a decision about where to land, taking into consideration the consequences of the hydraulic failure, which reduced braking capacity, a problem for the short runway and wet conditions at their designated alternate, Roanoke, VA. Landing gear and flaps had to be extended manually (an infrequently performed procedure), contributing to high workload en route to the alternate. In addition to the additional manual tasks, visibility was poor and mountains encircled the alternate airport. Weather was no better at other airports within diversion distance.

Communication in this flight was analyzed separately for the captain and the first officer, as well as for the normal and abnormal phases of the flight. We found significant differences between the high-performing and lower-performing crews, along with distinct patterns of communication for the captains and first officers associated with their rank on the flightdeck as they coped with the scenario challenges. Overall, captains' communication set the tone for the flight. They developed plans and provided direction with respect to critical event responses, assigned tasks, set priorities, and articulated decisions. First officers played a supporting role, even though they were sometimes "pilot flying." Typically, they monitored conditions and provided updates, communicated with ATC, and assisted the captain by gathering task-critical information from manuals and procedures.

In the following section we describe each of the five classes of communication that were associated with high levels of crew performance in this and other studies.

Build Shared Situation Models Building a shared model of the situation is essential so that all members of the team have up-to-date knowledge of the conditions under which they are functioning. It includes the state of the aircraft (c.f., the patient), the environment (c.f., availability of equipment), the aircraft's location (c.f., progress of the surgery or other procedure), and other crew members (c.f., status and availability of other staff). It is not enough that individual crew members have good "situational awareness" (Endsley 1995); the entire *team* must have good situational awareness, especially during high workload periods when individuals are focused on different activities (Orasanu 1995; Prince and Salas 1997). Communication is the means for keeping everyone up–to-date.

In our analysis of the B-737 crews, we found that situation updating in both normal and abnormal phases of flight was primarily the task of the first officers (more than twice as much as by the captains). This is not surprising given that the captain was usually the one flying the aircraft—an attention-demanding task. Much of the information communicated was routine SOP talk, such as target altitudes (for example, "*Coming up on 10,000*" [feet], a standard call, or "*Glide slope's captured*" on approach to landing). But other information was specific to emergent problems, such as updated weather conditions, in particular problematic ones, such as crosswinds. When the hydraulic system failed, it was the first officers who typically determined what functionality had been lost and what resources they still had. As Endsley (2000) has pointed out, situation awareness is not just recognition of cues, but also understanding their significance and projecting their implications so that plans can be made. For example, stating "*Looks like a cat-two up there*" indicates awareness of bad weather landing requirements; "*Pretty heavy to be landing there*" reflects concern with the length of the runway at an alternate airport.

While we found little explicit discussion of *risk* associated with various situations or courses of action, many evaluative utterances such as those just mentioned convey implicit risk judgments. A critical feature that crew members need to address is *time available* for dealing with problems. Tragic and avoidable accidents have occurred when flight crews failed to communicate temporal aspects of the situation.

For example, in 1990 a B-707 crashed following a missed approach at JFK in New York due to bad weather, after circling for several hours at various locations because of storms. The crew notified ATC that they were low on fuel, but were not specific about how long they could continue to fly, nor did they declare a "fuel emergency," which would have moved them to the front of the landing queue (NTSB 1991). Similarly, in the Portland, OR, crash described in the introduction, the flight engineer had warned the captain that they were running low on fuel but was not specific about how much longer they could fly (NTSB 1979).

First officers in the more effective simulator crews provided more situation reports in the abnormal phase of flight, when conditions were deteriorating, thereby supporting the captain's situation awareness and decision-making process (Orasanu 1990). In many cases they requested information from ATC without being asked for it by the captain, indicating that they appreciated the captain's information needs, a positive "anticipation ratio." (MacMillan et al. (2001) defined this as "the ratio of information transfers over requests for information.")

Address Plans and Decision Alternatives In contrast to the first officer's support role, captains provide the leadership essential for coping with emergent problems. In several simulator studies, the captain provided specific direction to the crew and set the tone for crew interaction. What distinguished captains in high-performing crews from those in lower-performing ones was their high level of planning, prioritizing and strategizing. When problems presented themselves, captains responded quickly, requesting essential information (for example, "*Call dispatch and ask them if any other airport is open*"), anticipating problems, and planning for how to cope with them. They did not rush to decision commitment, but provided themselves with a cushion of time so they could evaluate the situation and make the best plan, using resources both on the flightdeck and on the ground (for example, "*Let's see if the weather's improving ... Like to wait around a few minutes. We'll try it again*"). Captains in high-performing crews made 50 per cent more planning utterances than those in lower-performing crews. Many of the plans involved contingencies: *If x happens, we will do y.* As Miller, Galanter and Pribram (1960) noted, plans are the link between what one imagines will occur and actions taken to meet those events. Captains of lower-performing crews seemed to lack forward thinking, focusing instead on immediate tactics. Their behavior was reactive rather than anticipatory, involving many requests for information (that they might have anticipated earlier) and commands to other crew members (creating a rushed high-workload situation).

Captains in higher-performing crews articulated new goals that emerged along with the problems. For instance, instead of worrying just about getting to their destination, after the system failure they also had to cope with that malfunction, decide where to land, and manage their fuel status. We imagine that this situation might be analogous to one in the operating room when a patient responds differently than expected to a procedure and then a new problem is uncovered, but the duration of anesthesia is constrained by an underlying condition. In addition to contingency plans, more effective captains alerted their crew concerning things to watch for, made predictions about how the situation would evolve, and offered more explanations for what they were doing or thinking. These communications helped the crew to be forward-focused, prepared, and functioning as a unit.

Coping with high-consequence, time-limited situations in the simulator required significant crew coordination and workload management. Part of the planning process in the simulated flights involved prioritizing tasks and determining who would do what. In a three-person B-727 crew simulation (Chidester et al. 1990), the more effective captains turned over the job of flying the plane to the first officer while working on the decision problem themselves, in conjunction with the flight engineer (*"You fly this thing while I call the company"*). Structuring individual crew member activities, especially those that did not follow standard procedures, was evident in the communication of high-performing captains (*"You hold that lever down and I'll turn it"*). Non-standard procedures during high-workload phases of flight proved to be challenging. One way of preparing to meet the challenge was essentially to rehearse the procedure before it was needed. In the case of the manual gear and flap extension procedures, more effective captains instructed their crews to get out the abnormal procedures manuals, talk through the procedures, plan when they would begin the process, and who would do what. This prepared them to manage the process without a hitch, whereas crews that had not prepared found themselves under tremendous pressure to carry out these unfamiliar tasks during a high-workload phase of the flight (that is, while in approach to landing). Mackenzie et al. (1993) pointed out that problems associated with uncertainty in trauma treatment could be reduced by increased monitoring and preparation (Fletcher et al. 2002).

An interesting interaction appeared in the crew simulator performance: first officers in the less well-performing crews talked more than those in the higher-performing crews, especially in the abnormal phase of flight. Moreover, their communication included many of the same features as the higher-performing captains' talk: they suggested more plans, initiated more information requests, and offered more explanations. In general, first officers' talk was complementary to that of their captains: when the captain showed leadership, the first officer followed them; but when the captain was less assertive about handling the problems, their first officer frequently jumped in and tried to fill the leadership function, not always with success.

Use Briefings to Establish a Positive Crew Climate and Communication Norms One factor that clearly distinguishes more and less effective crews are briefings which set the stage for how the crew members interact with each other and especially how they manage difficult situations. In a field study, Ginnett (1987) observed 20 commercial air crews before they began a multi-day flight sequence, and described how the captains interacted with the crew members when they first met in the airport. Independent observers rated crew performance effectiveness during the flights. The bottom line: the quality of the captain's initial briefing was predictive of the crew's performance throughout the trip. Captains of effective crews clearly communicated a positive crew concept—that they were all working together toward one goal—and adopted a broad vision of the crew to include gate agents, baggage handlers, dispatch, and ATC. They established free and open communication and a positive crew climate, not just by talk but also by modeling it, setting the tone for safety, cooperation and effective communication. Modeling is a powerful learning approach, as Lingard and colleagues (2002) discovered in their analysis of stress in the OR. Novices were observed to mimic senior physicians' talk patterns—including the negative ones.

Effective captains in Ginnett's study did not dwell on task-specific instructions, but did point out issues that they might face during the flight, such as weather. They disavowed perfection (*"I just want you guys to understand that they assign seats[3] on this airplane based on seniority, not on the basis of competence. So anything you can see or do that will help out, I'd sure appreciate hearing about it"*). They used humor to make their points, invited questions, and demonstrated their competence rather than assuming it because of their status. Lingard and colleagues (2002) also found that senior physicians used jokes or stories to cajole cooperation from their surgical team or to hasten along a procedure.

The respect for the crew demonstrated by effective captains Ginnett observed during briefings is mirrored in the responses of effective captains in the simulation study that we analyzed. When first officers in the more effective simulator crews suggested plans or strategies, their captains frequently agreed or took the suggestions into account in their decisions. Even if they did not agree, they acknowledged the suggestions. In contrast, captains of the lower-performing crews frequently rejected suggestions offered by their first officers or just ignored them. Reinforcement theory clearly predicts that first officers whose captains took their suggestions into account are likely to continue to provide input and suggestions in the future.

Contrast the behavior of these effective captains with an ASRS report from pre-CRM days:

> The captain maintained 250 knots in violation of a speed restriction air traffic control had issued. When the first officer pointed out that ATC wanted them to "slow to 180 [knots]," the captain said "something to the effect of 'I'll do what I want.'" Shortly thereafter ATC cleared them to maintain 3,000 feet. The captain, however, "kept going to 2,500 feet." When the first officer told him their assigned altitude was 3,000 feet, the captain replied, "You just look out the damn window" (Foushee 1982, p. 1063).

Perry and her colleagues (2007) pointed out that some healthcare environments are characterized by "guilds" of specialized workers where communication across professional boundaries is strictly on a "need to know" basis. This may lead them to minimize their interdependencies and maintain a "cooperative distance." This type of silo thinking can get in the way of responding in a resilient manner when challenging patient care problems arise. Helmreich and Davies' (1996) observations in operating theaters found that 20–30 per cent of the briefings and team formation processes were unsatisfactory or met only minimal expectations. Ginnett's analysis of the benefits of briefings in establishing a positive and encompassing crew climate may prove a good model. While personality may influence captains' initial briefing strategies and team interaction patterns during the flight (and they do: see Chidester et al. 1990), briefing and team building are skills that can and are being taught.

---

3 "Seats" refer here to crew positions: captains sit in the left seat, first officers in the right seat.

Monitor and Manage Problems and Errors One critical reason for establishing a positive crew climate is to create an atmosphere in which crew members are willing to raise issues of concern that may influence safety. In the introductory section we cited several crashes in which failures of "monitoring and challenging" contributed to the accident. What needs to be monitored is not only the aircraft systems, weather, traffic, and ATC, but also the activities and apparent understanding of the other pilot. The current generation of CRM training emphasizes "threat and error management" (Helmreich, Klinect and Wilhelm 1999). Threats tend to be events in the aircraft or environment that pose a challenge to the crew, whereas errors typically are made by the flight crew, but also may be made by ATC or others in the system. (Monitoring external threats has been discussed already in the first section on building shared situation models.) Errors, which must be detected before they can be corrected, can be of several types: slips, lapses, mistakes, and violations (Norman 1981; Reason 1990). Slips include mishearing clearances, entering incorrect data into the flight management computer, or misreading a chart or a checklist item. Lapses include forgetting to enter data or make a call-out. Correcting these types of error may be straightforward since one can specify a clearly correct behavior. More difficult types of corrections involve mistakes that are grounded in professional judgment, or violations, willful disregard of the rules.

If another crew member has made an obvious error, calling it to their attention may involve a direct challenge to their status, judgment or skill. According to politeness theory (Brown and Levinson 1987), in situations like these speakers will seek to protect their addressee's "face" and use more indirect speech than in situations that are less face-threatening. However, by being indirect, subordinates run the risk of being misunderstood or of not being heard (Linde 1988). There is thus a tension between informative communication and socially successful ways of communicating. Our research suggests that effective communication attempts to optimize both informativeness and social appropriateness.

In two studies, we provided pilots with descriptions of aviation incidents involving errors by the pilot flying, either the captain or the first officer depending on the crew position of the study participant (Fischer and Orasanu 2000; Fischer, Rinehart and Orasanu 2001). Participants were asked to rate the effectiveness and directness of eight communication strategies that pilots in a previous study (Fischer 1999) had indicated that they would use in these situations. These strategies differed in terms of their focus (other-directed versus speaker-centered), explicitness, and structure (request only versus request plus reason).

Analyses revealed that both captains and first officers favored communications that appealed to the crew concept rather than to a status-based model (that is, captain commands, first officer suggests). Both pilot groups gave high effectiveness ratings to crew obligation statements (such as "*We need to deviate right about now*"), preference statements (for example, "*I think it would be wise to turn left*"), and hints (for example, "*That return at 25 miles looks mean*"). They consistently rated commands, the most direct communication strategy, as less effective. Common to these strategies is that they address a problem without disrupting the team climate. Like commands, they may explicitly state what should be done, but unlike commands they do not rely on status differences to assure compliance. While crew obligation statements seek compliance by appeal to a shared obligation, preference statements do so by referring to the solidarity between speaker and hearer. Hints are similar to crew obligation statements insofar as they too seek compliance by appeal to an external necessity. Many of the hints that pilots had produced in our earlier study were problem or goal statements that strongly implied what action should be taken (for example, *"Clearance was to 9,000!"* or *"I show you 15 knots slow"*). That is, once addressees acknowledge the problem, they are also committed to the appropriate action.

Effective communication strategies thus appeal to a crew's shared responsibility for coping with problem situations. This characteristic is also reflected in pilots' judgments of complex communications. Requests that were supported by problem or goal statements (for example, *"We need to bump the airspeed to Vref plus 15. There's windshear ahead"*) were rated as more effective than communications without supporting statements (that is, the first sentence alone in the previous example). Both constructions, however, were deemed comparable in the extent to which they specified a corrective action and enforced compliance. Pilots did not think that complex communications were less forceful than simple statements, but rather perceived them as more informative. Essentially, the complex structures contributed to building shared models and reducing the addressee's cognitive load.

Use Explicit, Efficient Communication   A final aspect of communication seen in effective crews is one that we imagine would be self-evident, yet sometimes eludes pilots, and probably medical personnel as well. That is the necessity of being explicit and using language efficiently. Explicitness and efficiency are two of Grice's maxims of communication, namely, to be clear in what we say and to say only as much as necessary to convey the message (Grice 1975). Failures of these maxims have contributed to aviation accidents. In 1985 the crew of an L-1011 approaching Dallas-Fort Worth faced a storm over the airport. The captain commented, *"Smell the rain. Smell it?"* The first officer replied, *"Yup. Got lightning in it too."* The captain did not pick up on the first officer's observation about the lightning, which could be read as an indirect warning. No discussion followed about whether to continue with the approach, which resulted in a windshear encounter and crash (NTSB 1986). Likewise, the use of non-specific individual words also may fail to communicate. Air traffic controllers tried to help the crew of a Lockheed L-1011 circling over Miami Airport as the aircraft began to descend in a slow circle toward the Everglades. All crew members were preoccupied with a malfunction of the nose landing gear position indicating system (a 59-cent light bulb), not realizing that the autopilot had inadvertently disengaged. The controller asked, *"How're things coming along up there?"* which the crew took to refer to the landing gear indicator, not to their altitude. By the time they realized the error, it was too late (NTSB 1973). We have already mentioned the lack of explicitness by the crew of a flight from Colombia to New York's JFK Airport in communicating their fuel status to ATC. Instead of using the word "Emergency," they simply stated that they were low on fuel, which did not convey the imminent catastrophe (NTSB 1991).

The reasons for lack of explicitness are many, including status differences, as mentioned in the previous section on monitoring and challenging. Goguen, Linde and Murphy (1986) noted that junior officers are likely to mitigate their challenges to captains. It is a form of politeness and less "face challenging" than less mitigated utterances. Yet those utterances place more of a burden on the recipient to figure out what the message is. However, the situation itself may be ambiguous. By using "hints" (Fischer and Orasanu 1999), the speaker leaves him- or herself some "wiggle room" instead of committing to an opinion. Colloquialisms, especially regional ones, may leave the addressee ignorant of the intended meaning (Cushing 1997), as in the Everglades crash. However, non-specific lexical choices or word retrieval difficulties may actually reflect fatigue or stress (Harrison and Horne 1997). While standardized vocabulary and phraseology has become the norm in aviation and has gone a long way toward reducing certain classes of communication errors, these strategies may only partly reduce lack of explicit communication due to stress.

Explicitness can also be defined at a level higher than lexical choices. It is also evident in how much one communicates about one's intentions and thinking about a problem. As Orasanu and Fischer (1992) noted, effective captains were more explicit in stating their goals, plans, and strategies, making predictions or warnings, and assigning crew tasks. In other words, they let their crews know what they were thinking. The degree of required explicitness varies with situational factors. Orasanu and Fischer (1992) found higher levels of explicitness in three-person crews than in two-person crews. This is not surprising given that when only two crew members are present on the flightdeck, they typically share a visual field and it is clear who the addressee is. When three crew members are present, the flight engineer sits behind the two pilots, typically facing the side of the aircraft. This situation demands greater explicitness to assure that the message gets to the proper person, that task assignments are clear, and that coordinated activities are not left to visual monitoring.

While explicitness may involve an increased level of communication, a countervailing force is communication *efficiency*. Communication takes mental effort, demands attention, and may interfere with carrying out other tasks, especially if it is not related to the task at hand. The aviation industry has adopted the "sterile cockpit" rule, which states that no unnecessary communication will take place when a flight is below 10,000 feet altitude. This was put into place to avoid the distraction associated with social interaction during take-off and climb or approach and landing, phases of flight during which there is considerable communication with ATC and during which attention must be focused on the task at hand (Loukopoulos, Dismukes and Barshi 2001). Similar concern with distractions and interruptions in medical environments was pointed out by Coiera and colleagues (Coiera et al. 2002; Coiera and Tombs 1998), who noted that nearly a third of healthcare providers' communications were interrupted by other demands. Parker and Coiera (2000) reported that a frequent consequence of such interruptions was failure to carry out intended actions or procedures.

Communication efficiency is also evident in what Kanki and Foushee (1989) called "closed-loop" communication: respondents close the loop with initiators by acknowledging or answering the initiating utterance, even if only with an "*uh huh*." The reply lets the initial speaker know that the utterance was heard and, hopefully, understood. If there is no reply, the speaker is left wondering, thereby increasing the speaker's cognitive burden, which may lead her or him to repeat the utterance, further burdening the communication environment.

Summary and Conclusions

In summary, certain features of effective communication on the flightdeck of airplanes appear to be applicable to the healthcare environment, whether it be the time-pressured and highly ambiguous milieu of the emergency department or the more planned but still dynamic operating room and its associated recovery environment. These include:

1. *Build shared mental models*: As unexpected dynamic conditions arise, it is essential that team members communicate to build a shared model of the emergent situation and how to cope with it: What is the problem? What is our plan? Who does what and when? What contingencies must be planned for? What cues or conditions must we look out for and what will we do? Only if all participants have a shared model will they be able to contribute efficiently to the shared goal.

2. *Establish a positive crew climate through briefings*: Briefings conducted by senior personnel go a long way to assure that team members understand their role in the effort and feel comfortable offering their contributions, which may be critical to patient safety and treatment success. Briefings set the tone or team climate; in both aviation and in medicine, team members "follow the leader," adopting the interactional style of the leader (Lingard et al. 2002). By establishing positive relationships, the leader can let the team know that she or he is not invincible and create a crew climate that is open and productive. This may be challenging in healthcare, given Flin et al.'s (2003) finding that senior anesthetists saw briefings as less important than did more junior physicians. Briefings may also be more challenging during 24-hour continuous operations such as in a trauma center.

3. *Monitor and challenge threats and errors*: Briefings set the stage for effective monitoring to prevent problems, errors, or conditions that could jeopardize the patient's well-being. While the leader creates a positive climate through briefings, team members must also learn appropriate ways to bring problems to the attention of senior personnel (called *advocacy* and *assertion* in early CRM parlance). These include being as specific as conditions allow, pointing out problems, suggesting solutions, and providing reasons for one's concerns. Our findings suggest the importance of crew-oriented communication in providing feedback and correcting errors. This certainly is consistent with Xiao et al.'s (2002) notion of building "transactive responsibility systems" in healthcare environments that are mindful of who has essential expertise and how to utilize it to support team resilience.

4. *Use explicit and efficient language*: Explicitness and efficiency reduce the mental load on message recipients and prevent errors. These factors are of greatest concern in high workload situations, where interruptions are frequent.

How explicit one needs to be depends on the level and type of expertise of the recipient. Equally important is the level of uncertainty in the patient situation. Xiao and Mackenzie (1998) found that explicit communication in trauma teams was especially likely to break down in non-routine situations, when creative thinking was required, and when responsibility was diffuse. Close the communication loop with acknowledgements and replies.

5. *Standardize and proceduralize communication*: This is not usually the responsibility of individuals or teams, but rather of the broader organization. By establishing standard procedures, the aviation industry has created an environment in which crew members who are strangers can climb into a flightdeck and fly a plane safely. This illustrates the mundane beauty of checklists and SOPs: the behavior of strangers becomes predictable and efficient.

These communication "lessons learned" from aviation are most likely practiced intuitively by many effective professionals in healthcare environments. What the aviation industry has demonstrated over the past 25 years is that these communication skills can be taught. The high level of safety in commercial aviation is a testament to the effectiveness of these practices, and perhaps will inspire adoption by the healthcare industry as well.

Acknowledgements

We wish to thank Gena Martin for her assistance with the preparation of this chapter. Support was provided by the NASA Behavioral Health and Performance Program and by Cooperative Agreement #NCC 9-58 with the National Space Biomedical Research Institute, for which we are grateful. The opinions expressed here are solely those of the authors and do not reflect official opinions of NASA.

References

Austin, J.L. (1962), *How to Do Things with Words* (London: Oxford University Press).

Baker, D.P., Beaubien, J.M. and Holtzman, A.K. (2006), *DoD Medical Team Training Programs: An Independent Case Study Analysis* (prepared by the American Institutes for Research under Contract No. 282-98-0029, Task Order No. 54 No. AHRQ Publication No. 06-0001) (Rockville, MD: Agency for Healthcare Research and Quality).

Bales, R.F. (1976), *Interaction Process Analysis: A Method for the Study of Small Groups* (Chicago, IL: The University of Chicago Press).

Billings, C.E. and Cheaney, E.S. (1981), *Information Transfer Problems in the Aviation System*, NASA Tech. Paper 1875 (Moffett Field, CA: NASA Ames Research Center).

Bogner, M.S. (ed.) (1994), *Human Error in Medicine* (Mahwah, NJ: Erlbaum).

Brown, P. and Levinson, S.C. (1987), *Politeness: Some Universals in Language Usage* (Cambridge: Cambridge University Press).

Chidester, T.R., Kanki, B.G., Foushee, H.C., Dickinson, C.L. and Bowles, S.V. (1990), *Personality Factors in Flight Operations: Volume 1. Leader Characteristics and Crew Performance in a Full-Mission Air Transport Simulation* (No. NASA Tech. Mem. 102259) (Moffett Field, CA: NASA Ames Research Center).

Coiera, E., Jayasuriya, R., Hardy, J., Bannan, A. and Thorpe, M. (2002), 'Communication Loads on Clinical Staff in the Emergency Department', *Medical Journal of Australia* 176:9, 415–18.

Coiera, E. and Tombs, V. (1998), 'Communication Behaviours in a Hospital Setting: An Observational Study', *British Medical Journal* 316:7132, 673–6.

Cooper, G.E., White, M.D. and Lauber, J.K. (eds) (1980), *Resource Management on the Flightdeck: Proceedings of a NASA/Industry Workshop (NASA CP-2120)* (Moffett Field, CA: NASA Ames Research Center).

Cushing, S. (1997), *Fatal Words: Communication Clashes and Aircraft Crashes* (Chicago, IL: The University of Chicago Press).

Donchin, Y., Gopher, D., Olin, M., Badihi, Y., Biesky, M., Sprung, C.L., Pizov, R.P. and Cotev, S. (1995), 'A Look into the Nature and Causes of Human Errors in the Intensive Care Unit', *Critical Care Medicine* 23:2, 294–300.

Dyer, J.L. (1984), 'Team Research and Team Training: A State of the Art Review', in F. Muckler (ed.), *Human Factors Review* (Santa Monica, CA: Human Factors Society).

Endsley, M.R. (1995), 'Toward a Theory of Situation Awareness', *Human Factors* 37:1, 32–64.

Endsley, M.R. (2000), 'Theoretical Underpinnings of Situation Awareness: A Critical Review', in M.R. Endsley and D.J. Garland (eds), *Situation Awareness Analysis and Measurement* (Mahwah, NJ: Erlbaum) 3–32.

Fischer, U. (1999). *Cultural Variability in Crew Discourse*, Final Report on NASA Cooperative Agreement NCC 2-933 (Atlanta, GA: Georgia Institute of Technology).

Fischer, U. and Orasanu, J. (1999), 'Say it Again, Sam! Effective Communication Strategies to Mitigate Pilot Error', in R.S. Jensen (ed.), *Proceedings of the 10th International Symposium on Aviation Psychology* (Columbus: Ohio State University) 362–6.

Fischer, U. and Orasanu, J. (2000), 'Error-challenging Strategies: Their Role in Preventing and Correcting Errors', *Proceedings of the International Ergonomics Association 14th Triennial Congress and the 41st Meeting of the Human Factors and Ergonomics Society* (San Diego, CA: HFES) 30–33.

Fischer, U., Rinehart, M. and Orasanu, J. (2001), 'Training Flight Crews in Effective Error Challenging Strategies', paper presented at the *Eleventh International Symposium on Aviation Psychology*, Columbus, OH.

Fletcher, G., McGeorge, P., Flin, R., Glavin, R.J. and Maran, N.J. (2002), 'The Role of Non-technical Skills in Anaesthesia: A Review of Current Literature', *British Journal of Anaesthesia* 88:3, 418–29.

Flin, R., Fletcher, G., McGeorge, P., Sutherland, A. and Patey, R. (2003), 'Anaesthetists' Attitudes to Teamwork and Safety', *Anaesthesia* 58:3, 233–42.

Foushee, H.C. (1982), 'The Role of Communications, Socio-psychological and Personality Factors in the Maintenance of Crew Coordination', *Aviation, Space and Environmental Medicine* 53, 1062–6.

Foushee, H.C. (1984), 'Dyads and Triads at 35,000 Feet: Factors Affecting Group Process and Aircrew Performance', *American Psychologist* 39:8, 885–93.

Foushee, H.C., Lauber, J.K., Baetge, M.M. and Acomb, D.B. (1986), *Crew Factors in Flight Operations: III. The Operational Significance of Exposure to Short-haul Air Transport Operations* (NASA Technical Memorandum 88322) (Moffett Field, CA: NASA Ames Research Center).

Foushee, H.C. and Manos, K.L. (1981), 'Information Transfer within the Cockpit: Problems in Intracockpit Communications', in C.E. Billings and E.S. Cheaney (eds), *Information Transfer Problems in the Aviation System*, NASA Report No. TP-1875. (NTIS No. N81-31162) (Moffett Field, CA: NASA Ames Research Center) 63–71.

Gaba, D.M. and Howard, S.K. (2002), 'Patient Safety: Fatigue Among Clinicians and the Safety of Patients', *New England Journal of Medicine* 347:16, 1249–55.

Ginnett, R.C. (1987), 'The Formation Process of Airline Flight Crews', in R.S. Jensen (ed.), *Proceedings of the 4th International Symposium on Aviation Psychology* (Columbus, OH: Ohio State University) 399–405.

Ginnett, R.C. (1993), 'Crew as Groups: Their Formation and Their Leadership', in E. Weiner, B. Kanki and R. Helmreich (eds), *Cockpit Resource Management* (San Diego, CA: Academic Press) 71–98.

Goguen, J., Linde, C. and Murphy, M. (1986), *Crew Communications as a Factor in Aviation Accidents* (Technical Memorandum No. A-86254) (Moffett Field, CA: National Aeronautics and Space Administration).

Grice, H.P. (1975), 'Logic and Conversation', in P. Cole and J.L. Morgan (eds), *Syntax and Semantics Volume 3: Speech Acts* (NY: Seminar Press) 225–42.

Grote, G. and Zala-Mezo, E. (2004), *The Effects of Different Forms of Coordination in Coping with Workload: Cockpit versus Operating Theatre*. Report on the psychological part of the project. GIHRE-Kolleg (Group Interaction in High Risk Environments) of the Daimler-Benz-Foundation (Zürich: Institut für Arbeitspsychologie).

Harrison, Y. and Horne, J.A. (1997), 'Sleep Deprivation Affects Speech', *Sleep* 20:10, 871–8.

Helmreich, R.L. (2005), 'What Crews Do: Context and Concepts of Threat and Error Management (TEM)', paper presented at the *Third ICAO/IATA LOSA/TEM Conference*, Kuala Lumpur, September 13.

Helmreich, R.L. and Davies, J.M. (1996), 'Human Factors in the Operating Room: Interpersonal Determinants of Safety, Efficiency and Morale', *Clinical Anaesthesiology* 10:2, 277–95.

Helmreich, R.L. and Foushee, C.H. (1993), 'Why Crew Resource Management? Empirical and Theoretical Bases of Human Factors Training in Aviation', in E.L. Weiner, B.G. Kanki and R.L. Helmreich (eds), *Crew Resource Management* (San Diego: Academic Press) 3–41.

Helmreich, R.L., Klinect, J.R. and Wilhelm, J.A. (1999), 'Models of Threat, Error, and CRM in Flight Operations', in R.S. Jensen (ed.), *Proceedings of the 10th*

Annual International Symposium on Aviation Psychology (Columbus, OH: Ohio State University) 677–82.

Helmreich, R.L. and Merritt, A. (1998), *Culture at Work in Aviation and Medicine: National, Organizational and Professional Influences* (Aldershot, UK: Ashgate Publishing).

Helmreich, R.L. and Sexton, J.B. (2004), 'Group Interaction under Threat and High Workload', in R. Dietrich and T.M. Childress (eds), *Group Interaction in High-risk Environments* (Burlington, VT: Ashgate Publishing) 9–23.

Kanki, B.G. and Foushee, H.C. (1989), 'Communication as Group Process Mediator of Aircrew Performance', *Aviation, Space, and Environmental Medicine* 60:5, 402–10.

Kanki, B.G. and Palmer, M.T. (1993), 'Communication and Crew Resource Management', in E. Weiner, B. Kanki and R. Helmreich (eds), *Cockpit Resource Management* (San Diego: Academic Press) 99–137.

Kayten, P.J. (1993), 'The Accident Investigator's Perspective', in E.L. Weiner, B.G. Kanki and R.L. Helmreich (eds), *Cockpit Resource Management* (San Diego: Academic Press) 283–314.

Keyton, J. (1999), 'Relational Communication in Groups', in L.R. Frey (ed.), *The Handbook of Group Communication Theory and Research* (Thousand Oaks, CA: Sage Publications) 192–222.

Klinect, J.R., Wilhelm, J.A. and Helmreich, R.L. (1999), 'Threat and Error Management: Data from Line Operations Safety Audits', in R.S. Jensen (ed.), *Proceedings of the 10th International Symposium on Aviation Psychology* (Columbus, OH: Ohio State University) 683–8.

Kluger, M. and Bullock, M. (2002), 'Recovery Room Incidents: A Review of 419 Reports from the Anaesthetic Incident Monitoring Study (AIMS)', *Anesthesia* 57:11, 1060–66.

Kohn, L., Corrigan, J. and Donaldson, M. (2000), *To Err is Human: Building a Safer Health System* (Washington, DC: National Academies Press).

Landrigan, C.P., Barger, L.K., Cade, B.E., Ayas, N.T. and Czeisler, C.A. (2006), 'Interns' Compliance with Accreditation Council for Graduate Medical Education Work-hour Limits', *Journal of the American Medical Association* 296:9, 1063–70.

Landrigan, C.P., Rothschild, J.M., Cronin, J.W., Kaushal, R., Burdick, E., Katz, J.T., Lilly, C.M., Stone, P.H., Lockley, S.W., Bates, D.W. and Czeisler, C.A. (2004), 'Effect of Reducing Interns' Work Hours on Serious Medical Errors in Intensive Care Units', *New England Journal of Medicine* 351:18, 1838–48.

Lauber, J.K. (1993), 'Foreword', in E.L. Weiner, B.G. Kanki and R.L. Helmreich (eds), *Cockpit Resource Management* (San Diego: Academic Press) xv–xviii.

Lauche, K., Ehbets-Müller, R. and Mbiti, K. (2001), 'Understanding and Supporting Innovation in Teams', *Proceedings of International Conference on Engineering Design* (Glasgow, UK: ICED) 395–402.

Lautman, L.G. and Gallimore, P.L. (1987), 'Control of Crew-caused Accidents: Results of a 12-operator Survey', in *Airliner* (Seattle: Boeing Commercial Airplane Co.) 1–6.

Leape, L., Bates, D., Cullen, D., Cooper, J., Demonaco, H.J., Gallivan, T., Hallisey, R., Ives, J., Laird, N., Laffel, G., Nemeskal, R., Petersen, L.A., Porter, K., Servi, D., Shea, B.F., Small, S.D., Sweitzer, B.J., Thompson, B.T. and Vander Vliet, M. (1995), 'Systems Analysis of Adverse Drug Events', *Journal of the American Medical Association* 274:1, 35–43.

Linde, C. (1988), 'The Quantitative Study of Communicative Success: Politeness and Accidents in Aviation Discourse', *Language in Society* 17:3, 375–99.

Lingard, L., Reznick, R., Espin, S., Regehr, G. and DeVito, I. (2002), 'Team Communications in the Operating Room: Talk Patterns, Sites of Tension, and the Implications for Novices', *Academic Medicine* 77:3, 232–7.

Loukopoulos, L.D., Dismukes, R.K. and Barshi, I. (2001), 'Cockpit Interruptions and Distractions: A Line Observation Study', in R. Jensen (ed.), *Proceedings of the 11th International Symposium on Aviation Psychology* (Columbus, OH: Ohio State University).

Mackenzie, C.F., Horst, R.L., Mahaffey, D.L. and the LOTAS Group (1993), 'Group Decision Making During Trauma Patient Resuscitation and Anesthesia', *Proceedings of the 37th Annual Meeting of the Human Factors and Ergonomics Society* (Santa Monica, CA: HFES) 372–6.

MacMillan, J., Paley, M.J., Levchuk, Y.N., Entin, E.E., Freeman, J.T. and Serfaty, D. (2001), 'Designing the Best Team for the Task: Optimal Organizational Structures for Military Missions', in M. McNeese, E. Salas and M. Endsley (eds), *New Trends in Cooperative Activities: Understanding System Dynamics in Complex Environments* (Santa Monica, CA: HFES) 284–99.

Miller, G.A., Galanter, E. and Pribram, K.H. (1960), *Plans and the Structure of Behavior* (NY: Holt, Rinehart and Winston).

Norman, D.A. (1981), 'Categorization of Action Slips', *Psychological Review* 88:1, 1–15.

NTSB (1972), *Aircraft Accident Report: Allegheny Airlines, Inc. Allison Prop Jet Convair 340/440, N5832, New Haven, CT, June 7, 1971* (No. NTSB-AAR-72-20) (Washington, DC: NTSB).

NTSB (1973), *Aircraft Accident Report: Eastern Airlines L-1011, N310EA, Miami, FL, Dec. 29, 1972* (No. NTSB-AAR-73-14) (Washington, DC: NTSB).

NTSB (1979), *Aircraft Accident Report: United Airlines, MD-DC8-61, N8082U, Portland, OR, Dec. 28, 1978* (No. NTSB-AAR-79-7) (Washington, DC: NTSB).

NTSB (1982), *Aircraft Accident Report: Air Florida, Inc., Boeing 737-222, N62AF, collision with 14th Street Bridge, near Washington national airport, Washington DC, January 13, 1982* (No. NTSB-AAR-82/08) (Washington, DC: NTSB).

NTSB (1986), *Aircraft Accident Report: Delta Airline, Inc., Lockheed L-1011-385-1, N726DA, Dallas/Fort Worth International Airport, Texas, August 2, 1985* (NTSB report No. 86/05) (Washington, DC: NTSB).

NTSB (1991), *Aircraft Accident Report: Avianca, The Airline of Colombia, Boeing 707-321B, HK2016. Fuel Exhaustion, Cove Neck, NY, January 25, 1990* (No. NTSB/AAR-91-04) (Washington, DC: NTSB).

NTSB (1994), *A Review of Flightcrew-involved, Major Accidents of U.S. Air Carriers, 1978–1990* (NTSB report No. PB 94-917001, NTSB/SS-94/01) (Washington, DC: NTSB).

Orasanu, J. (1990), *Shared Mental Models and Crew Decision Making* (No. CSL 46) (Princeton, NJ: Cognitive Science Laboratory, Princeton University).

Orasanu, J. (1995), 'Evaluating Team Situation Awareness Through Communication', in D. Garland and M. Endsley (eds), *Proceedings of International Conference on Experimental Analysis and Measurement of Situation Awareness* (Daytona Beach: Embry-Riddle Aeronautical University Press).

Orasanu, J. and Fischer, U. (1992), 'Distributed Cognition in the Cockpit: Linguistic Control of Shared Problem Solving', *Proceedings of the Fourteenth Annual Conference of the Cognitive Science Society* (Hillsdale, NJ: Erlbaum) 189–94.

Orasanu, J. and McDonnell, L. (1999), 'How Do Flight Crews Detect and Prevent Errors? I. Explanations for Failures to Correct Errors', in R.S. Jensen (ed.), *Proceedings of the 10th International Symposium on Aviation Psychology* (Columbus, OH: Ohio State University).

Orasanu, J. and Salas, E. (1993), 'Team Decision Making in Complex Environments', in G.A. Klein, J. Orasanu, R. Calderwood and C.E. Zsambok (eds), *Decision Making in Action: Models and Methods* (Norwood, NJ: Ablex) 327–45.

Parker, J. and Coiera, E. (2000), 'Improving Clinical Communication: A View from Psychology', *Journal of the American Medical Informatics Association* 7:5, 453–61.

Perry, S.J., Wears, R.L., Anderson, B. and Booth, A. (2007), 'Peace and War: Contrasting Cases of Resilient Teamwork in Healthcare', paper presented at the *Eighth International Naturalistic Decision Making Conference*, Pacific Grove, CA.

Prince, C. and Salas, E. (1997), 'Situation Awareness for Routine Flight and Decision Making', *International Journal of Cognitive Ergonomics* 1:4, 315–24.

Reason, J. (1990), *Human Error* (Cambridge, UK: Cambridge University Press).

Ruffell Smith, H.P. (1979), *A Simulator Study of the Interaction of Pilot Workload with Errors, Vigilance, and Decisions* (No. NASA Technical Memorandum 78482) (Moffett Field, CA: NASA Ames Research Center).

Sundstrom, E., De Muse, K.P. and Futrell, D. (1990), 'Work Teams: Applications and Effectiveness', *American Psychologist* 45:2, 120–33.

Watzlawick, P., Beavin, J.B. and Jackson, D.D. (1967), *Pragmatics of Human Communication: A Study of Interactional Patterns, Pathologies, and Paradoxes* (New York: Norton and Company).

Wilson, R., Runciman, W., Gibberd, R., Harrison, B.T., Newby, L. and Hamilton, J.D. (1995), 'The Quality in Australian Health Care Study', *The Medical Journal of Australia* 163:9, 458–71.

Xiao, Y., Hunter, W.A., Mackenzie, C.F., Jeffries, N.J., Horst, R. and the LOTAS Group (1996), 'Task Complexity and Emergency Medical Care and its Implications for Team Co-ordination', *Human Factors* 38:4, 636–45.

Xiao, Y. and Mackenzie, C.F. (1998), 'Collaboration in Complex Medical Systems', *Collaborative Crew Performance in Complex Operational Systems: NATO Human Factors and Medicine Symposium* (Neuilly sur Seine: NATO) 4–10.

Xiao, Y., Moss, J., Mackenzie, C.F., Seagull, F.J. and Faraj, S. (2002), 'Transactive Responsibility Systems', *Proceedings of the 46th Human Factors and Ergonomics Society Meeting* (Santa Monica, CA: HFES) 1428–32.

Chapter 4

Crew Resource Management (CRM) in the Aviation Industry

David M. Musson

Crew Resource Management, or CRM, has been a subject of considerable interest in healthcare circles for the last several years. An error reduction strategy, CRM can be described as a formal program of training in teamwork and other non-technical skills for pilots in multi-crew commercial and military flight operations. In recent years, aviation CRM has expanded to include non-pilot aircrew and other personnel whose actions impact upon flight safety. CRM programs typically include such elements as teamwork skills, leadership, and communication, as well as primary education in human factors and standardized procedures related to the safe operation of aircraft. In the United States, the Federal Aviation Administration (FAA) currently requires CRM training in commercial aviation, and guidelines for training design and implementation of such training are set out in FAA advisory circular AC 120-51E. CRM is a concept that has been embraced by global aviation safety, and outside of the United States, similar guidelines are provided by other governing and flight safety authorities, such as the International Civil Aviation Authority (ICAO 1998) and the Civil Aviation Authority in the United Kingdom (Safety Regulation Group 2003).

In general terms, CRM can be defined as the effective use of all available resources: human resources, hardware, and information in order to achieve a safe flight (Helmreich 1997; ICAO 1998). Such a definition, however, may not communicate the breadth or the complexity of current CRM training in commercial and military aviation. Properly executed training programs go beyond the basic concept of "team training," and are integrated with more conventional technical skills training, often using flight simulation as a key mode of delivery. In most progressive airlines, continual reinforcement of CRM skills is an essential element of ongoing airline or squadron line operations. This chapter will explore how the current conceptualization of CRM has been extended to include ongoing assessments of threats to safety by aircrew and the management of errors that are, to some extent, inevitable in technologically complex operational environments. CRM is referred to in a multitude of current patient safety initiatives, yet few personnel in healthcare have first-hand knowledge of these programs in other industries such as aviation. Few people with first-hand experience in aviation see CRM training as either completely ineffective, nor as a universal remedy for all matters related to flight safety. Furthermore, a general lack of understanding of CRM has perhaps led to increased skepticism about its potential effectiveness in healthcare among healthcare providers and researchers.

This chapter will also discuss the complexities of the question of validation for these training programs in an industry where major accidents are thankfully rare and improvements to flight safety are multi-factorial and complex, and where operational risks and complexities vary significantly from carrier to carrier. Finally, this chapter will explore the potential role of CRM in healthcare; how the lessons drawn from aviation may lead to the more rapid evolution of effective error reduction strategies, and how the complex questions of validation may be tackled.

Background

Crew Resource Management first appeared as a formal concept in the late 1970s and early 1980s under the name Cockpit (as opposed to Crew) Resource Management, also (and confusingly) represented by the acronym CRM. These early training programs were developed following a NASA meeting held in 1979 that was convened in response to growing concerns about the role of "pilot error" in aircraft accidents. Several of these crashes involved significant loss of life and received much public attention, both at the time and in resulting investigations. A review of some of these accidents provides a context for understanding the original development of CRM in that industry.

One accident that received much attention among both the general public and aviation safety experts alike was that of Eastern Airlines Flight 401. Flight 401 was a Lockheed L-1011 passenger jet arriving in Miami from New York late in the evening on December 29, 1972. The crew was highly experienced, and the flight was uneventful until final approach into Miami International Airport. When a gear down-and-locked confirmation light failed to illuminate, the crew abandoned the approach, executed a go-around, and attempted to resolve the problem. During the minutes that followed, the three crew members focused on the gear indicator light—they engaged the autopilot, turned their attention to the warning light, and even sent one crew member down into the avionics bay to check the physical status of the landing gear. Nine minutes after all of this started, and as the crew struggled to determine the cause, the aircraft unintentionally impacted the Everglades swamp at 227 knots. Of the 176 passengers and crew, 101 died on impact and two more died of their injuries in the following days. The National Transportation Safety Board (NTSB) investigation concluded that the autopilot had accidentally become disengaged during the final few minutes as the crew struggled with the indicator light problem, and that the crew failed to monitor the flight instruments during this critical period. In the wreckage, the gear was found in the down and locked position, and the failed indicator light was found to be due to a burned-out bulb (NTSB 1973).

Four years later, on March 27, 1976, a Royal Dutch Airlines (KLM) 747 and a Pan American Airlines (Pan Am) 747 collided on the runway in Tenerife. Between the two aircraft, 583 lives were lost in what is still the single worst aviation accident in history. The chain of events leading to this disaster is more complex than that of Eastern Flight 401, yet again the behavior of crew members during the final moments was determined by investigators to be a critical factor in the evolution of this accident. These two aircraft were among several jetliners that had been diverted to Los Rodeos Airport in northern Tenerife when a terrorist bomb blast temporarily closed the main airport, Gran Canaria International. This diversion, combined with long duty hours and bad weather, set the stage for confusion during taxiing and take-off when Gran Canaria reopened after several hours. Non-standard radio communication and the dangerous practice of clearing aircraft to taxi and depart when no one had clear visibility of aircraft positions were both felt to be contributory to this accident. The collision occurred as the KLM aircraft accelerated on its take-off roll and as the Pan Am jet taxied along the same runway, the Dutch jet attempting to lift off over the American aircraft as it emerged from the fog. This accident is significant to the history of CRM in that a steep command hierarchy and a lack of mutual agreement about the decision to proceed with take-off on the flight deck of the KLM 747 were felt to be key contributing factors to this accident (CAIAC 1978; International Civil Aviation Organization 1984).

One final accident that merits mention is that of United Airlines Flight 173 that occurred on December 28, 1978. Flight 173, a McDonnell Douglas DC-8, was on its approach to Portland International Airport on a flight from New York. As reported by crew during the accident investigation, the lowering of the landing gear prior to landing seemed abnormal, following which a gear down-and-locked indicator light failed to illuminate correctly. During the subsequent 50 minutes, the crew discussed emergency procedures, tried their best to verify gear status, briefed the cabin crew on the possibility of an emergency landing, contacted the company maintenance department in San Francisco to discuss the potential gear failure, and periodically checked fuel status as the plane circled. Fifty-four minutes after the crew first reported any concern about the landing gear, the first engine lost power due to exhausted fuel reserves, and within seven minutes Flight 173 lost all four engines as the aircraft ran out of fuel. Two minutes later the aircraft crash-landed in a wooded area six miles short of the airport. Eight passengers and two crew members died, and 180 people, including the captain and first officer, survived.

The NTSB, after investigating this crash, stated that a breakdown in cockpit management and teamwork was a significant factor in the evolution of this accident. In particular, they noted that while the captain is in command, it is the duty of the first officer to monitor the captain, and the duty of the flight engineer to monitor both the captain and the first officer. The failure of the captain to make timely decisions, his failure to consider the importance of time, distance and fuel while focusing almost entirely on gear status, and the failure of the first officer and flight engineer to voice any concern over fuel status until it was too late, were all critical factors in this accident (NTSB 1979).

In 1979, NASA convened a workshop entitled *Resource Management on the Flightdeck* to address aviation safety (Cooper, White and Lauber 1979). Accidents such as the ones described above were front and center at this meeting, and there was a growing awareness that the majority of airline accidents appeared to be due, at least in part, to issues of crew management as opposed to more typical cognitive human factors, or to mechanical or technical failures of the aircraft themselves. Data from accident investigations suggested that up to 70 per cent of major aviation accidents were due to flight crew actions (Helmreich and Foushee 1993). Helmreich and Hackman have theorized that deficiencies in pilot culture and training that led to this problem stemmed from the long-standing tradition of the lone, highly capable pilot that has its origins in the early days of aviation (Hackman and Helmreich 1987). This single pilot tradition manifests, they believe, in a naturally autocratic leadership style that fails to manage other flight crew to their maximum utility. The result of these meetings was the development of crew training aimed at giving pilots the skills to appropriately manage their crews, particularly during crises or safety critical phases of flight. This training was to be known as Cockpit Resource Management, though it can be argued that many of the concepts of CRM already existed in aviation, and were included under such umbrella concepts as airmanship, professionalism, and captaincy. CRM, however, represented the first attempt to formalize and codify such skills as leadership, decision making, conflict resolution, and communication.

The Early Years of CRM

A number of attempts to create CRM training programs arose in the early 1980s. As described by Helmreich, the earliest CRM programs had their roots in management training practices, drawing on the tools of business leadership consultants, and often involved philosophical exercises on teamwork, or role playing in small groups assigned such abstract tasks as identifying supplies necessary to survive in a lifeboat (Helmreich, Merritt and Wilhelm 1999). Such early attempts to teach pilots the importance of teamwork were largely unsuccessful, and may well have been responsible for some degree of push back from the flight community. Salas has noted that early programs had a tendency to focus on affective, personality, and attitudinal aspects of crew coordination, and that inadequate attention was paid to more trainable elements of crew coordination (Salas et al. 1999c).

In the mid 1980s, United Airlines became the first carrier to integrate CRM into full mission simulation training (Wiener, Kanki and Helmreich 1993). This program combined simulator-based training with theoretically driven management skills training based on the Blake and Mouton managerial grid (Blake and Mouton 1964). The Blake and Mouton grid contrasted *concern for people* with *concern for production*, with those scoring high on both dimensions being described as ideal *team style* individuals. Training and the encouragement of managers to focus on both people management skills and productivity was a fundamental principle of this approach. In adopting this philosophy to designing CRM, a key principle was that of identifying one's personal management style, and included the assessment of both one's own and one's peers' performance following simulation through the use of video recordings during formal debriefing. Psychologist Richard Hackman has since made the observation that real behavior change will only occur when people can practice their roles *in vivo*, hopefully gaining insight on later reflection, such as through videotape observation of themselves (Hackman 1993). Many of the fundamental elements of modern CRM evolved during this program, including such concepts as establishing expectancies for crew members to seek adequate information from each other, rational approaches to conflict resolution, and establishing clear guidelines for decision making in multi-person crews. Another key element of this program that was to become a hallmark of an effective CRM course was that of recurrent training, where concepts are reinforced and practiced in subsequent training sessions.

By the late 1980s, CRM programs were established in both commercial airlines and within military airlift command in the United States. Programs were built upon the kind of approaches exemplified by the United Airlines program discussed above, and often included both didactic educational components and application training in flight simulators. Some programs were expanded to include formal training for check airmen—the internal assessor pilots employed by airlines—so that CRM concepts could be reinforced during routine competency checks conducted in actual flight operations (Helmreich, Merritt and Wilhelm 1999). At some point during this process, the term shifted from Cockpit to Crew Resource Management, reflecting the awareness that personnel outside the cockpit also had significant roles to play in the safe operation of aircraft. Through the late 1980s and early 1990s, numerous variations on CRM developed, as the FAA mandated that while each airline was required to provide CRM training in some form, it was left to the airlines to design the specifics of these courses to match their operational needs. Helmreich has written extensively on the successive generations of CRM training, which will not be discussed in particular detail here. By the mid 1990s, most airline CRM programs shared many common elements, including: *Leadership*—responsibilities of the captain, lines of authority, responsibility for maintaining the appropriate cockpit environment; *Communication*—inquiry, assertiveness, crew participation in briefings and discussion, clarification of plans; *Decision Making*—dealing with such factors as gaining input from the crew when it becomes necessary to deviate from intended plans, as well as conflict resolution; *Situational Awareness*—including cross-monitoring, task delegation, and task fixation; *Interpersonal Skills*—mediation, cooperation; *Critique*—review of plans, debrief of flight; and *Stress Management*—including such issues as fatigue awareness and dealing with personal distractions.

By the late 1990s, CRM as a fundamental component of pilot competency was becoming a widely accepted concept. Thinking among CRM trainers and researchers began to shift beyond simple skills training to include such concepts as shared mental models, global situational awareness, and threat and error management. Mental models and shared mental models had become key in understanding how flight crews operate safely within the complex environment of aviation. A pilot's situational awareness, or their integrated understanding of the environment in which they operate is of fundamental importance to all decisions, actions, and communications. Whenever that model departs significantly from reality, there is the potential for disastrous consequences. In the Tenerife accident, for example, the KLM pilot's mental model included the erroneous belief that the runway was clear and that take-off clearance had been granted. Robertson and Endsley, leading researchers on situational awareness, have explored the conceptual relationship between CRM and situational awareness, and have argued that one of the fundamental values of CRM is to help maintain the accuracy of a pilot's mental model. Specifically, they argue, appropriately executed CRM ensures (1) accurate perception of physical elements in the flight environment, (2) comprehension of the current situation, and (3) accurate projection of future status (Robertson and Endsley 1995).

In addition to the mental model possessed by any one pilot, there is also the shared mental model possessed by the various crew members. The accuracy of this model, and its consistency between crew members, is also of great importance. Judith Orasanu, an organizational psychologist at NASA Ames Research Center, has written that shared situation models assure that all participants are solving the same problem and help exploit the cognitive capabilities of the entire crew (Orasanu 1990). She has found that when effective crews encountered high workload situations, co-pilots provided increased information in advance of problems, and pilots (in command) showed fewer requests for information. By contrast, less effective crews were characterized by a relative paucity of information from co-pilots, and increased requests for information from pilots (in command) during critical times. Presumably, a hallmark of effective crews was the awareness in advance of what information will be required—something that relies on shared expectations of what is to come. Additional studies conducted by researchers at the University of Central Florida have supported these findings (Stout et al. 1999), and shared mental models are generally considered now as fundamental to current conceptualizations of effective CRM.

Another recent concept in CRM is that of Threat and Error Management (TEM)—a model developed by the Human Factors Research Project at the University of Texas at Austin. To some extent, TEM is a reconceptualization of CRM as an ongoing, dynamic assessment and management of the various influences (or threats to safety) faced by aircrews (Klinect, Wilhelm and Helmreich 1999). This model draws heavily from the work of James Reason in that the continual management and minimization of external threats (overt and, where possible, latent) are key to minimizing the likelihood of an accident (Reason 1990, 1997). TEM draws on the work of Reason and others, such as Perrow's Normal Accident Theory (Perrow 1984), in that part of this model deals with the inevitability of consequential and inconsequential errors during complex operations. In doing so, TEM includes the active surveillance for errors and error outcomes, responses to, and management of, these errors as routine elements of safe cockpit operations.

Current Standards and Guidelines for CRM

As mentioned at the start of this chapter, the FAA lays out clear and comprehensive guidelines for airlines in the United States to follow in the design and delivery of CRM training in its advisory circular, AC 120-51E. This advisory circular provides background rationale, overall purpose, basic concepts in CRM, implementation guidelines for carriers, and detailed components of effective programs, as well as a list of specific curriculum topics. As a caution, the authors of these guidelines emphasize that in the safe operation of an aircraft, CRM does not compensate for a lack of technical proficiency. Similarly, the authors stress that technical proficiency in and of itself does not guarantee safe flight operations in the absence of effective crew coordination.

Two recent reviews by Salas at the University of Central Florida identified considerable variability in how various carriers have operationalized the guidelines set forth by the FAA (Salas et al. 1999b; Salas et al. 2006). Current FAA guidelines, however, suggest two major program elements, each associated with subcomponents and specific behaviors. The two major elements and their principal sub components are listed below in Table 4.1.

Table 4.1 Suggested curriculum topics for CRM training programs

Major Components	Specific Elements
Communication Processes and Decision Behavior	• Briefings • Inquiry/Advocacy/Assertion • Crew Self-critique • Conflict Resolution • Communications and Decision Making
Team Building and Maintenance	• Leadership/Follower-ship/Concern for Task • Interpersonal Relationships/Group Climate • Workload Management and Situation Awareness • Individual Factors/Stress Reduction

Source: FAA 2004

Three major components of effective training programs include initial indoctrination, recurrent training sessions, and a culture of continual reinforcement at every stage of training and in line operations. These are listed in AC 120-51E, but the concepts of recurrent training and operational reinforcement have been around since the initial iterations of the United Airlines CRM program described earlier in this chapter. An additional belief about the delivery of CRM is that programs must be customized to an organization's specific culture, needs, and operations. Such needs are outlined clearly in AC 120-51E, and Helmreich has written extensively on the topic (Helmreich 1993; Helmreich, Merritt and Wilhelm 1999). Early attempts to trade CRM programs between airlines met with mixed results, presumably because of differences in aircraft, routine operations, culture, and training department practices. Attempts to export specific CRM training packages outside of the US have been less than entirely successful. Differences in national culture, particularly as they relate to command authority and norms of socially appropriate communication, mandate that such training should most reasonably be developed within a given culture (Gregorich and Wilhelm 1993; Helmreich, Merritt and Wilhelm 1999).

The Question of Validation

In recent years, particularly with the increased interest in CRM in healthcare, the question of validation is frequently raised. This is reasonable; as a new concept for healthcare, the implementation of widespread CRM-like training presents a potentially enormous cost with unknown benefit. Similar concerns have been voiced within the aviation safety community (Besco 1997; Salas et al. 1999a), so the issue is not isolated to healthcare. Unfortunately the question of validation is complex and the answers are not straightforward. Salas has suggested applying Kirkpatrick's four levels of training evaluation in assessing the impact and effectiveness of resource management training (Salas et al. 1999b; Salas et al. 2006). In ascending order of validity, these levels of validation are: Reactions, Learning, Behavior, and Results (Kirkpatrick 1994). These two excellent reviews by the University of Central Florida research group applied Kirkpatrick's approach to 86 (58 and 28, respectively) accounts of CRM training and effectiveness evaluation in aviation as well as other work domains. As one might expect, the ease of validation diminishes as one ascends Kirkpatrick's levels of training effectiveness. Many studies have looked at reactions to CRM training, and while the results are somewhat mixed, reactions are generally positive and most pilots perceive that CRM training is a useful concept (Salas et al. 1999a; Salas et al. 2006). This may not be strong evidence of effectiveness, but it is significant in that negative reactions would tend to suggest both a lack of face validity to resource management training and a poor prognosis for actual behavior change following training.

More important than whether pilots like CRM training is whether or not they actually learn anything from such training. Research investigating this question has primarily focused on attitudinal change, typically assessed through the use of a self-report questionnaire. The most commonly used assessment tool has been a series of survey instruments developed by the University of Texas Human Factors research group. Both the Cockpit Management Attitudes Questionnaire, or CMAQ (Gregorich, Helmreich and Wilhelm 1990) and the subsequent Flight Management Attitudes Questionnaire, or FMAQ (Helmreich and Wilhelm 1991) have been used extensively by both trainers and researchers to assess pilot attitudes on a number of dimensions related to resource management. Findings have been somewhat mixed, but generally show positive attitudinal shifts following training (Helmreich, Merritt and Wilhelm 1999; Helmreich et al. 1990). There have also been interesting findings related to attitudinal change, training receptivity, and personality. Pilots with higher levels of interpersonal aggressiveness and poor attitudes towards key CRM concepts showed negative shifts in response to CRM training, suggesting that resource management skills may be more natural for some individuals than others, and forcing some concepts on a subset of pilots may be problematic (Chidester et al. 1991; Gregorich et al. 1989).

Several studies have examined knowledge and awareness changes following training, as opposed to attitudinal change. Surveys of pilots following attendance at CRM workshops has shown increased knowledge of human factors, and of the potential effects on performance caused by stressors such as fatigue and task load (Hayward and Alston 1991). Similar results have been found by Salas, who has shown that CRM training produced pilots with higher levels of knowledge on CRM fundamental principles when compared with those who had received no training (Salas et al. 1999b).

Earlier in this chapter, the concept of shared mental models was discussed as critical to the effectiveness of crew coordination. CRM programs stress this concept, and studies by Stout and others have demonstrated the positive impact of CRM training on the development of mental models in test subjects (Stout et al. 1999).

So, there is mounting evidence that CRM training is both positively viewed by aircrew and an effective means of providing relevant knowledge and producing desired changes in attitudes related to crew coordination. But does it produce the desired results in the cockpit? Several studies conducted to date seem to support that it does, but most of these have been quasi-experimental in design, and actual assessment of in-flight behavior is complicated by difficulty of access to the operational environment. In a series of laboratory experiments conducted in the 1990s, Salas was able to show that CRM training on a sample of pilots produced improved scores on teamwork and team coordination during a medium fidelity flight simulation evaluation. Pilots who did not receive CRM training showed no such improvement, though the effect sizes in this study were modest. The University of Texas at Austin has maintained a long-standing program of cockpit observation research. This program, the Line Operations Safety Audit, or LOSA, involves the structured observation of in-flight crew behavior. Early findings from this program showed significant improvements in CRM-related behaviors over time, in both simulation and actual flight operations following the implementation of CRM training (Helmreich et al. 1990). Subsequent studies confirmed these findings during an audit of in-flight crew performance following training at a major US carrier (Helmreich and Foushee 1993). More recently, this program has focused on examining threats and error management in the cockpit, and less so on the evaluation of training-induced behavioral changes. Further elaboration of LOSA can be found in FAA Advisory Circular 120-90.

The real question, of course, is whether CRM has actually made aviation safer as a result of its widespread implementation. This question is exceedingly difficult to answer with any certainty. The implementation of resource management training has been ubiquitous in aviation; indeed, the obligation to improve aviation safety through whatever appears to be the best route is the responsibility of both air carriers and the bodies that regulate them. CRM represents one element of that route, along with a multitude of other initiatives whose ultimate purpose is to reduce the frequency and severity of aircraft accidents. Improved weather radar, continuous engineering redesign and improvement, redundant operating systems, improved flight rules and regulations, collision warning systems, global positioning system navigation, and other advances have all been implemented simultaneously to CRM. No one intervention can be credited with accounting for aviation's impressive safety record, and none can solely be implicated in the failures that do occur. Anecdotal attributions to the effectiveness of CRM are not rare, and perhaps should not be dismissed as unscientific (as is sometimes done). These are similar to case reports in healthcare, and while they may not represent statistically significant findings, they do bring to light the impressions of experienced operators. The most cited of these case reports is that of United Airlines Flight 232, a McDonnell Douglas DC-10 flying from Denver to Chicago on July 19, 1989. A catastrophic failure of the number 2 engine during flight caused a rupture of three redundant hydraulic lines, leaving the aircraft with virtually no operating control surfaces. Despite expectations that the crew would find the aircraft impossible to fly, Captain Al Haynes, his crew, and a deadheading pilot who volunteered his assistance, managed to gain control of the aircraft and bring it to a crash landing at Sioux City Gateway Airport, saving 186 of the 298 passengers and crew on board. Following the crash, Captain Haynes attributed his success in part to the training he had received at United Airlines' CRM training program. The cockpit voice recorder (CVR) transcript for this accident has been examined in detail using a process called micro-coding, where individual lines and topics of communication are traced over time. Analysis showed that it was Haynes' ability to manage the crew without becoming overly focused on any one aspect of the crisis that likely allowed him to coordinate the crew under such complex conditions. In a systematic manner, he moved from problem to problem, delegating responsibility to other crew members while successfully maintaining appropriate global situational awareness— actions consistent with key objectives of CRM (Predmore 1995).

The Application of CRM to Healthcare

The idea that CRM concepts developed in aviation may have some applicability to healthcare goes at least as far back as 1990. At Stanford, anesthesiologist David Gaba saw parallels between aircraft emergency management and crisis management in anesthesia. This led to a program of high fidelity patient simulation and crisis management training that he termed Anesthesia Crisis Resource Management, or ACRM (Gaba, Fish and Howard 1994; Gaba et al. 1992). Development of ACRM has continued to the present day, and currently variants of ACRM are taught at multiple centers across the United States (Blum et al. 2004). At some centers, significant malpractice insurance premium reductions are granted to anesthesiologists who have undergone ACRM or ACRM-like training (Gaba, Howard and Fish 2001). While this is a positive move towards encouraging such training in an effort to reduce error and improve reliability, it may also serve as a disincentive for simulation centers and ACRM trainers to rigorously investigate the impact of their training on patient outcomes.

At around the same time that Gaba was developing ACRM, Swiss anesthesiologist Hans Gerhard Schaefer and psychologist Robert Helmreich pursued similar avenues to Gaba. Schaefer and Helmreich adapted existing CRM training and assessment methodology to operating room simulation, creating the Team Oriented Medical Simulation (TOMS) program at the University of Basel, in Switzerland. TOMS was a more team-based simulation, using full anesthetic and surgical elements, with a focus on team simulation and management (Helmreich and Schaefer 1994; Schaefer, Helmreich and Scheidegger 1995). The TOMS project also involved the development of the Operating Room Management Questionnaire (ORMAQ)—a healthcare version of the frequently used Flight Management Attitudes Questionnaire (FMAQ) discussed earlier in this chapter. The ORMAQ and subsequent variants have been used extensively in assessments of safety attitudes in healthcare (Schaefer, Helmreich and Scheidegger 1995; Sexton, Thomas and Helmreich 2000).

The 1990s also saw the first of several corporate training solutions that offered to implement CRM training in healthcare settings. MedTeams, developed by Dynamics Research Corporation, was based heavily on aviation CRM, and was derived largely from Helmreich's work on CRM behavioral markers (Musson and Helmreich 2004).

In a significant departure from the aviation model, this and subsequent healthcare CRM products developed by private industry are restricted in the degree to which their developers wish to share course content, making validation of such products problematic. Several validation studies have been attempted with MedTeams, and while reported results are promising, the bias in having suppliers of proprietary training products intimately involved in the evaluation of those products leaves such findings of questionable validity (Musson and Helmreich 2004).

Interest in the healthcare applications of CRM has grown steadily since the release in 2000 of the Institute of Medicine's landmark report on medical error, *To Err is Human: Building a Safer Health System*. The authors specifically pointed to resource management in fields such as aviation as a method that should be considered in efforts to reduce medical error in complex team environments in healthcare (Kohn, Corrigan and Donaldson 2000). However, it was quickly pointed out that validation of aviation's training practices was complex at best, and while it may hold promise, such training would need to be carefully evaluated before significant resources were expended in its implementation (Pizzi, Goldfarb and Nash 2001).

Multiple current efforts are underway to examine the potential for training based on CRM to improve team performance and reduce error in healthcare settings. One particularly impressive project has been the development of the Anesthesia Non Technical Skills (or ANTS) behavioral marker system at the University of Aberdeen in Scotland. ANTS represents a system of theoretically derived discrete and measurable behaviors, based conceptually on those of CRM, but derived in anesthesia through input from subject matter experts and the application of team management theory. This system of markers is grouped into the skill categories of Task Management, Team Working, Situation Awareness, and Decision Making (Fletcher et al. 2003). This system has been shown to be reliably assessable, once raters have been appropriately trained, though actual validation of these markers on patient outcomes has yet to be confirmed. While this project was designed to identify non-technical skill sets at the individual level among anesthesiologists, the methodological approaches used in its development serve as a model for this kind of research in healthcare.

Recently, the US Department of Defense (DoD), in collaboration with the Agency for Healthcare Research and Quality (AHRQ), has developed the TeamSTEPPS (Team Strategies and Tools to Enhance Performance and Patient Safety) program— a training system designed to improve teamwork and communication in military healthcare settings. This program draws extensively on lessons learned in aviation, and its implementation across the vast DoD healthcare system should hopefully include evaluative components that should further inform the question of whether CRM-like training actually leads to reductions in incidents and errors in healthcare.

Negative Responses to CRM

As mentioned earlier, CRM training in aviation has, at times, been characterized by a certain degree of pushback from pilots who perceive such training to be ineffective or even detrimental to running a good cockpit. Helmreich has addressed this point, describing what he terms "boomerang effects" where trainees emerge with measurable negative shifts in safety attitudes following training (Helmreich and Foushee 1993; Helmreich and Wilhelm 1991), and has suggested that similar problems may occur in healthcare (Helmreich, Musson and Sexton 2004). Such negative reactions may result from poorly designed CRM programs, or they may result from individual factors on the part of participants. At the group level, these reactions may be influenced by the presence of charismatic individuals who openly reject CRM concepts during training sessions (Helmreich and Foushee 1993). Additional work by Helmreich and his colleagues has found associations between aspects of personality, particularly low interpersonal orientation and sociability, and rejection of CRM training (Chidester et al. 1991; Gregorich et al. 1989). Such work fits intuitively with an expectation that those individuals who are lacking in their ability to work well with others may find training aimed at improving such skills to be particularly threatening. Continued research into these factors is warranted, and attempts to bring CRM-type training into healthcare would be well advised to heed the experiences of aviation in this area.

Conclusions

Crew Resource Management in aviation has evolved over the course of almost 30 years. From its inception, it was driven by efforts to reduce errors and accidents in the complex socio-technical work environment of commercial and military aviation. A common misinterpretation is that CRM is designed to improve teamwork; in actuality, CRM is designed to reduce accidents and improve safety. As such, it has been developed in concert with a myriad of other safety improvements over the same time period. The safety record of aviation is enviable—in recent years the US commercial aviation system has gone for periods of a full year without one fatality, despite the take-off and landing of thousands of aircraft every day. To attribute such success to one intervention is not possible, nor is it reasonable—CRM is likely neither a panacea for all problems encountered in aviation, nor is it likely useless. It is what it is—an attempt to give pilots the skills they require to manage their resources in the most optimal manner. Determining exactly what elements are most effective, and how best to teach and reinforce those elements, will most certainly continue to be the goal of researchers in this field.

The interest in CRM among healthcare providers will undoubtedly spur future studies on the nature, effectiveness, and evaluation of resource management training in that field. Certain lessons learned early in aviation are being relearned by healthcare providers—the ineffectiveness of one-shot training, perceptions of non-relevance when theoretical concepts are applied without consideration of operational realities, and the difficulties in validating something that is multifaceted, non-technical, and regionally specific. It is likely that while the fundamental concepts may be consistent from setting to setting, the specific nature of resource management programs will vary significantly in content, depending on whether they are applied in surgical centers, outpatient treatment facilities, or small rural clinics. Anecdotal accounts suggest that, as one would expect, borrowing training and assessment tools from aviation and applying them in medical settings without modification is not likely to be completely appropriate. Failures of such attempts are never published, but they do exist out there as failed pet projects, insignificant study findings, and frustration on the part of healthcare workers. Certain misconceptions are already arising that will self-correct over time—for example, the perception that CRM means a complete flattening of command hierarchies; in aviation, good CRM never means that the captain is not still in command of the aircraft. While this may be easily confused with open communication, freedom to voice dissent and request clarification, the abandonment of team structure and authority in crisis situations is not a desirable outcome of team training.

There are also intangible benefits to CRM that are seldom mentioned but of some significance. The effect that those programs have had on cockpit operational climate, pilot morale, and even organizational culture, as CRM-trained pilots rise through the ranks of airline management, are hard to assess but may well be among the more important outcomes of training that focuses on mutual respect, teamwork, and defining safety as a super-ordinate value. In healthcare, where issues of burn-out, professionalism, and poor teamwork are frequent points of contention, CRM-like training may have positive effects beyond that of improving patient safety. Researchers in the area of resource management in healthcare would do well to consider those outcomes in addition to improvements in patient safety.

References

Besco, R.O. (1997), 'The Need for Operational Validation of Human Relations-centered CRM Training Assumptions', presented at the *9th International Symposium on Aviation Psychology*, Columbus, OH.

Blake, R. and Mouton, J. (1964), *The Managerial Grid: The Key to Leadership Excellence* (Houston, TX: Gulf Publishing Co).

Blum, R.H., Raemer, D.B., Carroll, J.S., Sunder, N., Felstein, D.M. and Cooper, J.B. (2004), 'Crisis Resource Management Training for an Anaesthesia Faculty: A New Approach to Continuing Education', *Medical Education* 38:1, 45–55.

CAIAC (1978), Report A-102/1977 y A-103/1977, Madrid, Spain.

Chidester, T.R., Helmreich, R.L., Gregorich, S.E. and Geis, C.E. (1991), 'Pilot Personality and Crew Coordination: Implications for Training and Selection', *International Journal of Aviation Psychology* 1:1, 25–44.

Cooper, J.E., White, M.D. and Lauber, J.K. (1979), *Resource Management on the Flightdeck (NASA Conference Publication 2120, NTIS No. N80-22083)* (Moffett Field, CA: National Aeronautics and Space Administration – Ames Research Center).

FAA (2004), *Advisory Circular AC 120-51E Crew Resource Management* (Washington, DC: Federal Aviation Administration).

Fletcher, G., Flin, R., McGeorge, P., Glavin, R., Maran, N. and Patey, R. (2003), 'Anaesthetists' Non-Technical Skills (ANTS): Evaluation of a Behavioural Marker System', *British Journal of Anaesthesia* 90:5, 580–88.

Gaba, D.M., Fish, K.J. and Howard, K.M. (1994), *Crisis Management in Anesthesiology* (New York: Churchill Livingstone).

Gaba, D.M., Howard, K.M. and Fish, K.J. (2001), 'Simulation-based Training in Anesthesia Crisis Resource Management (ACRM): A Decade of Experiences', *Simulation and Gaming* 32:2, 174.

Gaba, D.M., Howard, S.K., Fish, K.J., Yang, G. and Sarnquist, F. (1992), 'Anesthesia Crisis Resource Management Training: Teaching Anesthesiologists to Handle Critical Incidents', *Aviation Space and Environmental Medicine* 63:9, 763–70.

Gregorich, S.E., Helmreich, R.L. and Wilhelm, J.A. (1990), 'The Structure of Cockpit Management Attitudes', *Journal of Applied Psychology* 75:6, 682–90.

Gregorich, S.E., Helmreich, R.L., Wilhelm, J.A., Chidester, T. and Jensen, R.S. (1989), 'Personality Based Clusters as Predictors of Aviator Attitudes and Performance', in *Proceedings of the 5th International Symposium on Aviation Psychology*, Volume II (Columbus, OH: Ohio State University) 686–91.

Gregorich, S.E. and Wilhelm, J. (1993), 'Crew Resource Management Training Assessment', in E.L. Wiener, B.G. Kanki and R.L. Helmreich (eds), *Cockpit Resource Management* (San Diego, CA: Academic Press) 173–98.

Hackman, J.R. (1993), 'Teams, Leaders, and Organizations: New Directions for Crew-oriented Flight Training', in E.L. Wiener, B.G. Kanki and R.L. Helmreich (eds), *Cockpit Resource Management* (San Diego, CA: Academic Press) 47–69.

Hackman, J.R. and Helmreich, R.L. (1987), 'Assessing the Behavior and Performance of Teams in Organizations: The Case of Air Transport Crews', in D.R. Peterson and D.B. Fishman (eds), *Assessment for Decision* (New Brunswick, NJ: Rutgers University Press) 283–316.

Hayward, B.J. and Alston, N. (1991), 'Team Building Following a Pilot Labor Dispute: Extending the CRM Envelope', presented at the *6th International Symposium on Aviation Safety*, Columbus, OH.

Helmreich, R.L. (1993), 'Fifteen Years of the CRM Wars: A Report from the Trenches', *Proceedings of the Australian Psychology Symposium*, Sydney, Australia, 73–87.

Helmreich, R.L. (1997), 'Managing Human Error in Aviation', *Scientific American* 276:5, 62–7.

Helmreich, R.L. and Foushee, H.C. (1993), 'Why Crew Resource Management? Empirical and Theoretical Bases of Human Factors Training in Aviation', in E.L. Wiener, B.G. Kanki and R.L. Helmreich (eds), *Cockpit Resource Management* (San Diego, CA: Academic Press) 3–45.

Helmreich, R.L., Merritt, A.C. and Wilhelm, J.A. (1999), 'The Evolution of Crew Resource Management Training in Commercial Aviation', *International Journal of Aviation Psychology* 9:1, 19–32.

Helmreich, R.L., Musson, D.M. and Sexton, J.B. (2004), 'Human Factors and Safety in Surgery', in P.F. Nora and B. Manuel (eds), *Surgical Patient Safety: Essential Information for Surgeons in Today's Environment* (Chicago, IL: American College of Surgeons).

Helmreich, R.L. and Schaefer, H.G. (1994), 'Team Performance in the Operating Room', in M. Bogner (ed.), *Human Error in Medicine* (Hillsdale, NJ: LEA) 225–53.

Helmreich, R.L. and Wilhelm, J.A. (1991), 'Outcomes of Crew Resource Management Training', *International Journal of Aviation Psychology* 1:4, 287–300.

Helmreich, R.L., Wilhelm, J.A., Gregorich, S.E. and Chidester, T.R. (1990), 'Preliminary Results from the Evaluation of Cockpit Resource Management Training: Performance Ratings of Flightcrews', *Aviation, Space and Environmental Medicine* 61:6, 576–9.

ICAO (1998), *Human Factors Training Manual* (Montreal, Quebec: International Civil Aviation Organization).

International Civil Aviation Organization (1984), 'Human Factors Report on the Tenerife Accident', ICAO Accident Digest Circular 153-AN/56, Montreal, Canada, 22–68.

Kirkpatrick, D.L. (1994), *Evaluating Training Programs: The Four Levels* (San Francisco, CA: Berret-Koehler).

Klinect, J.R., Wilhelm, J. and Helmreich, R.L. (1999), 'Threat and Error Management: Data from Line Operations Safety Audits', in R.S. Jensen (ed.), *Proceedings of the 10th International Symposium on Aviation Psychology* (Columbus, OH: Ohio State University) 683–8.

Kohn, L.T., Corrigan, J. and Donaldson, M.S. (2000), *To Err is Human: Building a Safer Health System* (Washington, DC: National Academies Press).

Musson, D.M. and Helmreich, R.L. (2004), 'Team Training and Resource Management in Healthcare: Current Issues and Future Directions', *Harvard Health Policy Review* 5:1, 25–35.

NTSB (1973), *Accident Investigation Report NTSB-AAR-73-14* (Washington, DC: National Transportation Safety Board).

NTSB (1979), *Accident Investigation Report NTSB-AAR-79-07* (Washington, DC: National Transportation Safety Board).

Orasanu, J. (1990), 'Shared Mental Models and Crew Performance', paper presented at the *34th Annual Meeting of the Human Factors and Ergonomics Society*, Orlando, Florida.

Perrow, C. (1984), *Normal Accidents: Living with High-Risk Technologies* (New York, NY: Basic Books).

Pizzi, L., Goldfarb, N.I. and Nash, D.B. (2001), 'Crew Resource Management and its Applications in Medicine', in *Evidence Report/Technology Assessment No. 43 – Making Healthcare Safer: A Critical Analysis of Patient Safety Practices, AHRQ Publication Number 01-E058* (Washington, DC: AHRQ).

Predmore, S. (1995), 'Microcoding of Communications in Accident Investigation: Crew Coordination in United 811 and United 232', in B. Kanki and O.V. Prinzo (eds), *Methods and Metrics of Voice Communications* (San Antonio, TX: Federal Aviation Administration) A45–A50.

Reason, J.T. (1990), *Human Error* (Cambridge, UK: Cambridge University Press).

Reason, J.T. (1997), *Managing the Risks of Organizational Accidents* (Burlington, VT: Ashgate Publishing).

Robertson, M. and Endsley, M. (1995), 'The Role of Crew Resource Management (CRM) in Achieving Situation Awareness in Aviation Settings', in R. Fuller, N. Johnson and N. McDonald (eds), *Human Factors in Aviation Operations* (Aldershot, UK: Avebury Aviation, Ashgate Publishing) 281–6.

Safety Regulation Group (2003), *CAP 737 – Crew Resource Management (CRM) Training Guidance for Flight Crew, CRM Instructors (CRMIs) and CRM Instructor-Examiners (CRMIEs)* (West Sussex, UK: Civil Aviation Authority).

Salas, E., Burke, C.S., Bowers, C.A. and Wilson, K.A. (1999a), 'Team Training in the Skies: Does Crew Resource Management (CRM) Training Work?', *Human Factors* 43:4, 641–74.

Salas, E., Fowlkes, J.E., Stout, R.J., Milanovich, D.M. and Prince, C. (1999b), 'Does CRM Training Improve Teamwork Skills in the Cockpit? Two Evaluation Studies', *Human Factors* 41:2, 326–43.

Salas, E., Prince, C., Bowers, C.A., Stout, R.J., Oser, R.L. and Cannon-Bowers, J.A. (1999c), 'A Methodology for Enhancing Crew Resource Management Training', *Human Factors* 41:1, 161.

Salas, E., Wilson, K.A., Burke, C.S. and Wightman, D.C. (2006), 'Does Crew Resource Management Training Work? An Update, an Extension, and Some Critical Needs', *Human Factors* 48:2, 392–412.

Schaefer, H.G., Helmreich, R.L. and Scheidegger, D. (1995), 'Safety in the Operating Theatre – Part 1: Interpersonal Relationships and Team Performance', *Current Anaesthesia and Critical Care* 6:1, 48–53.

Sexton, J.B., Thomas, E.J. and Helmreich, R.L. (2000), 'Error, Stress, and Teamwork in Medicine and Aviation: Cross Sectional Surveys', *British Medical Journal* 320:7237, 745–9.

Stout, R.J., Cannon-Bowers, J.A., Salas, E. and Milanovich, D.M. (1999), 'Planning, Shared Mental Models, and Coordinated Performance: An Empirical Link is Established', *Human Factors* 41:1 61–71.

Wiener, E.L., Kanki, B.G. and Helmreich, R.L. (1993), *Cockpit Resource Management* (San Diego, CA: Academic Press).

PART 2
Advances in Team Communication

Chapter 5

Safety Event Reporting Systems: Problem Detection in Distributed Systems

Charles E. Billings, Philip J. Smith and Amy L. Spencer

This chapter looks at lessons learned from a safety event reporting system used as part of the National Aviation System (NAS) in the United States and its potential applicability to the design of healthcare systems (Tamuz and Thomas 2006). This perspective is guided by the fact that both healthcare and aviation represent distributed work systems. They are both systems in which people with different responsibilities, expertise, and data access must work together to make these respective systems work, and in which coordination and collaboration are sometimes completed synchronously and sometimes asynchronously.

In the NAS, this work is distributed across a number of different organizations and individuals, a number of them within the Federal Aviation Administration (FAA) and others within the air carriers and general aviation community. Within the FAA, air traffic controllers and traffic flow managers are located at facilities across the United States, including the Air Traffic Control Systems Command Center (with responsibility for coordination of flows at a national level), 21 regional enroute centers with responsibility for the airspace in their surrounding regions, and airport traffic control towers. Within an air carrier, responsibility is distributed among people with a variety of roles, including ATC coordinators (who collaborate with FAA traffic flow managers and help manage schedules), dispatchers (who share responsibility with the pilots for the conduct of the flight, and who complete both flight planning and flight following activities), maintenance staff, and pilots.

In a healthcare system, work is similarly distributed across a number of different specialists, ranging from doctors and nurses to medical technologists, each with different areas of expertise. In this system, except when automated, information concerning patients and resources is often less centrally available than in aviation, even though any one of several subsystems may contain unique information critical to care.

Thus, in both domains, as in many other dynamic decision-driven systems involving risk, the management and control of data and information is critical. In addition, aviation and healthcare systems both need to be resilient operations that can cope with unanticipated problems. Finally, both types of systems are able to function only because they contain feedback loops which are designed to make needed information available quickly and efficiently, thus helping the practitioners in those systems to learn and adapt.

Below, we review lessons learned from the design and use of a system to provide feedback within the NAS, and then discuss the potential applicability of these lessons to healthcare systems. More specifically, we discuss a model underlying this critical incident reporting system and give a brief description of the methods that have been used as part of its design and functioning. Then, based on over 30 years of experience with error reporting, we discuss some fundamental principles and axioms that should govern the architecture and operation of systems that accept sensitive or confidential data concerning functional breakdowns in human performance in usually reliable systems that involve risk for the humans served by these systems.

A Motivating Incident

In December, 1974, a Trans World Airlines Boeing 727 crashed into Mt Weather, west of Dulles International Airport, while executing an approach to the airfield in bad weather (National Transportation Safety Board 1975). During the accident investigation, the National Transportation Safety Board learned that another aircraft, a Douglas DC-8 belonging to United Airlines, had very nearly hit the same mountain six weeks earlier for the same reason while executing the same approach procedure. The crew reported the incident to their airline, which conducted an investigation. At that time, however, there was no national mechanism for disseminating safety-critical information to the aviation community.

Following the accident, a Special Air Safety Advisory Group was impaneled to advise the Congress. Among its recommendations, this body pointed out the need for systematic feedback of safety-critical aviation information. The FAA quickly established an Aviation Safety Reporting Program to collect and disseminate such data, with the promise of immunity from enforcement action for pilots and other aviation professionals who reported such problems. These aviation professionals, however, did not feel secure about reporting this sort of information to the agency responsible for enforcing aviation regulations, and the program received few useful reports. The FAA then asked the National Aeronautics and Space Administration (NASA), an organization with no enforcement or regulatory authority, for its assistance.

NASA rapidly put together a small group of aviation-oriented human factors researchers and supported them in the creation and implementation of an independent Aviation Safety Reporting System (ASRS) to collect, analyze and distribute safety-critical information (Billings and Reynard 1984; Reynard et al. 1986; Hardy 1990). The information received was collected in confidence, but the system also guaranteed immunity from enforcement action to pilots and other persons reporting to it. The NASA ASRS received enthusiastic support from the US aviation community and reports began coming in rapidly in April, 1976. Over time since then, several other nations have established similar incident reporting systems modeled on the ASRS; 11 national aviation incident reporting systems are presently in operation on every continent. More recently, other domains, notably healthcare, have also begun to focus on adverse event reporting as a potentially effective way to secure better information concerning patient safety lapses.

The NASA ASRS as a Model of an Information Feedback Process

The Aviation Safety Reporting System was designed to improve the feedback of safety-critical information in a very large, widely distributed, service system. In brief, the ASRS was designed to accept narrative data from practitioners in aviation in order to provide useful data concerning system and human problems that can compromise safety. Thus, to help ensure its effectiveness, its design was strongly focused on safety in order to avoid potential diversions that could have resulted from a broader charter, including consideration of quality, efficiency, and cost. By structurally separating safety concerns from consideration of these other (still important) issues, this design helps to ensure that the safety message will not be watered down. If safety–cost trade-offs, for example, need to be considered, they are dealt with through other organizations and therefore forced to be discussed explicitly.

The system is *confidential*. Its data and information are only released after they have been de-identified in ways that ensure that the reporters have become anonymous. The system is *non-punitive*, as the FAA, the regulatory agency over aviation, has indicated both in information releases and in Federal Aviation Regulations (FARs) that it will not undertake enforcement action against persons who have reported inadvertent violations of the regulations. The system is *voluntary*, in that no person is required to report any incident to it. In this respect it differs from the functioning of the National Transportation Safety Board (NTSB), whose mandate is to investigate aircraft and other aviation system accidents, although the two systems cooperate extensively and routinely share de-identified data and knowledge with each other. The critical features of the ASRS, then, are aimed toward encouraging the release and sharing of safety-related information which had not previously been made widely available because of fear of repercussions to the holders of the information. The importance of these features has been similarly noted in the development and use of medical safety reporting systems (Leape 2002; Schuerer et al. 2006).

Another important feature that has generally been advocated for all such safety reporting systems is an emphasis on reporting near misses, "on the assumption that errors that do not harm patients are signals of weaknesses in the system that may ultimately result in harm" (Clarke 2006: 1089). Because in resilient systems like aviation and healthcare near misses are likely to occur with higher frequency than actual adverse events, their inclusion can substantially increase the chances of detecting issues in a timely fashion. This consideration has been further supported by a one-year study of a critical incident reporting system by Frey et al. (2002) in which they concluded: "Most of the system changes were based on minor critical incidents which were often detected only after a longer period of time. This shows the value of our 'low-threshold' critical incident monitoring. Repeated checks along the drug delivery process (prescription, preparation, administration) are an important means to reduce adverse drug events" (Frey et al. 2002: 594).

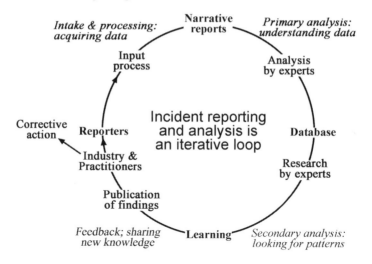

Figure 5.1 The incident reporting and analysis process

Figure 5.1 illustrates the principal ASRS methods. The figure is best read from the nine o'clock point clockwise and it is described in that order.

Input Process

Reporters may be any persons who are involved in or observe an aviation-related event which they believe may potentially compromise aviation system safety. They submit narrative reports to a central ASRS office. At that office, the identified reports are logged in, date- and time-stamped, and scrutinized by one or more expert analysts.

The analysis staff is comprised of retired pilots, air traffic controllers, flight engineers, and mechanics, all of whom have had many years of professional experience in one or more aviation specialties. The analysts code the reports to facilitate retrieval. They also provide brief summaries of the information contained. Since the reports are still identified at this point, the analysts have the discretion to telephone the reporter to gather additional information or to expand on the information provided. Each report is then made anonymous by physically removing a dedicated section, which is thereupon returned to the sender by US mail. (The time-stamped identification strip thereafter serves as proof that a report was sent and received by the ASRS, and serves to activate the immunity provision of the FARs if the FAA learns about an incident by other means and decides to investigate it.)

Analysis by Experts

The narrative reports are then scrutinized to determine whether they contain time-critical information which needs to be communicated to the FAA and/or other organizations in the aviation industry for safety reasons. If so, an ASRS Alert

Bulletin (or for less safety-critical information, an Information Report) is prepared, reviewed, and sent to recipients selected by ASRS staff by mail or electronically (see Figure 5.2). This is usually accomplished within 24–48 hours, or more quickly if necessary.

ALERT
BULLETIN

AB 2003:64/3-32
7/16/03
579835, 582798, 584752

TO: Embraer-Empressa Brasileira Aeronautica S/A

INFO: FAA (ASY-300, AFS-200, AFS-300, AFS-900, MKC-AEG, ACO CE115W ICT,
AEU-100, ANM-100), AASC, ASAP, ALPA, APA, ATA, IAM, IATA, ICAO. ICASS,
IFALPA, NBAA, NTSB, PAMA, RAA

FROM: Linda J. Connell, Director
NASA Aviation Safety Reporting System

SUBJ: EMBRAER COCKPIT SEAT ANOMALY

We recently received an ASRS report describing a safety concern which may involve your area of operational responsibility. We do not have sufficient details to assess either the factual accuracy or possible gravity of the report. It is our policy to relay the reported information to the appropriate authority for evaluation and any necessary follow-up. We feel you should be aware of the following:

ASRS has received several reports from EMB135 and EMB145 flight crews concerning continued instances of cockpit seat movement during take off. An EMB145 captain's seat slid back to the full aft position during takeoff to where the control wheel was out of reach. The captain had the first officer take control of the aircraft and abort the takeoff. Apparently, the adjustment pin did not lock securely into the seat rails. The flight returned to the gate and company maintenance subsequently installed a newer type of seat rails. (ACN 579835) Other reporters claim that a number of first officer seats have malfunctioned before and that improved seat rails should be installed in all their EMB 135 and 145 aircraft. (ACN's 582798, 584752)

(Keywords: Cockpit Seats, Seat Locks/Stops)

To properly assess the usefulness of our AB service, we would appreciate it if you would take the time to give us your feedback on the value of the information that we have provided. Please contact Michael Jengo at (650) 969-3969 or mjengo@mail.arc.nasa.gov.

     Aviation Safety Reporting System
625 Ellis Street * Suite 305 * Mountain View * CA * 94043

Figure 5.2 A sample ASRS Alert Bulletin

The reports are then provided to research analysts with appropriate expertise, who evaluate the contained information in some depth, add a further summary and appropriate key words or phrases, and give the annotated report to the information staff, which prepares and readies the report and any ancillary data for database entry (see Figure 5.3). During this process, analysts may consult together, provide summaries of the data to each other, and so on. They also hold frequent meetings to ensure that the technical staff remains conversant with the information flowing into the system, since not all analysts will have time to see all of the report intake (which totals slightly more than 715,000 reports over 30 years of operation).

Secondary Analysis by Experts

The de-identified, coded reports are available to any interested persons for research or other purposes. Most reports are prepared by analysts or the information staff at the ASRS, who conduct searches of the database in response to queries from the public, other persons or aviation organizations, or by the ASRS management proactively in order to provide needed data to the NTSB, FAA, or aviation security personnel. Regular teleconferences are also held by FAA, ASRS and NASA experts to discuss problems as they occur, or trends observed in ASRS data. The conferences regularly lead to further searches of the data as the ASRS becomes aware of developing trends in civil aviation. They may also lead to the preparation by the ASRS of technical reports which are then made available to the general public. A large part of the secondary analysis activity involves trend-seeking and analysis in search of new findings, because civil aviation is rapidly evolving as new technologies are introduced, many of which have important implications for aviation operations. All of these activities are important parts of the learning and feedback processes that are the primary motivators for the ASRS' existence as part of the nation's ongoing aviation safety surveillance apparatus.

Sharing New Knowledge: Publication of Findings

The ASRS publishes various documents in support of its mission, from two-page summaries of data and safety information that are sent monthly to nearly 100,000 persons, to more highly technical summaries of ASRS studies that are shared with all segments of the US aviation industry. In addition, the system may develop and disseminate information relevant to one or more classes of aviation practitioners (mechanics, flight attendants, and so on) which is distributed to and through organizations that serve these specific elements of the aviation community. The ASRS hopes that, among the persons who see and read its various reports, at least some will choose to provide reports to the system themselves about incidents they have observed. When this occurs, the iterative loop has been closed. The ASRS has found that this has been a fairly effective stimulus to potential reporters over the years.

ACN:579835

Time
Date: 200304
Day: Tue
Local Time of Day: 1801 - 2400
Place
Locale Reference Airport: BOS Airport
State Reference: MA
Altitude AGL Single Value: 0
Aircraft/ 1
Controlling Facilities Tower: BOS Tower
Make Model: EMB ER 135 ER&LR
Person/ 1
Function. Oversight: PIC
Function. Flight Crew: Captain
ASRS Report: 579835
Person/ 2
Function. Flight Crew: First Officer
Person/ 3
Function Controller: Local
Events
Anomaly. Aircraft Equipment Problem: Critical
Anomaly. Other Anomaly: Loss Of Aircraft Control
Anomaly. Other Anomaly. Other Capt Seat Slid Back on Tkof
Independent Detector. Other. Other: Flight CrewA: 1
Resolutory Action. Flight Crew: Rejected Takeoff
Resolutory Action. None Taken: Detected After the Fact
Resolutory Action. Other: FO Assumed Ctl of Acft
Consequences. Other: Company Review

Narrative
ABORTED TKOF DUE TO CAPTS SEAT (PF) SLIDING BACK FAR ENOUGH TO BE UNABLE TO CTL
THE ACFT. FO TOOK CTL AT DIRECTION OF CAPT. THIS HAPPENED AT APPROX 80 KTS. THE
SEAT SLID BACK 4-5 SEAT SLOTS. WE PERFORMED THE REQUIRED CHKLISTS AND FOUND
THAT CHKLIST STATES... CAPT WILL ASSUME CTL OF THE ACFT... THIS IS NOT ALWAYS
POSSIBLE CALLBACK CONVERSATION WITH RPTR REVEALED THE FOLLOWING INFO: THE
CREW WAS FLYING AN EMBRAER 135 ACFT. CAPT INDICATED HE IS ONLY 5 FT 6 INCHES IN HT.
HE ADJUSTS HIS SEAT FULL FWD. HE HAD A VERY SHARP FO WHO ASSUMED CTL OF THE
ACFT DURING THE ABORTED TKOF. THE FO HAD JUST CALLED 80 KTS. CAPT STATES THE SEAT
RAILS HAVE HOLES THAT AN ADJUSTMENT PIN LOCKS INTO SIMILAR TO THOSE ON CESSNA
ACFT. THE CAPT SAID HE HAS HAD THIS HAPPEN BEFORE, BUT THE SEAT HAS ONLY SLIDE
BACK ONE NOTCH ADJUSTMENT BEFORE LOCKING. THIS TIME IT SLIDE FULL BACK. AFTER THE
ABORT THE CREW TAXIED BACK TO THE GATE. THE CREW LISTED THE SEAT PROB IN THE
ACFT MAINT LOG. THE COMPANY REPLACED THE SEAT RAILS WITH THE NEW BROWN
COLORED RAILS. THE CAPT WOUL DLIEK TO SEE ALL ACFT MODIFIED WITH THE NEW RAILS AS
SOON AS POSSIBLE. THE CAPT HAS FLOWN CESSNA ACFT AND WAS AWARE OF THEIR PROB.
HE SAID THE ONLY THING HE COULD THINK OF WHEN THE SEAT WAS SLIDING BACK, WAS
DON'T FULL ON THE CTL WHEEL OVER AND OVER AGAIN. THE CAPT STATES THE OLDEST
ACFT IN THE ACR FLEET WAS DELIVERED IN 1997.

Synopsis
E-135 CAPT'S SEAT SLID BACK ON TKOF ROLL, TO THE POINT THAT THE FO HAD TO ASSUME
CTL OF THE ACFT

Figure 5.3 An example of a de-identified ASRS report

Corrective Action

It will be noted that corrective action lies outside the closed circle in the diagram above. This structural separation of reporting from regulation is deliberate. The ASRS has tried to remain objective in every respect, in a domain which has at least its share of interest groups, as well as political and policy concerns. The ASRS staff and its advisors (a formally instituted group of 15–20 people consisting of aviation technical and management experts that has been active since the first days of the ASRS in 1975) have recognized the perils inherent in "taking sides" in controversies whose solutions may have enormous potential costs for the industry or the government. It therefore makes a practice of bringing the best available evidence to bear on problems it discovers, and suggesting possible solutions when it has evidence that suggests they might be helpful, but it does not make recommendations about potential solutions for identified problems, preferring to allow such solutions to be developed by industry and its knowledgeable practitioners, and the government, who usually are more able to explore all benefits and costs of such changes.

Axioms to Guide the Design of Safety Reporting System Operations

Based on experience with the ASRS, a number of guiding principles can be abstracted for consideration in the design of other such incident reporting systems. These are described below.

The Need for Consensus Among System Stakeholders

The ASRS Advisory Committee is mentioned above. The need for such an advisory group was identified very early in the course of system development. The developers, a small group of aviation human factors researchers, knew that the data that they hoped to collect would in many cases be sensitive and that they could subject reporters to risks up to and including loss of employment and income if they were not protected. The same data might expose aviation employers and service providers to economic risks. It was felt that the most honest approach to these risks would be to involve as many segments of the aviation community as possible in the planning for and development of the ASRS.

As soon as the sponsor of the program, the FAA, had approved its basic concept and design, the developers instituted a process of briefings for as many segments of the community as could be identified. In those briefings, the developers shared in as much detail as possible the risks and benefits that they believed could accrue from national operation of such a venture. During this process, they were able to identify representative organizations that might be willing to assist them by providing guidance and counsel concerning the risks, and expertise regarding system problems and their solutions. All of these organizations were asked to nominate representatives to serve on an Advisory Committee for the ASRS.

No attempt was made to limit the potential representatives to persons or organizations that were likely to be favorably inclined toward the ASRS concept. In fact, the developers were especially anxious to identify and enlist persons and groups who might not be supportive of such an idea. The briefed organizations therefore included labor organizations that represented employees in the aviation industry, manufacturers of aircraft and equipment, representatives of the public served by aviation, special interest groups, attorneys involved in aviation litigation, and organizations representing pilots at many levels, from pleasure through commercial and airline pilots.

The final Advisory Committee included representatives of all of these types of interests. The group provided a great deal of advice and counsel, both during the development process and thereafter. The developers believed, and still believe, that constituting the Advisory Committee in this manner served several purposes: it made stakeholders out of groups which otherwise might have been hostile to the concept, gave them an active role in the success of the operation, and made advocates that might otherwise have been neutral or negative to what needed to be accomplished. Members of the Advisory Committee have supported the ASRS in many cases when other organizations or governmental bodies have found the system to be an inconvenient or threatening mechanism for truth-seeking.

System Security

The developers gave much attention to designing the intake, handling, and storage of data in ways that could effectively guarantee the safety and security of the data and thus the confidentiality and safety of reporters. Because the system was operated under the aegis of the United States government, government practices for the management of sensitive and classified information were instituted, and government policies for secure physical facilities were used throughout. ASRS employees were screened for reliability and were frequently re-briefed concerning the importance of system security. Finally, Advisory Committee members from employee representative organizations were asked to form a subcommittee to conduct periodic evaluations of ASRS security policies and processes; they were the only persons aside from cleared ASRS staff who were given *carte blanche* to scrutinize every aspect of system operations at any time, day or night. They took this responsibility seriously. As a result, to our knowledge, there has been no security breach of any importance during 30 years of operations.

Preserving Raw Data

When the ASRS was designed, its developers were adamant that the raw report texts be saved in order to preserve intact as much potentially useful information as possible. This approach was criticized because of its cost, but over the years, the raw narratives of certain reports have been invaluable aids to understanding the system problems that were reported. The de-identified but otherwise intact report texts remain available if needed.

Ability to Retrieve Reports Through Comprehensive Indexing

When reports are analyzed, analysts are free to add explanatory material. The analysts also add key words and descriptors from lists that have been used and revised over many years. These descriptors have appreciably aided in the retrieval of reports, though it should be said that the ASRS was designed to avoid missing needed reports, even at the expense of the retrieval of a substantial number of "false positives." This approach appears to have been correct. Given that failures of a given type are uncommon in the largely reliable aviation system, there are often only one or a few reports describing a given serious problem. Retrieval of all of them may be necessary for the understanding of a problem, necessitating a bias in terms of recall rather than precision in retrievals.

Assistance in the Search Process

Though ASRS data are in the public domain after they enter the ASRS databases, searching this very large body of data can be difficult. The ASRS maintains a staff of qualified persons who can help users to define their requests, then perform the requests and send the results in the form of a written report. This has proved to be a more economical and efficient method of using the data.

Objectivity, Neutrality, and Credibility

It is absolutely necessary that any adverse event reporting system be perceived by its community as objective, in view of the often politically sensitive issues that may be raised by reporters. The system's output of reports and other information will allow it to be evaluated against this goal, but the system's personnel must exercise continual care to ensure that nothing it disseminates can be perceived as slanted.

The system must also maintain strict neutrality among opposing views within its community; such views will often be strongly held by labor, management, or other interested parties. The system must remain in contact with its stakeholders to ensure that this position is clear to them; an advisory group (see above) is one excellent resource for this purpose.

Finally, it is necessary that the reporting system be perceived as credible. The expertise of its analysts and other staff will do more to ensure this than any other factor. Furthermore, in a highly dynamic environment, it may be necessary to rotate analysts and perhaps other personnel at intervals to be certain that these critical persons remain current and proficient in their profession or trade.

Responsiveness to System Needs

When information is needed in the aviation system, it is often needed in a hurry. This is particularly true when an aircraft accident has occurred, but it may be just as true after a "near miss," when the system is trying to make improvements to obviate another similar occurrence which could have more severe consequences. The ASRS database was designed to make retrieval of important information fairly simple, and the coding system has gone through several major revisions to make it more responsive to user needs. Though de-identified system data are publicly available, most users have found it quicker and more efficient to utilize ASRS personnel to make such data searches, both because of the wide expertise within the analysis group and because of their familiarity with the coding conventions and ways to get to needed information quickly.

The Uses and Limitations of Safety Data

It is important to realize that data of the sort collected by the ASRS are voluntarily submitted in the interests of safety by a wide variety of persons who have various levels of expertise. For that reason, among others, it is difficult to ascertain precisely the characteristics of the population submitting reports, and equally difficult to characterize the population of incidents and other data from which the submitted sample is drawn (Clarke 2006). Because of the large body of data, many researchers have attempted to use the ASRS to characterize the aviation population in a number of respects, not realizing that it is usually not possible to describe the population from which the sample came. Over time, investigators have found a number of approaches that limit this uncertainty, but it can never be obviated.

As an example, some researchers have attempted to construct matched control populations that can be used to circumscribe a sample of interest. This technique has been very useful, particularly for studies of environmental or other stressors known to affect many members of the flying population, such as fatigue (Lyman and Orlady 1981) or toxins such as carbon monoxide. In other cases, researchers have assumed that certain characteristics of the reporting population are similar enough to non-reporters to permit careful extrapolation from the available sample to the population from which it came (Billings and Cheaney 1981).

There is always a potential risk in simply accepting a body of data as probably true, without regard to its sources, so certain cautions and assumptions must always be made with regard to the data sources. The staff of the ASRS, however, bearing in mind the ease of submitting a valid report, have been impressed by the care taken by many reporters to go beyond the minimum information that suffices to support a claim for immunity. The system routinely receives reports containing considerable detail, thoughtful self-analyses of incidents, diagrams, supporting data, taped narratives, and even offers to come to the ASRS to discuss complex incidents. No reporter to the ASRS has to do this much, but several complex cases have provided invaluable data enrichment through reporters' efforts.

It is the belief of ASRS staff that reporters by and large support what the ASRS is trying to do and feel a responsibility to support its safety improvement efforts. They are therefore inclined, in the absence of data to the contrary, to accept these careful reports at their face value, although they are able, for a short period of time, to add to the data originally provided. When the structure of the NASA Aviation Safety Reporting System was designed, it was explicitly required that the data that the system hoped to receive be kept intact so that the raw reports submitted remain available. ASRS staff still believe that those reporters are truthful, know much more about what happened than they do, and therefore deserve to be listened to carefully. This information has helped the aviation community to understand all sorts of human and system problems. And, as Clarke (2006) notes, in spite of the limitations of safety event reporting systems from a traditional epidemiological or statistical sampling perspective, "an accurate count of all the instances of a specific problem is not necessary. One needs only enough reports to know there is a problem" (Clarke 2006: 1090). Once a problem has been identified, other methods can be applied to further evaluate the underlying nature, causes, and significance. The significance of this conceptual approach cannot be highlighted strongly enough. The ASRS is designed to enhance rapid detection of potential problems before they lead to a serious accident, placing an emphasis on the importance of a small number of reports. While large-scale epidemiologic studies have a role as well, in an application area where early detection is vital, investigations can and should be motivated by even a single near miss.

If, therefore, analysts can generally trust what their reporters are trying to tell them, and if they observe even a relatively small incidence of a given type of report, they are inclined to believe that the events described did occur. Given the relative rarity of most kinds of serious errors among professional aviators, it is believed that such clusters of reports deserve very careful attention. An example was a relatively small number of reports of serious upsets in smaller aircraft following Boeing 757 or 767 aircraft on final approaches encountering severe wake turbulence. If these reports had been ignored because there "weren't enough of them," the ASRS would almost certainly have contributed to a small but significant number of fatal accidents. It is necessary to have a high index of suspicion as well as good data to be a good analyst in a safety reporting system.

Safety Reporting in Other Domains: Healthcare

Many of the agencies responsible for healthcare delivery and oversight first learned about the ASRS in 1996 and believed that similar systems could help them learn more about errors in the healthcare system. The Veterans Health Administration (VHA), a healthcare delivery system with a good deal of autonomy, started inquiring about the ASRS and similar systems and moved toward establishment of an adverse event reporting and analysis system rather more quickly than most others in this country. Its research arm instituted measures designed to look more carefully into errors in its healthcare system, and utilized the knowledge and experience of the ASRS staff to help it get started, using the ASRS as a model. The Institute of Medicine report, *To Err is Human* (Kohn, Corrigan and Donaldson 2000), cited the ASRS in its report, which led others in the healthcare field to also consider whether the data obtained by systems analogous to the ASRS might be of assistance in their safety efforts. The data thus far obtained by VHA and other healthcare reporting systems have been encouraging to patient safety experts.

Through 2005, there were eight states in the US that had created "patient safety reporting systems that aggregate reports, analyze them, and provide some feedback" (Clarke 2006). As one of the longer standing examples, the Institute for Safe Medication Practices has a program that has been in effect for over 20 years. Pennsylvania has a mandatory program in all hospitals and gets over 10,000 reports each month; two outside independent organizations perform their analyses. The United States Pharmacopoeia, which analyzes Pennsylvania's data, operates a successful confidential system for hospitals, and the Joint Commission for Accreditation of Healthcare Organizations gets a few hundred reports a year, although it must deal with potential distrust by the medical organizations which are required to be periodically reaccredited. There is still, however, substantial distrust of such reporting systems by healthcare workers, and especially the senior managers of hospitals and other facilities which are constantly worried about litigation problems, sometimes with good reason.

The biggest problem in healthcare safety reporting, as it was in aviation, is a matter of *trust*. As Schuerer et al. (2006) note, error reporting can be incomplete for a variety of reasons "including fear of data discovery, fear of job loss for admitting mistakes, and apathy from the perception that no changes result from the reporting" (Schuerer et al. 2006: 881). Healthcare is not the tidy, rule-based organization that aviation is, and it has a great many stakeholders. Safety reporting in healthcare has a long way to go—but significant progress continues to be made, guided in part by the lessons learned in aviation.

References

Billings, C.E. and Cheaney, E.S. (eds) (1981), *Information Transfer Problems in the Aviation System* (NASA TP-1875).

Billings, C.E. and Reynard, W.D. (1984), 'Human Factors in Aircraft Incidents: Results of a Seven-Year Study', *Aviation, Space and Environmental Medicine* 55: 960–65.

Clarke, J.R. (2006), 'How a System for Reporting Medical Errors Can and Cannot Improve Patient Safety', *American Surgeon* 72:11, 1088–91.

Frey, B., Buettiker, V., Hug, M., Waldvogel, K., Gessler, P., Ghelfi, D., Hodler, C. and Baenziger, O. (2002), 'Does Critical Incident Reporting Contribute to Medication Error Prevention?', *European Journal Of Pediatrics* 161:11, 594–9.

Hardy, R. (1990), *NASA's Aviation Safety Reporting System* (Washington, DC: Smithsonian Institute Press).

Kohn, L., Corrigan, J. and Donaldson, M. (2000), *To Err is Human: Building a Safer Health System* (Washington, DC: National Academies Press).

Leape, L.L. (2002), 'Reporting of Adverse Events', *New England Journal of Medicine* 347:20, 1633–8.

Lyman, E.G. and Orlady, H.W. (1981), *Fatigue and Associated Performance Decrements in Air Transport Operations*, NASA Contractor Report 166167 (Moffett Field, CA: NASA).

National Transportation Safety Board (1975), *Aircraft Accident Report: Trans World Airlines Boeing 727-231, Berryville, VA, Dec. 1, 1974* (Washington, DC: National Transportation Safety Board Report Number NTSB-AAR-75-16).

Reynard, W.D., Billings, C.E., Cheaney, E.S. and Hardy, R. (1986), *The Development of the NASA Aviation Reporting System* (NASA Reference Publication 1114).

Schuerer, J., Nast, P., Harris, C., Krauss, M., Jones, R., Boyle, W., Buchman, T., Coopersmith, C., Dunagan, W.C. and Fraser, V. (2006), 'A New Safety Event Reporting System Improves Physician Reporting in the Surgical Intensive Care Unit', *Journal Of The American College Of Surgeons* 202:6, 881–7.

Tamuz, M. and Thomas, E. (2006), 'Classifying and Interpreting Threats to Patient Safety in Hospitals: Insights from Aviation', *Journal of Organizational Behavior* 27:7, 919–40.

Chapter 6

Voice Loops: Engineering Overhearing to Aid Coordination

Emily S. Patterson, Jennifer Watts-Perotti and David D. Woods

The seemingly disparate domains of space shuttle mission control and healthcare share the need for distributed personnel to coordinate in order to manage interdependencies. Given potentially high consequences for failure, personnel in both domains need to be continuously ready to quickly respond in a coordinated fashion to anomalous or otherwise surprising events (Woods and Hollnagel 2006). Communication "groupware" technology that supports "overhearing" may support this need.

In healthcare, audio devices are typically used for direct, synchronous communication between practitioners who are not co-located; for example, a floor nurse calls a resident physician to relay a patient's request to increase the dose of a narcotic in order to better control pain. Many "telehealth" applications have a similar function of enabling direct, synchronous communication between physically separate parties, albeit often with video data and patient–provider communication.

In NASA space shuttle mission control, a sophisticated audio-based tool called "voice loops"[1] supports multi-channeled, direct, synchronous communication between personnel who are physically separate. It has been argued that the primary benefit of voice loops is the ability for NASA personnel to overhear potentially relevant conversations[2] in order to aid coordination. How the voice loops support coordination in space shuttle mission control is detailed in Patterson, Watts-Perotti and Woods (1999). Audio devices with similar coordination functions exist in aviation, ambulance, railroad, and airline dispatching centers, emergency call centers, and the military. A visual display based upon automatically processed voicemail serves a similar function in telecommunications network monitoring (Whittaker and Amento 2003). The use of voice loops has also been explored for primarily social communication in an office setting with few surprising events and relatively low consequences for failure (Singer et al. 1999).

Vuckovic, Lavelle and Gorman (2004) found that overhearing was a social norm that was explicitly taught in a cardiac intensive care unit in order to aid

---

1 The system is also called digital voice communication system (DVCS).

2 Overhearing tends to be a secondary task that is conducted while focal attention is given to a primary task. Therefore, the voice loops support so-called pre-attentive reference (Woods 1995), in that controllers do not obviously listen to the voice loop until something unusual captures their attention.

interdisciplinary team coordination. The quality of physician–nurse communication is believed to contribute to variation in risk-adjusted outcomes in intensive care units (ICUs) (Knaus et al. 1986; Baggs et al. 1999; Schmitt 2001, Render et al. 2005; Higgins 1999). In particular, rounds have been identified as an opportunity to improve interdisciplinary communication (Gurses and Xiao 2006; Provonost et al. 1999). Interventions that foster interdisciplinary communications during rounds have been associated with 1) an increased understanding by interdisciplinary team members of the long-term plan in a medical-surgical ICU (Dodek and Raboud 2003), and 2) decreased mortality, increased patient satisfaction, and increased quality of work life in a surgical ICU (Uhlig et al. 2002).

This chapter explores how some of the benefits of "overhearing" that are realized on a daily basis in space shuttle mission control (Patterson et al. 1999) might theoretically be achieved in several settings, including the ICU, operating room, outpatient clinic, acute care, pharmacy, emergency department, and electronic ICU.[3] Specifically, this chapter explores potential trade-offs in design and implementation choices with relation to:

* Overhearing updates to a primary decision maker
* Supervisors overhearing detailed team discussions
* Peer to peer hand-off updates
* Interdisciplinary negotiations on key decisions
* Specialist consult communications
* Front line supervisors or coordinators listening remotely to detect escalations
* Overhearing by indirect audiences

The Voice Loop System

A voice loop is a real-time auditory channel that connects physically distributed people, such as a person in the so-called "Front Room" (Figure 6.1) with his or her support personnel in the "Back Rooms." A controller who speaks on a loop broadcasts to all controllers who are listening in on that loop. A controller monitoring a loop hears any communication among other controllers connected to that loop.

During shift changes, incoming personnel monitor voice loops upon arrival, but they only "plug in" their headset to their dedicated console position after the release of the prior shift. Therefore, it is always clear who is responsible for a particular position, including responding to communication requests on the loops. The official end of the shift is broadcast by the incoming Flight on the Flight Director loop following updates from all incoming Front Room personnel to the incoming Flight. By scheduling a one-hour overlap across shift changes, the outgoing personnel can provide detailed updates to incoming personnel as well as monitor the accuracy of their shorter updates to the incoming Flight.

---

3 To the authors' knowledge, voice loops have not yet been implemented in a healthcare setting, so many issues would need to be considered prior to implementation. To reduce the risk of negative, unanticipated side effects, experimentation in a simulated setting would be prudent.

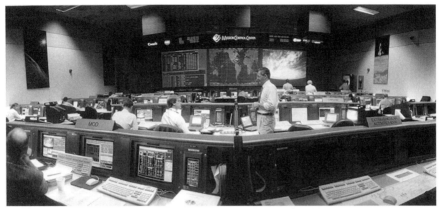

Figure 6.1 The Front Room in the Mission Control Center

Multiple voice loops can be monitored at the same time. The multiple loops require a mechanism for controllers to select and modify which loops they are monitoring and which they can speak on. The interface is a map of the available loops. Any controller can choose to monitor any of the available communication channels by directly manipulating this representation of the space of channels. Generally, most of the loops lie dormant until a need arises to use them, with the exception of the Front-to-Back loops that connect the Front Control Room (FCR) controllers with their support personnel.

By formal communication protocols in mission control, flight controllers have privileges to speak on only a subset of the loops they can listen in on. In the voice loop control interface, each channel can be set either to monitor or talk modes. Only one channel at a time can be set to the talk mode, although many channels can be monitored at the same time. In order to talk on a loop set to the talk mode, a controller presses a button on a hand unit or holds down a foot pedal and talks into a headset.

Each controller customizes the set of loops they monitor by manipulating the visual representation of the loops at their console. The controllers can save a configuration of multiple voice loops on "pages" under their identification code. The most commonly used loops are grouped together onto a primary page. The controllers then reorganize and prioritize the loops to fit the particular operational situation going on at that time by changing the configuration of loops that are being monitored and by adjusting the relative volume levels on each loop.

The voice loop interface is generally considered to be easy to use and an appropriate communication tool for a dynamic environment like space shuttle mission control. The fundamental display units are visual representations of each auditory loop, which captures the way controllers think about the system. In addition, if individual loops are analogous to windows in a visual interface, then the pages of sets of loops are analogous to the "room" concept in window management (Henderson and Card 1986). Controllers are able to customize the interface by putting their most commonly used loops together on a single "page." Active loops on these pages can be dynamically reconfigured in response to the constantly changing environment. Dynamic allocations of which loops to listen to are done by directly selecting loops to turn off and on. These loops are labeled by the console position title, not the individuals' names, making them easier to interpret, remember, and use consistently across shifts. Controllers increase or decrease the salience of particular loops by using loop volume controls to adjust relative loudness to create a foreground/background effect.

Loops Reflect Mission Control Organization

The voice loop system design reflects the cooperative structure in mission control (Figure 6.2). A primary voice loop, the Flight Director loop, is dedicated to communications between the Flight Director and the primary controllers in the Front Room. All controllers continuously monitor the Flight Director loop, but only direct communications between the Front Room controllers and the Flight Director are allowed. Because of the importance of this loop, only issues of high significance are discussed on it, and communication is kept clear and concise.

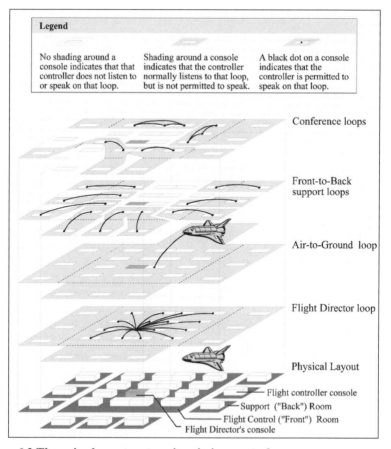

Figure 6.2 The voice loop structure in mission control

Similarly, most controllers monitor the Air-to-Ground loop between mission control and the astronauts during low communication periods. Only one controller, CAPCOM, is authorized to communicate with the astronauts. CAPCOM is an astronaut and physically sits next to the Flight Director because the Flight Director makes the final decisions on what should be communicated on this loop. Despite their ability to interact face-to-face, most of the communications between Flight and CAPCOM are done on the Flight Director loop so that other controllers can listen in.

Interactions between Front Room controllers and their support staff are conducted on Front-to-Back support loops. These are the loops that are normally set to the "talk" setting and are often not monitored by other subsystem controllers. Discussions on these loops are much more detailed and less formal than communications on higher priority loops. For example, unexpected telemetry data values and factors that might account for them would be discussed on these loops.

Conference loops are continuously monitored but lie unused until a situation arises that requires coordination across subsystem controllers. By having dedicated conference loops, groups of subsystem controllers that would need to interact during predictable failure scenarios can be quickly formed without tying up communications on the other loops. When a meeting between controllers who do not have a dedicated conference loop needs to be formed, a Front Room controller announces on the Flight Director loop for specific controllers to meet on an ad hoc conference loop.

Monitoring Multiple Loops in Parallel

Each controller typically monitors a minimum of four loops in parallel: the Flight Director loop, the Air-to-Ground loop, the Front-to-Back loop, and a conference loop. These loops are only a small subset of the potentially available loops. For example, 164 voice loops were used during the STS-76 space shuttle mission. When communications escalate following an unexpected event, Back Room support personnel are generally assigned overlapping configurations of loops to monitor and report significant communications on the Front-to-Back loop, because it is judged too difficult to listen to all of the relevant ones at once.

While it may seem difficult to monitor multiple loops in parallel, this ability is essential to controllers' activities and goals. For example, during an observed simulation, the Front Room mechanical systems controller noticed an abrupt change in the data on her telemetry screens. In order to determine the cause of this change, she monitored and interacted with four loops in parallel. By listening for deviations in standard communications on the Air-to-Ground loop, she could track whether the astronauts were experiencing any abnormal circumstances aboard the shuttle. Listening to the Flight Director loop kept her aware of whether or not other controllers were also seeing strange data patterns. She contacted a related controller on a conference loop to give him a "heads up" that her systems were functioning abnormally, and she discussed the details of the data with her Back Room staff to determine what might have caused the change in the data. Eventually, she heard the electrical controller inform the Flight Director on the Flight Director loop that an electrical bus had failed. This failure would account for the unexpected changes in her system data. She contacted the electrical controller on a conference loop to find out whether the bus could be fixed, and then discussed the impact of this failure with her support staff over the Front-to-Back loops.

Healthcare: Overhear Updates to a Primary Decision Maker

In mission control, arguably the most important coordination function of the voice loops technology is the ability for all controllers to overhear most of the updates provided to the primary decision maker, the Flight Director. It is noteworthy that controllers in the Front Room use the voice loops to communicate, which requires pushing a button, even when it is possible to easily communicate face to face. By overhearing these updates, practitioners can:

- Anticipate unexpected events, planned responses, potential hazards
- Synchronize planned events
- Be aware of major modifications to plans
- Know the rationale for non-routine requests

In the ICU, observational studies suggest that there are opportunities to improve interdisciplinary communications, and in particular provide nursing personnel with greater insight into the decision-making processes employed by resident and attending physicians. First, Donchin et al. (1995) found that most communications occurred within so-called disciplinary "stovepipes," and that nurses did not participate in physician rounds. Second, Lamb and Napodano (1984) found from transcript analysis that there was little interaction between practitioners and minimal physician initiation of information exchange on the team. Third, Coiera and Tombs (1998) found that nursing staff did not always have contact information for individuals in other disciplines, in which cases they were observed to infer the intent of messages based on insufficient information.

One translation strategy (Table 6.1) would be to allow ICU nurses to listen to audiotapes of physician rounds. It is currently possible for nurses to participate in rounds in ICUs, and doing this could enable full participation in rounds, including proactively raising issues and participating in discussions. Nevertheless, Patterson et al. (2006) observed that in two out of four ICUs, nurses did not believe that they were allowed to speak during rounds. In addition, four ICU nurses from different hospitals participated in bedside rounds for a total five out of eleven patients (45 per cent), even though all reported that they intended to participate in rounds during the observations. They primarily missed rounds to pursue patient care activities that were judged to be a higher priority. These data suggest that ICU nurses might listen to audiotapes of physician rounds on their patients at a later time if they are busy with other tasks during rounds. This strategy would require an infrastructure that enabled easy taping and placement of audio data while also protecting private patient data. In addition, it might be important to minimize the burden on physicians to support the taping process, given that they might not directly benefit from taping rounds. Note that a common barrier to technology use when one group does the work for another's benefit is commonly referred to as "Grudin's Law" (Norman 1993).

A similar strategy would be to enable pharmacists who are rounding with one physician team to either simultaneously or asynchronously overhear rounds of other physician teams. Adverse drug events were found to be reduced in the ICU when pharmacists participate in physician rounds (Leape et al. 1999). In this situation, multiple channels might be a beneficial feature, although that would probably depend on the timing and frequency of communications for the various groups. Note that pharmacists likely should not overhear rounds communications while verifying medications or doing other cognitively challenging primary tasks.

Outside the ICU, nursing participation in rounds is often judged to be prohibitive due to time pressure associated with a higher patient: nurse ratio. It is unclear whether an audio capture of rounds communications would be listened to. It is possible that features that increase efficiency, such as "quick playback," markers at the beginning of patient discussions, and tailored selection of text to listen to would increase adoption (cf., Whittaker and Amento 2003).

In order to better support "on-call" functions where nurses can help other nurses' patients in critical situations, such as a patient unintentionally disconnected from a ventilator, nurses might be able to listen in real-time to all the communications made to a charge nurse either by listening to his or her cell phone traffic or by having the charge nurse wear a microphone. In this situation or others where headsets or other equipment is continuously worn, it might be important to minimize weight and size, have an easy "off" button, and also employ infection control protocols.

An extension of the idea of having a charge nurse "loop" is for functions that cut across units within a hospital, such as bed allocations (or nursing staff, housekeeping, infection control, engineering,and so on), to listen to that loop, primarily without talking on the loop. Ideally, the design would be multi-channeled, where all of the charge nurse "loops" could be monitored simultaneously.

Instead of overhearing all updates to a particular decision maker, this strategy could instead be applied to all updates from a particular individual or group. For example, to aid transitions from ambulances to the Emergency Department, all ambulances might be equipped with voice loop communications that enable low-cost ("lightweight") updates to someone who is responsible for direct communications, while relevant groups can listen in to aid anticipation. For example, in recent observations (Anders et al. 2006), an Emergency Department was surprised that two patients (a mother and child) arrived from a single ambulance, which necessitated scrambling for resources (a bed, a pediatric specialist) that would have been able to be proactively anticipated had the information been known earlier. One challenge would be to assign consistent responsibility for direct communications and for indirect overhearing, given the unpredictable nature of the number of incoming patients. In addition, a critical design decision would likely include how to avoid negatively impacting performance by practitioners reasonably concerned about the implications of currently private communications being made observable to indirect parties such as lawyers in the event of a poor outcome.

Table 6.1 Translating (inferred) benefits of voice loops to healthcare settings

Coordination Function	(Inferred) Benefit in Mission Control	Function Translated to Healthcare Setting
Overhear updates to a primary decision maker	Anticipate unexpected events, planned responses, potential hazards	ICU nurses listen to audiotapes of physician rounds
	Synchronize planned events	Pharmacists listen to selected portions of automatically transcribed physician rounds
	Be aware of major modifications to plans	Floor nurses use "quick playback" of selected portions of automatically summarized audio from physician rounds to answer specific questions
	Know the rationale for non-routine requests	Nurses use voice loop to hear all communications with charge nurse
		Bed schedulers use multi-channeled voice loops to hear all communications with all charge nurses simultaneously
		Emergency Department team hears ambulance updates about critically ill incoming patients
		Intake nurses listen to multiple physician–patient conversations to estimate how much time before the room will become available
		Operating room scheduler monitors communications in multiple operating rooms to predict when rooms will be available

Supervisors overhear detailed team discussions	Identify redundant activities Reallocate tasks	Nursing or physician supervisors occasionally "lurk" on loops to overhear detailed team communications
Peer to peer hand-off updates	Detect erroneous assessments, assumptions, missed opportunities Verify "hanging" activities not dropped across handovers of responsibility	Incoming personnel monitor relevant voice loops to prepare for hand-off update Nurse supervisors listen to hand-off updates Attending physician listens to physician sign-outs Electronic ICU intensivist physician listens to resident sign-outs for selected patients Electronic ICU nurse listens to hand-off updates
Interdisciplinary negotiations on key decisions	Monitor communication of key decisions and stances Broadcast impasse resolutions (from face-to-face meetings) Mediate communication across communities with different languages	Care managers for infectious disease patients listen to communications between patient and physician, and hand-off updates Patient advocates or caregivers review automatically transcribed interactions with primary care physician prior to written order Log for major changes to plan posted and updated by anyone in temporary space on front page of electronic medical record
Specialist consult communications	Support efficient and effective addition of specialist "on call" resource Support follow-up requests for information	Specialist resource (e.g., respiratory therapist, dietician, Rapid Response Team, social worker, infection control, IV site therapy, electronic ICU) reviews summarized transcriptions of communications in the last day
Front line supervisors listen remotely to work for which they are directly responsible	Quickly detect escalation of activities	Attending anesthesiologist or surgeon orchestrating multiple simultaneous operations Telemetry nurse monitoring multiple patients simultaneously

Another potential application is for nurses to better prioritize intake tasks based on more accurate assessments of when physician and room resources will become available. For example, we have observed intake nurses drop filling out clinical reminders (Saleem et al. 2005) in order to avoid a physician having to wait to see a patient, when later it became evident that more time was available. In this situation, nurses could likely monitor multiple channels at once because the majority of the content would not be important to hear in detail, and the risk of missing important information is low. Rather, the nurse would be "keeping an ear out" for words, tones or sounds like a door opening that signaled an impending conclusion to the visit.

A similar approach would be for operating room schedulers to monitor in parallel communications in multiple operating rooms in order to predict when rooms will become available. For this particular application, video technology might be more effective since it is unclear if there are clear auditory cues that signal the end of an operation. If audio is employed, it is likely that a single microphone permanently attached to the room itself could be used, thereby avoiding issues with keeping the surgical area uncontaminated.

Healthcare: Supervisors Overhear Detailed Team Discussions

In space shuttle mission control, the Flight Director will occasionally listen in on detailed Front-to-Back loops to gain a sense of how things are going at a more detailed level. With the voice loop system design in mission control, it is not possible to know if anyone is "lurking" on a loop, but the experienced controllers were aware of the practice because Flight would occasionally talk on their private loop in a way that made it clear that he had been listening to their conversations. Given the centrality of the system in operations, users did not have the option to avoid using the loops. However, when particularly sensitive information was conveyed, they were observed to use other means such as the telephone, or in one case, there was a private "hidden" loop that was used.

In healthcare, similar strategies have been observed by nurse supervisors who occasionally "walk the floors" and attending physicians who show up in an unscheduled fashion to be available to physicians in training. The primary difference is that the subordinates are aware of the observation, which could be inferred to mean that the supervisor is concerned about the quality of their performance. With voice loop technology, physician or nursing supervisors could occasionally "lurk" on existing voice loops to overhear detailed team communications. In the absence of voice loop technology, this function could be employed with similar stealth by reviewing electronic health record information.

There is a trade-off with this function in that if users perceive a potential threat to reputation or privacy, they might be less willing to use the loops. These issues were seen in two other audio-based systems. First, with the Thunderwire system used by a software development team in an office setting (Singer et al. 1999), a primary complaint was not knowing who was listening on the loop. The next iteration of the system was planned to make observable the users who were listening (not just who was allowed to listen). Second, Whittaker and Amento (2003) found that supervisors in a network telecommunications customer call center found it highly beneficial to have a tailored view of the automatically transcribed audio data in order to identify unnecessarily redundant activities and reallocate tasks to better distribute workload. End users also judged it beneficial in order to eliminate the need to interrupt others to verbally broadcast what problems were being worked on. They did not want anyone to be able to see the working drafts until they were released, however, to reduce the possibility of somebody acting on something that might change. The trade-off was managed by providing a summary display that hid the detailed content until the problem was resolved.

Healthcare: Peer to Peer Hand-off Updates

In space shuttle mission control, the voice loop technology supports shift handovers in a number of ways. The primary benefits of using voice loops to support hand-offs are improved collaborative cross-checking (Patterson, Roth and Render 2005) in that all personnel hear hand-off updates to the Flight Director, which helps in detecting erroneous assessments, assumptions, and missed opportunities. In addition, it is easier to verify that "hanging" activities are not dropped across transitions of responsibility and authority, in that outgoing personnel monitor the updates provided by the incoming replacement to the incoming Flight Director and the loops generally make work observable throughout the shift.

A specific "warm up" tactic used by all Front Room and Back Room controllers was to monitor their typical loops upon arrival, as well as review log entries and data screens, prior to the hand-off update. In this way, the hand-off could be more effective and efficient (Patterson, Roth et al. 2004). If voice loop technology was used, it is likely that this strategy could directly translate to support hand-off updates.

On one acute care floor, a nurse manager was observed to listen to audiotaped shift change updates in order to identify opportunities to improve the system in general, as well as identify opportunities to improve patient care for particular patients (Patterson, Roth and Render 2005). Similar strategies could be employed with voice loop technologies, but with the benefit of removing the need to be physically present and have all of his or her resources dedicated to the task while listening.

Similar strategies could be employed by attending physicians for the sign-out process. For this application, it is likely that the ability to capture and queue the review, particularly with a quick playback function or automated transcription, might aid adoption.

The electronic intensive care unit (e-ICU) is believed to enable more timely decisions about patient care for the critically ill by increasing access to specialized ICU knowledge (Becker 2000). In one e-ICU, critical care nurses staffed during the day remotely monitor data for ICU patients from five hospitals. It is possible that e-ICU nurses could listen to hand-off audio data either in real-time or after-the-fact for a subset of critical patients, in order to better understand the care plan. An intensivist physician who is staffed at night could monitor resident sign-outs for particular patients, in order to gain insight into the intent behind particular orders.

Healthcare: Interdisciplinary Negotiations on Key Decisions

In space shuttle mission control, every observed hand-off update about 16 decisions (for example, they decided to land a day early because there is a leak) was associated with the team's "stance" towards the decision (for example, we think that they should land as soon as possible to reduce the chances that the leak will get worse, Patterson and Woods 2001). By conveying this information, the team members can push for change in a coordinated fashion if the decision was "reopened" for negotiation across disciplines (in mission control, this is primarily the operational and engineering communities).

During observations of nursing shift change hand-offs on four acute care wards (Patterson, Roth and Render 2005), there were 71 instances of stance information conveyed during the hand-off updates. This information was not captured elsewhere in official paperwork, so listening to audio data from hand-off updates seems like a promising avenue to detect this information for a number of potentially interested parties. In this study, the stance of the nurse, the physician, and the patient were often communicated, as well as occasional references to the family and other specialists such as respiratory therapists.

During the observed STS-76 mission (Watts-Perotti and Woods, forthcoming), negotiations between the operations and engineering communities in mission control were conducted in a series of face-to-face meetings. It was considered important to conduct these off of the loops in order to facilitate the negotiation process, and it is possible that the same need for private negotiations across disciplines might be necessary in healthcare. However, following the meetings, the resolutions to resolve particular impasses (for example, we will land one day early) were broadcast over the loops. Therefore, it might be important to be able to turn "off" the ability for others to listen in on certain interdisciplinary meetings for a period of time until a resolution has been reached on a critical decision (for example, whether or not to proceed with surgery).

A mediator facilitates conversations between the operational and engineering communities in mission control. This position primarily serves the function of restricting and queuing requests from the engineering community that might disrupt time-critical and high-consequence operations in order to facilitate longer term goals such as maintaining shuttle integrity over multiple flights. An additional function was to help translate across the different languages and cultures of the two communities. Although the mediator was never observed to speak during observations, he was expected to monitor several operational and engineering loops simultaneously. In addition, it was expected that he would "lurk" on ad hoc conferences. It is possible that patient advocates, such as caregivers with medical training, case managers or social workers could serve similar functions in provider–patient communications.

Healthcare: Specialist Consults

In situations where specialist resources might be needed to be quickly and effectively "called in," having those resources gain an advance understanding might be valuable.

This might be particularly true for resources which are likely to be used somewhere in the hospital, such as IV site therapy, with the main uncertainty being for which patients. If electronic data that make it easier to predict the need for a specialist resource are available, tools might be developed to enable automated prediction of patients likely to need a specialized resource. Then the specialist resources could "listen in" on these likely patients to anticipate, without interrupting the care team, whether they will be needed, to do what, and when.

In the network telecommunications call center system described in Whittaker and Amento 2003, peripheral team members (for example, facilitators for customer interactions) were the primary people that had follow-up requests for information some time after the problem was resolved. In these cases, the people who had directly done the work were often unavailable. System features of automatically transcribed audio data that facilitated search and identification by header and timestamp information in a summary view were helpful in answering these questions, and were primarily done by supervisors.

Healthcare: Front Line Supervisors or Coordinators Listen Remotely to Detect Escalations

In mission control, front line supervisors, defined as people with principal authority and responsibility for tasks that have resources that augment their capabilities (for example, Front Room controllers with Back Room controller support), were highly sensitive to cues that indicated an escalation of activities (see Woods and Patterson 2001 for an example). Generally, these cues were detected on background loops from overall tone, emotion, and tempo of communications. When this occurred, the observed personnel frequently would "turn up the volume" on a particular loop and listen intently. A decision to escalate was also considered a critical one that required mutual awareness in the network telecommunications call center. In healthcare, potential applications of this function might include attending anesthesiologists or surgeons orchestrating multiple simultaneous operations or a telemetry nurse monitoring multiple patients simultaneously. It is also possible that information such as a request for a code team or news of an incoming critical patient to the Emergency Department might automatically trigger a loop to turn "on" for particular personnel to listen to. The design of when to turn the loop "off" after a problem is resolved, or at least change from "talk" to "monitor," might also be considered. In the case of the Thunderwire system in Singer et al. (1999), users requested that loops automatically turn off when there is an incoming phone call.

Healthcare: Overhearing by Indirect Audiences or Stakeholder Representatives

In space shuttle mission control, most of the voice loops are archived permanently and are available upon request by the Freedom of Information Act. In addition, some of the voice loops are able to be heard live on NASA TV. Although rare, use of the archived data for other purposes has been observed in mission control, primarily after an unfortunate outcome.

The difference between the accessibility of voice loops data and patient data is a key difference to consider in the translation of the voice loops concept to healthcare. Although no voice loop systems are known to exist currently in healthcare, speculation suggests that some or all of the following indirect audiences might be interested in the use of the data for other purposes:

- Patient (caregiver)
- Quality assurance
- Finance/administration
- Insurance companies
- Regulators
- Lawyers

Explicit translation of the data into a format geared to meet the needs of these indirect parties might be necessary prior to implementation for direct users. In addition, protection of data from parties such as lawyers might need to be considered in order to reap the potential benefits of the system, such as policies to delete all audio data after two days. Note that failure to consider potential indirect audiences for data has contributed to failures to adopt other systems, so it is recommended that they be considered explicitly during design and implementation, even if the use is not one that is intended to be supported.

This chapter explored how coordination benefits of "overhearing" that are realized on a daily basis in space shuttle mission control through the use of voice loop technology might theoretically be achieved in several healthcare settings, including the ICU, operating room, outpatient clinic, acute care, pharmacy, Emergency Department, and electronic ICU. The illustrative examples discussed in this chapter are not exhaustive by any means.

For such a relatively simple technology, there are a remarkable number of potential uses and benefits to be reaped, including:

- Anticipating unexpected events, planned responses, potential hazards
- Synchronizing planned events
- Being aware of major modifications to plans
- Knowing the rationale for non-routine requests
- Identifying redundant activities
- Reallocating tasks
- Detecting erroneous assessments, assumptions, missed opportunities
- Verifying "hanging" activities not dropped across handovers of responsibility
- Monitoring communication of key decisions and stances
- Broadcasting impasse resolutions (from face-to-face meetings)
- Mediating communication across communities with different languages
- Supporting efficient and effective addition of specialist "on call" resource

- Supporting follow-up requests for information
- Quickly detecting escalation
- Translating to and answering follow-up requests from stakeholder audiences

It is hoped that discussion of possible translation of uses and benefits of voice loop technology will inspire innovative uses of audio technology to improve team coordination, particularly across disciplines, in healthcare. Clearly, there are a variety of distinctions between mission control and healthcare that will necessitate tailoring the use of voice loop technology. This chapter has attempted to make some preliminary "best guesses" as to potential leverage points and resolutions of competing goals in a trade-off space. Nevertheless, seemingly insignificant design and implementation details can derail an otherwise useful concept. The use of well-known scenario-based iterative design methods in a simulated setting are highly recommended to reduce the risk of unintended side effects on performance, and to facilitate adoption of a new system that has the potential to fundamentally alter the nature of work (cf., bar coding studies described in Patterson, Rogers and Render 2004).

Acknowledgements

Research support was provided by NASA Johnson Space Center under Grant NAG9-390, Dr Jane Malin technical monitor. A VA HSR&D Merit Review Entry Program Award supported Dr Patterson. The views expressed in this article are those of the authors and do not necessarily represent the views of the Department of Veterans Affairs.

References

Anders, S., Woods, D.D., Wears, R.L. and Perry, S.J. (2006), 'Limits on Adaptation: Modeling Resilience and Brittleness in Hospital Emergency Departments', in E. Rigaud and E. Hollnagel (eds), *Second Symposium on Resilience Engineering*, Juan-les-Pins, France, November 8–10, 2006.

Baggs, J.G., Schmitt, M.H., Mushlin, A.I., Mitchell, P.H., Eldrege, D.H., Oakes, D. and Hutson, A.D. (1999), 'Association Between Nurse–Physician Collaboration and Patient Outcomes in Three Intensive Care Units', *Critical Care Medicine* 27:9, 1991–8.

Becker, C. (2000), 'Telemedicine System Helps Manage ICUs', *Modern Healthcare* 30:37, 62.

Coiera, E. and Tombs, V. (1998), 'Communication Behaviours in a Hospital Setting: An Observational Study', *British Medical Journal* 316:7132, 673–6.

Dodek, P.M. and Raboud, J. (2003), 'Explicit Approach to Rounds in an ICU Improves Communication and Satisfaction of Providers', *Intensive Care Medicine* 29:9, 1584–8.

Donchin, Y., Gopher, D., Olin, M., Badihi, Y., Biesky, M., Sprung, C.L., Pizov, R. and Cotev, S. (1995), 'A Look into the Nature and Causes of Human Errors in the Intensive Care Unit', *Critical Care Medicine* 23:2, 294–300.

Gurses, A.P. and Xiao, Y. (2006), 'A Systematic Review of the Literature on Multidisciplinary Rounds to Design Information Technology', *Journal of American Medical Informatics Association* 13:3, 267–76.

Henderson, D. and Card, S. (1986), 'Rooms: The Use of Multiple Virtual Workspaces to Reduce Space Contention in a Window-based Graphical User Interface', *ACM Transactions on Graphics* 5:3, 211–41.

Higgins, L.W. (1999), 'Nurses' Perceptions of Collaborative Nurse–Physician Transfer Decision Making as a Predictor of Patient Outcomes in a Medical Intensive Care Unit', *Journal of Advanced Nursing* 29:6, 1434–43.

Knaus, W.A., Draper, E.A., Wagner, D.P. and Zimmerman, J.E. (1986), 'An Evaluation of Outcome from Intensive Care in Major Medical Centers', *Annals of Internal Medicine* 104:3, 410–18.

Lamb G.S. and Napodano, R.J. (1984), 'Physician–Nurse Practitioner Interaction Patterns in Primary Care Practices', *American Journal of Public Health* 74:1, 26–9.

Leape, L., Cullen, D.J., Clapp, M.D., Burdick, E., Demonaco, H.J., Erickson, J.I. and Bates, D.W. (1999), 'Pharmacist Participation on Physician Rounds and Adverse Drug Events in the Intensive Care Unit', *Journal of the American Medical Association* 282:3, 267–70.

Norman, D.A. (1993), *Things That Make us Smart* (Reading, MA: Addison Wesley).

Patterson, E.S., Hofer, T., Brungs, S., Saint, S. and Render, M.L. (2006), 'Structured Interdisciplinary Communication Strategies in Four ICUs: An Observational Study', *Proceedings of the Human Factors and Ergonomics Society 50th Annual Meeting* (Santa Monica, CA: HFES) 929–33.

Patterson, E.S., Rogers, M.L. and Render, M.L. (2004), 'Simulation-based Embedded Probe Technique for Human–Computer Interaction Evaluation', *Cognition, Technology and Work* 6:3, 197–205.

Patterson, E.S., Roth, E.M. and Render, M.L. (2005), 'Handoffs During Nursing Shift Changes in Acute Care', *Proceedings of the Human Factors and Ergonomics Society 49th Annual Meeting* (Santa Monica, CA: HFES).

Patterson, E.S., Roth, E.M., Woods, D.D., Chow, R. and Gomes, J.O. (2004), 'Handoff Strategies in Settings with High Consequences for Failure: Lessons for Health Care Operations', *International Journal for Quality in Health Care* 16:2, 125–32.

Patterson, E.S., Watts-Perotti, J. and Woods, D.D. (1999), 'Voice Loops as Coordination Aids in Space Shuttle Mission Control', *Computer Supported Cooperative Work: The Journal of Collaborative Computing* 8:4, 353–71.

Patterson, E.S. and Woods, D.D. (2001), 'Shift Changes, Updates, and the On-call Model in Space Shuttle Mission Control', *Computer Supported Cooperative Work: The Journal of Collaborative Computing* 10:3–4, 317–46.

Patterson, E.S., Woods, D.D., Cook, R.I. and Render, M.L. (2007) 'Collaborative Cross-Checking to Enhance Resilience', *Cognition, Technology and Work* 9:3, 155–62.

Provonost, P.J., Jenckes, M.W., Dorman, T., Garret, E., Breslow, M.J., Rosenfeld, B.A., Lipsett, P.A. and Bass, E. (1999), 'Organizational Characteristics of Intensive Care Units Related to Outcomes of Abdominal Aortic Surgery', *Journal of the American Medical Association* 281:14, 1310–17.

Render, M.L., Kim, H.M., Deddens, J., Sivaganesin, S., Welsh, D.E., Bickel, K., Freyberg, R., Timmons, S., Johnston, J., Connors Jr, A.F., Wagner, D. and Hofer, T. (2005), 'Variation in Outcomes in Veterans Affairs Intensive Care Units with a Computerized Severity Measure', *Critical Care Medicine* 33:5, 930–39.

Saleem, J.J., Patterson, E.S., Militello, L., Render, M.L., Orshansky, G. and Asch, S.A. (2005), 'Exploring Barriers and Facilitators to the Use of Computerized Clinical Reminders', *Journal of American Medical Informatics Association* 12:4, 438–47.

Schmitt, M. (2001), 'Collaboration Improves the Quality of Care: Methodological Challenges and Evidence from US Health Care Research', *Journal of Interprofessional Care* 15:1, 47–66.

Singer, A., Hindus, D., Stifelman, L. and White, S. (1999), 'Tangible Progress: Less is More in Somewire Audio Spaces', *Proceedings of the SIGCHI Conference on Human Factors in Computing Systems: the CHI Is the Limit* (Pittsburgh, Pennsylvania, United States, May 15–20, 1999), CHI '99 (New York: ACM Press) 104–11.

Uhlig, P.N., Brown, J., Nason, A.K., Camelio, A. and Kendal, E. (2002), 'System Innovation: Concord Hospital', *Joint Commission Journal on Quality Improvement* 28:12, 666–72.

Vuckovic, N.H., Lavelle, M. and Gorman, P. (2004), 'Eavesdropping as Normative Behavior in a Cardiac Intensive Care Unit' (JHQ Online) W5-1 to W5-6, September–October.

Watts-Perotti, J. and Woods, D.D. (forthcoming), 'How Anomaly Response is Distributed Across Functionally Distinct Teams in Space Shuttle Mission Control'.

Whittaker, S. and Amento, B. (2003), 'Seeing What You Are Hearing: Co-ordinating Responses to Trouble Reports in Network Troubleshooting', *Proceedings of European Conference on Computer Supported Cooperative Work* (Netherlands: Kluwer) 219–38.

Woods, D.D. (1995), 'The Alarm Problem and Directed Attention in Dynamic Fault Management', *Ergonomics* 38:11, 2371–93.

Woods, D.D. and Hollnagel, E. (2006), *Joint Cognitive Systems: Patterns in Cognitive Systems Engineering* (Boca Raton, FL: Taylor and Francis).

Woods, D.D. and Patterson, E.S. (2001), 'How Unexpected Events Produce an Escalation of Cognitive and Coordinative Demands', in P.A. Hancock and P.A. Desmond (eds), *Stress Workload and Fatigue* (Hillsdale, NJ: Lawrence Erlbaum Associates) 290–304.

Chapter 7

Building Shared Situation Awareness in Healthcare Settings

Melanie C. Wright and Mica R. Endsley

Safe effective delivery of healthcare is a team effort. It requires the coordination of many individuals with different roles, different training, differing experience, and even different perspectives on care. Information sharing is integral to the coordination of these teams. The care and outcome of patients relies on the healthcare team's knowledge and understanding of both the patient's current state or presenting illness and past medical history. Of course, providers must have a strong knowledge base related to their specialty to provide effective care. However, without an adequate understanding of the dynamic information associated with each individual patient, healthcare teams will fail in their efforts to appropriately diagnose, treat, and otherwise care for patients.

The term situation awareness (SA) describes an individual's awareness and understanding of the dynamic information that is relevant to their current environment and task. SA is a critical precursor to effective decision making. This dynamic knowledge is especially important in the healthcare environment where misinformation can result in catastrophic consequences. The theory of SA has also been extended to include such team environments, and addresses the need for both team SA and shared SA as forming a basic foundation for needed coordination and team performance. In this chapter, we present a model of team SA that describes the critical foundations upon which high levels of shared SA are developed in team environments, including the role of communications. We also describe devices and processes that facilitate the development of high levels of team SA.

Situation Awareness and Team SA Defined

Situation awareness (SA) can be thought of as an internalized mental model of the current state of a healthcare provider's environment (Endsley 2001). All of the incoming data from information systems, paper-based communications, the outside environment, fellow providers, and others (for example, patients, family) must be brought together into an integrated whole. This integrated picture forms the central organizing feature from which all decision making and action takes place. A major portion of a healthcare provider's job is involved in developing SA and keeping it up to date in a rapidly changing environment. This is a task that is not simple in light of the complexity and many factors that must be taken into account in order to make effective care decisions.

The formal definition of SA defines three distinct levels of SA (Endsley 1995a). The first level is perception, which involves perceiving critical factors in the environment such as patient vital signs, lab values, and awareness of other team member activities. The second level is comprehension or an understanding of what those factors mean, particularly when integrated together in relation to the care provider's goals. For example, a provider will integrate and synthesize information about past medical history, present illness, and treatments to understand the significance of elevated laboratory values and know if it represents an expected and temporary event or some other problem that requires additional attention. The third and highest level of SA is projection—an understanding of what will happen with the system in the near future. Providers will use their knowledge and understanding of the current situation to predict, for example, a patient's response to drug delivery. This type of projection is critical in allowing them to be proactive, rather than reactive in responding to both expected and unexpected events.

The process of achieving SA, or situation assessment, is sometimes described as "sensemaking," or making sense of the information or of events in the environment (Weick 1995; Klein, Moon and Hoffman 2006). While people sometimes engage in effortful, intentional deliberation and assessment to make sense of the data to form Level 2 SA, evidence suggests that situation recognition is frequently instantaneous and reflexive (Kaempf, Wolf and Miller 1993, 1107–11). Active sensemaking is engaged in when needed, but represents only a portion of the picture. A detailed model of the factors involved in achieving and maintaining SA is provided in Endsley (1995a), as shown in Figure 7.1. In addition to representing the three levels of SA, key factors in the model include: (1) the role of goals and goal-directed processing in directing attention and interpreting the significance of perceived information; (2) the role of expectations (fed by the current model of the situation and by long-term memory stores) in directing attention and interpreting information; (3) differing methods of processing information (for example, deliberate effortful processing requiring working memory versus automated pattern recognition based on experience) to achieve SA; and (4) the importance of feedback in attaining and maintaining SA. As an individual begins to make sense of the world, achieving higher levels of SA, this information then drives further information seeking and direction of attention. Individuals are then able to distinguish important and relevant perceptual data from that which may be distracting and inconsequential.

Team Situation Awareness

Just as SA is critical to the performance of an individual, team SA is critical to the performance of teams. Team SA is "… the degree to which each team member possesses the SA required for his or her responsibilities" (Endsley 1995a). A team can be considered to have high team SA when all of the individuals on the team possess the SA required for their respective roles. If each of two team members needs to know a piece of information, it is not sufficient that one knows it perfectly but the other does not. For instance, in the operating room, if the scrub nurse is aware

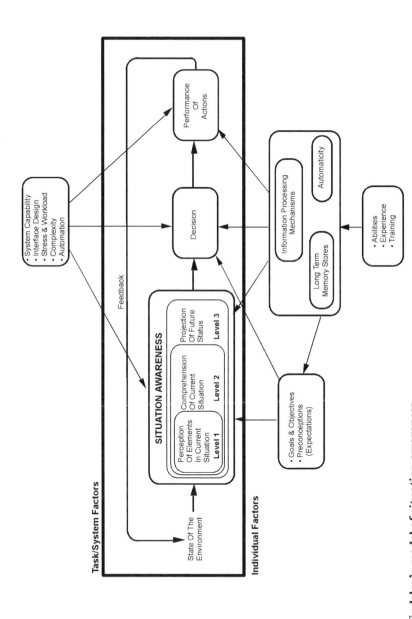

Figure 7.1 Endsley's model of situation awareness

Source: Endsley 1995a. (Reprinted with permission from *Human Factors*. Copyright 1995 by the Human Factors and Ergonomics Society. All rights reserved.)

of certain information, but not the surgeon who also needs it, the SA of the team is deficient and performance may suffer unless the discrepancy is corrected. The state of team SA (from poor to perfect) will vary over time in much the same way that individual SA varies over time.

In a team, each team member has a subgoal pertinent to his or her specific role that feeds into the overall team goal. Associated with each team member's subgoals are a set of SA elements about which he or she is concerned—the SA requirements for that team member's job (Endsley 1989; Endsley 1995a). As the members of a team are essentially interdependent in meeting the overall team goal, some overlap between team members' subgoals and, therefore, their SA requirements will be present. It is this subset of information that necessitates much of team coordination. That coordination may occur as a verbal exchange, as duplication of displayed information, or by some other means.

Team SA can be divided into two types: (1) complementary SA, in which the team members have SA that does not overlap but is complementary, resulting in the needed team SA; and (2) shared SA, in which team members share the same SA. A major part of teamwork involves the area where SA requirements overlap (see Figure 7.2), or shared SA. Shared SA requirements exist as a function of the essential interdependency of the team. For example, in an emergency room environment, nurses and physicians will each have unique functions for which they will have unique SA requirements. Yet it is also clear that they must operate on a common set of data and that the assessments and actions of one can have a large impact on the assessments and actions of the other. This interdependency will create a high need for shared SA. A high level of team SA, like individual SA, is a critical precursor to effective team decisions and actions (see Figure 7.3).

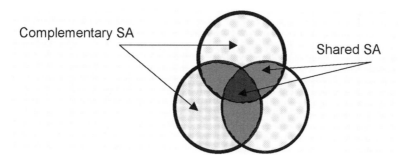

Figure 7.2 Complementary and shared SA requirements

COMMUNICATION

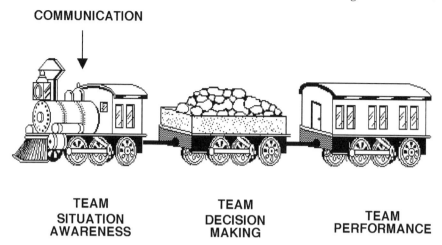

TEAM	TEAM	
SITUATION	DECISION	TEAM
AWARENESS	MAKING	PERFORMANCE

**Figure 7.3 Communication and team SA as critical precursors to team
decision making and performance**

There are different possible states of shared SA between two team members: (1)
both correct, (2) one correct and one incorrect, and (3) both incorrect. Clearly, the
goal is for all team members to have correct shared SA. In the case where two
team members both have incorrect SA, it is possible that their SA be incorrect and
different or that they both have common, but incorrect, SA. A dangerous situation
occurs when team members share common but incorrect SA. In one study of SA
incidents in commercial aviation, it was noted that 60 per cent involved losses of
SA by both crew members (Jentsch, Barnett and Bowers 1997, 1379). In this case,
there is no dissonance between team members that may lead to the identification
and resolution of a problem. Team members may remain locked into their incorrect
picture of the situation until some external event occurs to alter it. For example,
if a blood pressure monitor in the operating room is not calibrated properly (for
example, after bed movement), surgeons, anesthesia providers, and nurses may all
proceed to treat the patient based on inaccurate data.

Problems in Team Situation Awareness

Teams have been found to suffer from SA problems in a number of different ways, as
shown in Figure 7.4. First, the needed information may not be passed clearly between
team members. For example, critical patient information may not be included on the
chart, may be illegible, or may not be communicated from one clinician to another.
Secondly, when the information is passed, different team members may interpret the
information differently, based on differing goals or mental models. For example,
one specialist who reads a particular test result may not necessarily reach the same
conclusions as another specialist who has a different reservoir of knowledge about a
particular disease. Finally, even with the same understanding of the current state of

the patient, different care providers may have different projections of what is likely to occur in the near future. One provider may think the patient will remain stable, while another realizes that the patient is likely to get worse. The different mental models that different team members bring with them have a significant effect on the projections they will make. In addition, the more heterogeneous the teams, the more likely they are to have different mental models, and thus the more likely they are to reach very different comprehension and projections. These teams are also more likely to be separated and have less direct communication and access to shared information than collocated teams from the same department.

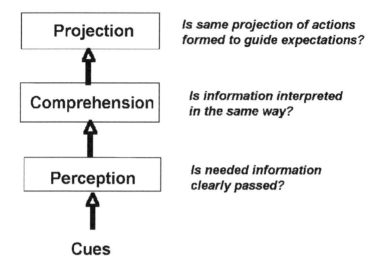

Figure 7.4 Failures in team SA

If teams are communicating effectively, then they can overcome these potential disconnects in SA. In examining failures in team SA in other domains, however, several problems have been found that limit this outcome (Endsley and Robertson 2000). Often certain teams are not aware that other teams do not have the required information or that they need certain information, and thus do not attempt to communicate it. Teams also tend to communicate at the level of data or observations (Level 1 SA), rather than at higher levels, under the assumption that others will inherently reach the same conclusions or projections as they have, which is often not the case.

Another failure in team SA is that feedback loops are often very poor between different organizations or departments, reducing the opportunity for learning and thus improving mental models and SA. For example, when a patient is misdiagnosed by one physician and later correctly diagnosed, the first physician may never be made aware of the misdiagnosis. Thus, for that physician, the wrong diagnosis may be reinforced and the error perpetuated for the next patient. Hand-offs and shift turnover are critical areas for potential failures in team SA. Not only can critical information about patient state be missed, but providers also may not pass on factors such as changes over time or other events that seem insignificant, but can be important to understanding and interpreting what occurs in the next shift.

Measuring Teamwork and Team Situation Awareness

Measuring teamwork is important for assessing both the teamwork skills of individuals and teams and for assessing the effectiveness of interventions such as training programs, new equipment designs, or new team communication processes. Current tools or methods for assessing teamwork skills in healthcare generally involve the use of observer-based rating scales, which often are specific to the healthcare task at hand (Fletcher et al. 2003; Healey, Undre and Vincent 2004; Thomas, Sexton and Helmreich 2004). These scales typically incorporate a component of situation awareness or situation assessment (observable actions that enhance team SA). Problems with these types of scales may include: (1) a high degree of domain-specific knowledge required for the individuals doing the observations; (2) difficulty in achieving high degrees of inter-observer agreement; and (3) the need to focus on only teamwork skills that are "observable." We recently evaluated a general behaviorally anchored team coordination rating scale (Wright et al. 2006). Two observers rated medical students' teamwork on two simulated emergent care tasks based on the exhibition of team skill behaviors that would support the maintenance and development of a high degree of shared SA. We were able to establish moderate inter-observer agreement regarding overall team skill ratings.

An alternative to measuring team skills using behaviorally based observations is the objective measure of situation awareness using the Situation Awareness Global Assessment Technique (SAGAT). This technique involves the presentation of specific task-relevant queries to assess an individual's SA at a given point in time (Wright, Taekman and Endsley 2004). While SAGAT generally requires a simulation or otherwise artificial evaluation environment (see Jones and Endsley 2000 for an alternative), it can be used to objectively assess whether participants in a task have a high level of SA. An objective measure of SA such as SAGAT can provide unique insight into team performance. Queries can be designed to assess specific SA requirements for each team member role. More importantly, however, responses to queries related to common SA requirements can be compared across team members, identifying SA differences between team member roles. In addition, specific responses can be compared to determine whether the same responses (correct or incorrect) are made across team member roles. This type of analysis can provide diagnostic information regarding the source of breakdowns in team SA. For example, common incorrect responses may be indicative of problems that affect the entire team in a similar way (such as poorly designed information display). Alternatively, a mix of correct and incorrect responses or different incorrect responses across team member roles may be indicative of breakdowns in team coordination.

Healthcare Team Communications and SA

In healthcare, research involving the assessment of SA is limited (Wright, Taekman and Endsley 2004). A study by Zhang et al. incorporated the measurement of SA using a variation on SAGAT to compare two anesthesia displays (Zhang et al. 2002). They found significant differences in SA due to type of display for Level 1 and Level 2 SA for some of the scenarios tested. More recently, researchers have begun to incorporate theoretical models of SA into the analysis of medical errors (Reader et al. 2006; Singh, Petersen and Thomas 2006). Because of the critical importance of teamwork in healthcare, most SA research in healthcare is focused on issues of teamwork and team SA.

There is limited research in healthcare defining a direct link between measures of team SA and clinical team performance. One exception is recent research in our laboratory that revealed strong correlations ($r = 0.97$ and $r = 0.65$) between a measure of clinical team performance (ordering appropriate tests, selecting appropriate treatments) and subjective ratings of team communication and SA in two simulated emergent care tasks by teams of first-year medical students (Wright et al. forthcoming). There is, however, broad evidence to support the importance of good team communication and coordination to quality clinical care (Joint Commission 2006). And there is evidence in healthcare and other work environments to support an assertion that high levels of team SA are required for effective team communication and coordination.

For example, research in other work environments has shown that high performing teams provide unsolicited information to team members (Urban et al. 1993, 1233–7; Johannesen, Cook and Woods 1994, 225–9). In addition to providing unsolicited reports, experienced team members provided additional information in their reports (Johannesen, Cook and Woods 1994, 225–9). When asked a question, rather than simply answering the question, they often provide additional details based on the context of the question. Urban et al. (1993, 1233–7) found that good teams appeared to be more efficient in their use of questions, asking fewer questions (yet still receiving all the necessary information). Jentsch et al. (1995) found that teams that were faster in detecting a problem used more standard communications, made more leadership statements, and vocalized more situation awareness observations than did slow teams.

In an observational study of cognitive and collaborative demands in the operating room, the researchers identified information loss or degradation as an emerging theme related to system vulnerabilities (Roth et al. 2004). The source of information loss was frequently related to the transfer of pre-operative information, such as the pre-operative assessment and information specified in a pre-operative "case booking" by the surgical team. Either critical information was missing from the relevant pre-operative documents or the team members receiving the information failed to perceive or act on that information.

As another example, successes related to the use of "briefings" and checklists may be attributed to the promotion of better team SA. Einav, Gopher and Donchin (2006) found that the use of pre-operative briefings significantly decreased the number of operations in which one or more team members revealed a lack of knowledge regarding the patient or procedure. The cardiac surgery team at Concord Hospital in Concord, NH designed and implemented start-of-day collaborative care rounds to share information and develop a plan for each patient (Uhlig et al. 2002). The briefing process includes a structured communication protocol and is conducted at the patient's bedside (including the patient and family in the process). Following the implementation of this protocol, Concord Hospital's cardiac surgery patients had a significant reduction in mortality from expected rates.

Situation Awareness Research and Applications in High Hazard Sectors

Research in aviation and other environments where SA has been measured supports a link between SA and task performance or outcomes. Measures of SA have correlated with performance in aviation (Venturino, Hamilton and Dvorchak 1989, 4/1–4/5; Endsley 1990, 41–5). In a study of major airline accidents, 88 per cent of accidents involving human error were linked to problems with SA (Endsley 1995b, 287–92). SA measures have been shown to be sensitive to both task difficulty and experience in aviation and in power plant operations (Selcon, Taylor and Koritsas 1991, 57–61; Collier and Folleso 1995, 115–22). With respect to a relationship to decision making, Bell and Lyon found that fighter pilots with lower observer ratings of SA during a combat scenario had a greater number of decision errors than pilots with more highly rated SA (Bell and Lyon 2000, 129–46).

Beyond this, research has also shown measures of SA to be sensitive to differences between system or design characteristics that were not reflected by performance measures. This is particularly interesting for complex fields where errors occur rarely but have high consequences, such as both aviation and healthcare. In one example, Endsley conducted a study comparing the SA of pilots using a new avionics system with that of pilots using the old system (Endsley 1988, 789–95). Pilots subjectively believed the new system to be better, but mission performance measures showed no differences. Endsley used SAGAT to evaluate the new system. She found that the new system provided pilots with better SA regarding knowledge of enemy aircraft location and other critical factors compared to the old system.

In another example, concern about the effects of a new form of air traffic control known as "free flight" on the ability of the air traffic controllers to track and monitor aircraft led to a comparison of performance and SA between the new and old systems (Endsley et al. 1997). Performance tests with the new system showed trends toward performance differences regarding separation errors, although the results were not significant. SAGAT measures in this experiment were able to provide more diagnostic detail, showing that controllers were aware of significantly fewer aircraft under free flight conditions (Level 1 SA), that controllers had a significantly reduced understanding of what was happening in the traffic situation (Level 2 SA), and that controllers had reduced knowledge of where aircraft were going (Level 3 SA). These studies suggest that, within the limited sensitivity, scope, or time involved in a laboratory study, measures of SA can have diagnostic powers beyond measures of performance that may be predictive of performance problems or errors that would otherwise remain unseen. In healthcare, where "gold standard" outcome measures may fail to predict infrequent but catastrophic errors or events, such diagnostic and predictive measures can be an important addition.

Devices, Mechanisms, and Processes to Support Shared Situation Awareness

The development of high levels of shared SA and overall team SA involve a number of external devices such as written communications or shared displays, internal mechanisms such as a shared understanding of one another's tasks, and deliberate processes such as briefings or hand-off checklists (Endsley, Bolte and Jones 2003).

Shared SA Devices

Shared SA devices are those that are used to share or communicate real-time dynamic information related to shared SA requirements. Verbal communication is the most obvious device, and research has shown that teams that use verbal communication effectively outperform teams that do not. Research on verbal communication patterns of teams described earlier revealed that there are discernable differences in verbal communication between low and high performing teams. Other verbal communication techniques that serve to enhance information exchange and the development of shared SA may include acknowledging information received, repeating back or summarizing information received, and the use of standard terminology.

Other devices used to communicate dynamic information related to shared SA requirements include written communications and information displays (visual, auditory, or other forms). In healthcare, written communications such as patient charts, physician orders, and lab results contain critical information for supporting shared SA. Recent research has revealed that these devices can be a source of error (Roth et al. 2004) and it is clear that careful design of written communications is critical to enhancing team SA.

Visual displays such as patient physiological monitors also display information that is required by multiple team members. Low technology shared displays such as white boards or other large shared information displays may also serve as critical shared SA devices in healthcare (Nemeth et al. 2004; Xiao 2005). For example, Moses Cone hospital in Greensboro, NC has recently developed and implemented two forms of low technology shared information displays that support the development and maintenance of shared SA. First, they created "hall passes," affixed to the top of a patient's chart, traveling with patients that are being transported throughout the hospital. These short printed documents contain a small set of critical shared SA information (such as whether the patient is on oxygen or has communication barriers) that is relevant to transporting and receiving units. Secondly, they created white boards for patient rooms containing line items for critical shared SA information relevant to anyone entering the room, such as current medications, daily goals, and contact information for both the patient's nurse and the patient's family (Fillipo 2006). Wears and colleagues have studied the use and development of status boards in the emergency department (Wears et al. 2007). They suggest that the success and continued use of such low-tech devices is because they are locally owned and designed, easily reconfigurable, informal, and widely accessible to the team. Features of the boards that are useful are initiated easily and adopted, while ineffective features are quickly dropped.

Shared SA Mechanisms

Shared SA mechanisms are internal mechanisms that aid the development of SA. In particular, the presence of shared or common mental models is believed to support shared SA. The term "mental model" is used to describe internal models, stored in long-term memory, that represent a person's underlying knowledge about specific systems or environments. Serfaty, Entin and Volpe (1993, 1228–32) found that discrepancies between the mental model of a team leader and the mental model of subordinates on the cost of errors generated non-trivial patterns of error making in teams. Cross-training team members on other team member tasks may support the development of common or shared mental models and has led to improved team performance and communication (Travillian et al. 1993, 1243–7; Volpe et al. 1996). Orasanu (1993, 137–72) found that effective flight crews had captains that exhibited planning behavior that facilitated the development of shared mental models between crew members.

Bolstad and Endsley (1999; 2000) have explored the effect of shared displays on fostering shared mental models and shared situation awareness. They found that performance was best when subjects were able to view one another's displays initially and then perform without viewing one another's displays (Bolstad and Endsley 1999). This suggests that sharing the displays allowed them to develop similar mental models, but that during task performance, viewing both displays provided excess information that was detrimental to performance. In a separate study, teams performed better under high workload when team members used displays that abstracted pertinent information from the other team member's display, compared to fully shared displays or displays that did not provide the additional information (Bolstad and Endsley 2000). They also found that communication shifted from verbal communication to more implicit coordination (due to shared situation awareness) with the shared displays. At high levels of workload, the shared displays provide advantages by reducing communication requirements. Bolstad and Endsley (2000) caution that shared displays should be designed carefully because excess information provided on shared displays can slow performance.

Shared SA Processes

Lastly, shared SA processes refers to specific processes that effective teams use to support the development of shared SA. These processes may: (1) support real-time sharing of dynamic data (for example, means of effective communication); (2) promote the development of a shared understanding of the goals of the team and the problem at hand; or (3) serve to foster an environment where information sharing is promoted. Examples of processes that support the development of shared SA may include the use of hand-off checklists, multidisciplinary rounds, briefings, time-outs, and debriefings. Research described previously has shown the benefits of these processes on clinical outcomes (Lingard et al. 2005; Einav, Gopher and Donchin 2006, 954–8; Uhlig et al. 2002). As another example, Leonard, Graham and Bonacum (2004) describe the benefits of specific communication tools or processes that support information sharing. They describe the success of two of these: (1) the use of a structured language process that follows the acronym "SBAR" for situation, background, assessment, recommendation; and (2) the use of a specific critical language phrase (that is, "I need clarity") as a means of stressing an important or critical situation. Both of these processes have been adopted into practice within the Kaiser health system.

Implications for Design and Training to Support Healthcare Team Communications

Implications for Design

There are a number of implications that a model of team SA has on the design of healthcare equipment and processes. First, a model of team SA makes it clear that the identification of critical shared SA requirements is key to the design of effective information displays and information sharing tools (for example, checklists or forms). Human factors methods such as cognitive task analyses may be used for eliciting these requirements (see, for example, Endsley, Bolte and Jones 2003; Crandall, Klein and Hoffman 2006). Clearly, however, these methods must focus attention on the SA requirements that must be shared between individuals or team member roles. This process will thus require a multidisciplinary approach with subject matter expertise related to each of the team member specialties and roles.

Second, it is important to consider the design and use of displays or communication tools with the primary purpose of promoting and maintaining a high degree of shared SA. Several healthcare interventions described earlier—start-of-day briefings (Uhlig et al. 2002), pre-operative briefings (Lingard et al. 2005; Einav, Gopher and Donchin 2006, 954–8), structured communications (Leonard, Graham and Bonacum 2004), "hall passes" (Fillipo 2006)—support this assertion. In addition to processes such as these that directly involve the sharing of information, processes that promote an environment of information sharing are also beneficial. This may be as simple as a leader who routinely greets team members, introduces his or herself, and acknowledges and requests input from all team members, regardless of "rank" or experience.

Third, a model of shared SA implies that equipment and processes for individual roles should also be designed with interactions with other team members in mind. For example, displays that abstract small subsets of information from the domain of another team member could foster the development and maintenance of shared mental models that will support shared SA (Bolstad and Endsley 2000). In addition, designers must also consider that displays that may primarily be used by one provider (for example, an anesthesia provider) may also be used by other providers (for example, a surgeon), and that the presentation of information should support both purposes (see Endsley, Bolte and Jones 2003 for a detailed description of specific principles regarding the design of systems to support shared SA).

Implications for Healthcare Team Training and Assessment

A model of team SA also has a number of implications for training and assessment of healthcare teams. First, training and assessment of teamwork should incorporate behaviors that serve to develop and maintain shared SA. A number of healthcare team training programs have been developed and implemented in recent years (see Baker et al. 2003 for a review). A publicly available healthcare team training program, titled TeamSTEPPS, incorporates a model of team behavior that involves knowledge, skills, and attitudes associated with leadership, communication, situation monitoring, and mutual support (Department of Defense Patient Safety Program and Agency for Healthcare Research and Quality 2006). Examples of specific behaviors that enhance the development and maintenance of shared SA include: (1) communication skills such as the use of standard terminology, acknowledgement and repeat back of information received, the use of structured communication, and the use of critical language; and (2) the knowledge and practice of specific processes such as planning, briefing, and time-outs that support the development and maintenance of shared SA.

Related to this, the second implication of a model of team SA on training is that training of teamwork should include relevant practice in realistic training environments. Behaviors such as the use of structured communication and the conduct of effective briefings require not only the knowledge of these tools, but also practice or experience to attain skill in their use (Dreyfus 2004). Practice in these skills should be incorporated into the important and relatively common on-the-job healthcare provider training. In addition, practice in these skills should include multidisciplinary simulation-based training that can focus on critical scenarios that might otherwise be rarely encountered during training (Hamman 2004; Wilson et al. 2005). It is also possible to integrate the training of shared SA processes and communication skills into simulated clinical skills training. A model of team SA suggests that a meaningful understanding of shared SA requirements will likely require practice environments that incorporate all of the complexity of the relevant healthcare work environment. Helmreich, Merritt and Wilhelm (1999) describe how team training in aviation has evolved over the past 25 years into a more integrated approach, with teamwork skills being integrated into all flight training, rather than being presented as a stand-alone training module.

Third, a model of team SA implies that training of healthcare providers should incorporate effective cross-training and multidisciplinary training. For members of a team to have a shared understanding of the environment and their goals, it is critical that they have an understanding of the tasks, goals, and information requirements of other members of the team. This will require greater depth of training than lecture-based discussion of the goals and roles of other healthcare team members. Effective cross-training and multidisciplinary training should include on-the-job exposure to the requirements and demands of providers or specialties with which individuals will have close collaboration. Similarly, multidisciplinary simulation training will provide the opportunity for evaluating both shared SA processes and requirements.

Finally, a model of team SA also implies that assessment of team SA should be completed in realistic practice environments. Traditional assessment measures such as written examinations and oral examinations generally assess the "knows" and "knows how" aspects of Miller's pyramid of clinical competence (Miller 1990). While these methods can be applied to principles of good team coordination, the higher levels of clinical competence including "shows how" and "does" are likely to be more important for assessing skills that support shared SA. Assessment in simulation or real world environments is essential for evaluating the success of both training and design approaches to enhancing team SA. Assessment can be attained through a number of techniques including: (1) observation of behaviors that support shared SA, (2) direct measurement of SA, or (3) measurement of clinical team performance or patient outcomes.

Conclusions

Research focused on measuring individual and team SA provides insight into the effect of SA on both individual and team performance. Behaviors that support the development of shared SA such as planning and frequent situation assessment updates have been shown to be associated with more effective team performance. Techniques such as cross-training in different team member roles and the design of collaborative information displays can also support the development of shared SA. Theories of individual and team SA can support healthcare team communication by providing a basis for better understanding the SA requirements within different healthcare roles and environments. This understanding then serves to inform system design, training, and assessment to enhance healthcare team communication.

Acknowledgements

Dr Wright's research is currently funded by grants from the Agency for Healthcare Research and Quality, NIH (K02 HS015704-01) and the Anesthesia Patient Safety Foundation. The efforts described in assessing the team skills of medical students were funded by grant #0304-101 of the Edward J. Stemmler, MD Medical Education Research Fund at the National Board of Medical Examiners. The authors would like to thank Jeffrey Taekman, Robert Wears, and Christopher Nemeth for their valued reviews and input.

References

Baker, D.P., Gustafson, S., Beaubien, J., Salas, E. and Barach, P. (2003), *Medical Teamwork and Patient Safety: The Evidence-Based Relation* (Washington, DC: American Institutes for Research).

Bell, R.H. and Lyon, D.R. (2000), 'Using Observer Ratings to Assess Situation Awareness', in M.R. Endsley and D.J. Garland (eds), *Situation Awareness Analysis and Measurement* (Mahwah, NJ: Lawrence Erlbaum Associates).

Bolstad, C.A. and Endsley, M.R. (1999), 'Shared Mental Models and Shared Displays: An Empirical Evaluation of Team Performance', *Proceedings of the 43rd Meeting of the Human Factors and Ergonomics Society* (Santa Monica, CA: HFES).

Bolstad, C.A. and Endsley, M.R. (2000), 'The Effect of Task Load and Shared Displays on Team Situation Awareness', *Proceedings of the 44th Annual Meeting of the Human Factors and Ergonomic Society* (Santa Monica, CA: HFES).

Collier, S.G. and Folleso, K. (1995), 'SACRI: A Measure of Situation Awareness for Nuclear Power Plant Control Rooms', in D.J. Garland and M.R. Endsley (eds), *Experimental Analysis and Measurement of Situation Awareness* (Daytona Beach, FL: Embry-Riddle University Press).

Crandall, B., Klein, G. and Hoffman, R.R. (2006), *Working Minds: A Practitioner's Guide to Cognitive Task Analysis* (Cambridge, MA: The MIT Press).

Department of Defense Patient Safety Program and Agency for Healthcare Research and Quality (2006), 'Team Strategies and Tools to Enhance Performance and Patient Safety', [website] (updated November 6, 2006): <http://www.usuhs.mil/cerps/teamstepps.html>, accessed November 12, 2006.

Dreyfus, S.E. (2004), 'The Five-Stage Model of Adult Skill Acquisition', *Bulletin of Science, Technology and Society* 24:3, 177–81.

Einav, Y., Gopher, D. and Donchin, Y. (2006), 'Briefing in the Operating Room – A Tool for Enhancing Coordination and Enriching Shared Knowledge Bases', *Proceedings of the Human Factors and Ergonomics Society 50th Annual Meeting* (Santa Monica, CA: HFES).

Endsley, M.R. (1988), 'Situation Awareness Global Assessment Technique (SAGAT)', *Proceedings of the National Aerospace and Electronics Conference (NAECON)* (New York: IEEE).

Endsley, M.R. (1989), *Final Report: Situation Awareness in an Advanced Strategic Mission* (Hawthorne, CA: Northrop Corporation).

Endsley, M.R. (1990), 'Predictive Utility of an Objective Measure of Situation Awareness', *Proceedings of the Human Factors Society 34th Annual Meeting* (Santa Monica, CA: HFES).

Endsley, M.R. (1995a), 'Toward a Theory of Situation Awareness in Dynamic Systems', *Human Factors* 37:1, 32–64.

Endsley, M.R. (1995b), 'A Taxonomy of Situation Awareness Errors', in R. Fuller, N. Johnston and N. McDonald (eds), *Human Factors in Aviation Operations* (Aldershot, UK: Ashgate).

Endsley, M.R. (2001), 'Designing for Situation Awareness in Complex Systems', *Proceedings of the Second International Workshop on Symbiosis of Humans, Artifacts and Environment*, Kyoto, Japan.

Endsley, M.R., Bolte, B. and Jones, D.G. (2003), *Designing for Situation Awareness: An Approach to Human-Centered Design* (London: Taylor and Francis).

Endsley, M.R. and Garland D.J. (eds) (2000), *Situation Awareness Analysis and Measurement* (Mahwah, NJ: Lawrence Erlbaum Associates).

Endsley, M.R., Mogford, R., Allendoerfer, K., Snyder, M.D. and Stein, E.S. (1997), *Effect of Free Flight Conditions on Controller Performance, Workload, and Situation Awareness: A Preliminary Investigation of Changes in Locus of Control Using Existing Technology* (Atlantic City, NJ: Federal Aviation Administration William J. Hughes Technical Center).

Endsley, M.R. and Robertson, M.M. (2000), 'Training for Situation Awareness in Individuals and Teams', in M.R. Endsley and D.J. Garland (eds), *Situation Awareness Analysis and Measurement* (Mahwah, NJ: Lawrence Erlbaum Associates).

Fillipo, B. (2006), 'Communication and Teamwork: Essentials for Patient-centered Care', presented at the *North Carolina Quality and Patient Safety Conference* (Chapel Hill, NC: North Carolina Center for Hospital Quality and Patient Safety).

Fletcher, G., Flin, R., McGeorge, P., Glavin, R., Maran, N. and Patey, R. (2003), 'Anaesthetists' Non-Technical Skills (ANTS): Evaluation of a Behavioural Marker System', *British Journal of Anaesthesia* 90:5, 580–88.

Fuller, R., Johnston, N. and McDonald, N. (eds) (1995), *Human Factors in Aviation Operations* (Aldershot, UK: Ashgate).

Garland, D.J. and Endsley, M.R. (eds) (1995), *Experimental Analysis and Measurement of Situation Awareness* (Daytona Beach, FL: Embry-Riddle University Press).

Hamman, W.R. (2004), 'The Complexity of Team Training: What We Have Learned from Aviation and its Applications to Medicine', *Quality and Safety in Healthcare* 13:Suppl. 1, i72–9.

Healey, A.N., Undre, S. and Vincent, C.A. (2004), 'Developing Observational Measures of Performance in Surgical Teams', *Quality and Safety in Healthcare* 13:Suppl. 1, i33–40.

Helmreich, R.L., Merritt, A.C. and Wilhelm, J.A. (1999), 'The Evolution of Crew Resource Management Training in Commercial Aviation', *International Journal of Aviation Psychology* 9:1, 19–32.

Jentsch, F., Barnett, J.S. and Bowers, C.A. (1997), 'Loss of Aircrew Situation Awareness: A Cross Validation', *Proceedings of the Human Factors and Ergonomics Society Annual Meeting* (Santa Monica, CA: HFES).

Jentsch, F.G., Sellin-Wolters, S., Bowers, C.A. and Salas, E. (1995), 'Crew Coordination Behaviors as Predictors of Problem Detection and Decision Making Times', *Proceedings of the Human Factors and Ergonomics Society 39th Annual Meeting* (Santa Monica, CA: HFES).

Johannesen, L.J., Cook, R.I. and Woods, D.D. (1994), 'Cooperative Communications in Dynamic Fault Management', *Proceedings of the Human Factors and Ergonomics Society 38th Annual Meeting* (Santa Monica, CA: HFES).

Joint Commission (2006), 'Sentinel Event Statistics – June 30, 2006', [website] (updated June 30, 2006): <http://www.jointcommission.org/SentinelEvents/Statistics/>, accessed February 6, 2007.

Jones, D.G. and Endsley, M.R. (2000), 'Can Real-time Probes Provide a Valid Measurement of Situation Awareness?', in D.B. Kaber and M.R. Endsley (eds),

Human Performance, Situation Awareness, and Automation: User-Centered Design for the New Millennium (Atlanta: SA Technologies, Inc.).

Kaber, D.B. and Endsley, M.R. (eds) (2000), *Human Performance, Situation Awareness, and Automation: User-Centered Design for the New Millennium* (Atlanta: SA Technologies, Inc.).

Kaempf, G.L., Wolf, S. and Miller, T.E. (1993), 'Decision Making in the AEGIS Combat Information Center', *Proceedings of the Human Factors and Ergonomics Society 37th Annual Meeting* (Santa Monica, CA: HFES).

Klein, G., Moon, B. and Hoffman, R.R. (2006), 'Making Sense of Sensemaking 1: Alternative Perspectives', *IEEE Intelligent Systems* 21:4, 70–73.

Leonard, M., Graham, S. and Bonacum, D. (2004), 'The Human Factor: The Critical Importance of Effective Teamwork and Communication in Providing Safe Care', *Quality and Safety in Healthcare* 13:Suppl. 1, i85–90.

Lingard, L., Espin, S., Rubin, B., Whyte, S., Colmenares, M., Baker, G.R., Doran, D., Grober, E., Orser, B., Bohnen, J. and Reznick, R. (2005), 'Getting Teams to Talk: Development and Pilot Implementation of a Checklist to Promote Interprofessional Communication in the OR', *Quality and Safety in Healthcare* 14:5, 340–46.

Miller, G.E. (1990), 'The Assessment of Clinical Skills/Competence/Performance', *Academic Medicine* 65:9, S63–7.

Nemeth, C., O'Connor, M., Cook, R., Wears, R. and Perry, S. (2004), 'Crafting Information Technology Solutions, Not Experiments, for the Emergency Department', *Academic Emergency Medicine* 11:11, 1114–17.

Orasanu, J. (1993), 'Decision-making in the Cockpit', in E.L. Wiener, B.G. Kanki and R.L. Helmreich (eds), *Cockpit Resource Management* (San Francisco: Academic).

Reader, T., Flin, R., Lauche, K. and Cuthbertson, B.H. (2006), 'Non-technical Skills in the Intensive Care Unit', *British Journal of Anaesthesia* 96:5, 551–9.

Roth, E.M., Christian, C.K., Gustafson, M.L., Sheridan, T.B., Dwyer, K., Gandhi, T.K., Zinner, M.J. and Dierks, M.M. (2004), 'Using Field Observations as a Tool for Discovery: Analysing Cognitive and Collaborative Demands in the Operating Room', *Cognition, Technology and Work* 6:3, 148–57.

Selcon, S.J., Taylor, R.M. and Koritsas, E. (1991), 'Workload or Situational Awareness? TLX vs. SART for Aerospace Systems Design Evaluation', *Proceedings of the Human Factors Society 36th Annual Meeting* (Santa Monica, CA: HFES).

Serfaty, D., Entin, E.E. and Volpe, C. (1993), 'Adaptation to Stress in Team Decision-making and Coordination', *Proceedings of the Human Factors and Ergonomics Society 37th Annual Meeting* (Santa Monica, CA: HFES).

Singh, H., Petersen, L.A. and Thomas, E.J. (2006), 'Understanding Diagnostic Errors in Medicine: A Lesson from Aviation', *Quality and Safety in Healthcare* 15:3, 159–64.

Thomas, E.J., Sexton, J.B. and Helmreich, R.L. (2004), 'Translating Teamwork Behaviours from Aviation to Healthcare: Development of Behavioural Markers for Neonatal Resuscitation', *Quality and Safety in Healthcare* 13:Suppl. 1, i57–64.

Travillian, K.K., Volpe, C.E., Canon-Bowers, J.A. and Salas, E. (1993), 'Cross-training Highly Interdependent Teams: Effects on Team Processes and Team Performance', *Proceedings of the Human Factors and Ergonomics Society 37th Annual Meeting* (Santa Monica, CA: HFES).

Uhlig, P.N., Brown, J., Nason, A.K., Camelio, A. and Kendall, E. (2002), 'John M. Eisenberg Patient Safety Awards. System Innovation: Concord Hospital', *Joint Commission Journal on Quality Improvement* 28:12, 666–72.

Urban, J.M., Bowers, C.A., Monday, S.D. and Morgan, B.B. (1993), 'Effects of Workload on Communication Processes in Decision-making Teams: An Empirical Study with Implications for Training', *Proceedings of the Human Factors and Ergonomics Society 37th Annual Meeting* (Santa Monica, CA: HFES).

Venturino, M., Hamilton, W.L. and Dvorchak, S.R. (1989), 'Performance-based Measures of Merit for Tactical Situation Awareness', *Situational Awareness in Aerospace Operations (AGARD-CP-478)* (Neuilly Sur Seine, France: NATO-AGARD).

Volpe, C.E., Cannon-Bowers, J.A., Salas, E. and Spector, P.E. (1996), 'The Impact of Cross-training on Team Functioning: An Empirical Investigation', *Human Factors* 38:1, 87–100.

Wears, R.L., Perry, S.J., Wilson, S., Galliers, J. and Fone, J. (2007), 'Emergency Department Status Boards: User-evolved Artefacts for Inter- and Intra-group Coordination', *Cognition, Technology and Work* 9:3, 163–70.

Weick, K.E. (1995), *Sensemaking in Organizations* (Thousand Oaks, CA: Sage Publications).

Wiener, E.L., Kanki, B.G. and Helmreich, R.L. (eds) (1993), *Cockpit Resource Management* (San Francisco: Academic).

Wilson, K.A., Burke, C.S., Priest, H.A. and Salas, E. (2005), 'Promoting Healthcare Safety Through Training High Reliability Teams', *Quality and Safety in Healthcare* 14:4, 303–9.

Wright, M.C., Taekman, J.M. and Endsley, M.R. (2004), 'Objective Measures of Situation Awareness in a Simulated Medical Environment', *Quality and Safety in Healthcare* 13:Suppl. 1, i65–71.

Wright, M.C., Taekman, J.M., Griffin, K., Hobbs, G.W. and Petrusa, E.R. (2006), 'Assessment of Team Coordination Skills in Medical Education and Clinical Practice', presented at the *2006 Research in Medical Education Annual Meeting* (Seattle, WA: American Association of Medical Colleges).

Wright, M.C., Petrusa, E.R., Griffin, K.L., Phillips-Bute, B.G., Hobbs, G.W. and Taekman, J.M. (forthcoming), 'Assessing Teamwork in Medical Education and Practice: Validity of Behaviorally Anchored Ratings'.

Xiao, Y. (2005), 'Artifacts and Collaborative Work in Healthcare: Methodological, Theoretical, and Technological Implications of the Tangible', *Journal of Biomedical Informatics* 38:1, 26–33.

Zhang, Y., Drews, F.A., Westenskow, D.R., Foresti, S., Agutter, J., Bermudez, J.C., Blike, G. and Loeb, R.G. (2002), 'Effects of Integrated Graphical Displays on Situation Awareness in Anaesthesiology', *Cognition, Technology and Work* 4:2, 82–90.

PART 3
Healthcare Team Communication in the Field

Chapter 8

Factors Affecting Team Communication in the Intensive Care Unit (ICU)

Tom Reader, Rhona Flin and Brian Cuthbertson

The intensive care unit (ICU) is a high-risk, acute medical environment that requires multidisciplinary teams to provide life-saving care for critically ill patients. Although a relatively new speciality, intensive care medicine is now an integral part of patient care in most health services (Halpern, Pastores and Greenstein 2004). Patients in the ICU are admitted according to the severity of their illnesses, with the majority suffering from multiple organ dysfunctions that require intensive and immediate treatment. Due to the serious nature of patient illnesses in the ICU, the outcomes of treatment interventions are often difficult to predict. However, research investigating the management of ICUs has shown that the organizational characteristics of an intensive care unit, and in particular the quality of communication amongst team members, have a considerable impact upon patient outcomes (Carson et al. 1996; Shortell et al. 1994). Additionally, studies measuring instances of critical incidents in the ICU (events in which a patient was, or could have been, unintentionally harmed) have frequently shown a link between team communication failures and breakdowns in patient safety (Wright et al. 1991). These findings are consistent with patient safety research showing communication failures to be a key causal factor underlying adverse events (Schaefer and Helmreich 1994).

Communication failures are not peculiar to healthcare settings, they are everyday occurrences in all types of working environments (Flin, O'Connor and Crichton forthcoming). However, in safety-critical industries they can have serious consequences—for example, the loss of the *Piper Alpha* oil platform (with 167 fatalities) was partly attributable to key information not being transferred at a shift handover (Cullen 1990). In order to improve communication within and between teams, it is necessary to understand exactly how teams in particular work environment exchange information and what factors affect the level of individual and shared understanding. This type of research is most advanced in the aviation industry where flightdeck communications have been studied by aviation psychologists for many years (Kanki and Palmer 1993; Kanki and Smith 2001). For example, research has shown that patterns of communication (e.g. closed-loop communications) are related to flight team performance (Bowers et al. 1998; Orasanu 1990), and that junior flight officers are less assertive at communicating information compared to pilots (Jentsch et al. 1999). Such research findings are used to inform not only workplace design and operating procedures but also the specialised Crew Resource Management (CRM) training that is used to enhance crew performance, principally by improving communication skills (CAA 2006). In order to design appropriate interventions (such as CRM training) to enhance team communication in the ICU, it is necessary to examine empirically the communication skills associated with high levels of safety and patient care, and also to understand the factors that affect how team members normally communicate with one another. The current chapter reviews ICU team communication research, as well as introducing the results from two studies of team communication recently conducted in the UK intensive care environment.

Framework of Teamwork and Performance in the ICU

Researchers have long attempted to understand group behavior and its effect upon performance. Frequently, the "input–processes–output" framework model has been used to describe the relationship between teamwork and team effectiveness (Hackman 1990; McGrath 1984; Salas, Weaver and Cannon-Bowers 2002; Steiner 1972; Unsworth and West 2000). This takes the perspective that "inputs" such as the composition of team members and the types of tasks being performed affect teamwork processes (for example, communication), which in turn influence team effectiveness. Figure 8.1 uses a simplified "input–processes–outcomes" framework to describe a variety of factors that affect the effectiveness of ICU teams (Flin, O'Connor and Crichton forthcoming).

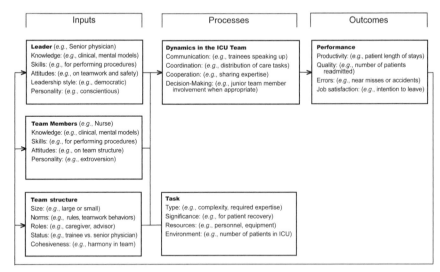

Figure 8.1 ICU team performance framework
Source: Adapted from Flin, O'Connor and Crichton (forthcoming).

A range of inputs have been found to affect team processes. These include the attitudes and abilities of team members, the combination of personalities within the team, and the degree to which the team leader can influence team members to complete both their individual and team objectives (Unsworth and West 2000). Also important is the structure of the team in terms of size, the norms of acceptable behavior, the roles of team members during specific tasks, status differences and influence between team members, and the cohesiveness of team members (Steers 1988). The properties of the tasks being performed by the team must also be considered (Kent and McGrath 1969). For example, the complexity and importance of tasks will likely affect how decisions are made during the task and the level of communication and coordination needed between team members for completing the task. It is notable that the various team inputs are interdependent, as the skills, abilities and personality of individual team members will affect the structure of the team (for example, the role and status of team members) depending on the type of task being performed. The team inputs affect the team processes (for example, complex tasks being performed with inexperienced trainee team members will likely result in increased emphasis on decisions being made by team leaders), with this in turn affecting both task performance and individual levels of job stress and satisfaction. Lastly, the performance of the team will feedback to affect the team inputs, with successful team performance likely increasing team cohesiveness and improving individual knowledge and skills.

Using the framework discussed above as a guide, the following sections draw on both published ICU team research and work recently conducted by our group at the University of Aberdeen to discuss: (1) the relationship between team processes and ICU outcomes, and (2) the relationship between team inputs and team processes. The following subjects are discussed:

- Team communication and patient safety
- Team communication and patient outcomes
- Status differences and communication
- Status, communication and decision making
- Interruptions during team communications
- Patterns of communication amongst the ICU team

Team Processes and ICU Outcomes

A number of studies have examined the relationship between team processes and patient outcomes in the ICU. These have typically focused on both the relationship between team member communication failures and patient safety, and effective team communication and patient outcomes.

Team Communication and Patient Safety

The importance of effective team communication for patient safety has been demonstrated in various medical domains (Gaba 1989; de Leval et al. 2000).

A review of 11 studies analyzing 2,677 critical incidents revealed 49 per cent of contributory factors underlying incidents to be associated with poor non-technical skills. These are social and cognitive skills that are crucial for maintaining safety, and are often taught and assessed in aviation and medical CRM courses (Fletcher et al. 2004; Gaba, Fish and Howard 1994; O'Connor, Flin and Fletcher 2002). Of the contributory factors identified as being associated with poor non-technical skills, approximately 20 per cent were cited as originating from poor communication and teamwork (Reader et al. 2006). Similarly, root-cause analyses of ICU adverse events have identified particular team communication failures leading to patient harm. For example, a reluctance of nursing staff to speak up on the observation of errors, and lack of communication and understanding regarding medication handovers between nurses and doctors, have been found to contribute directly to the occurrence of preventable adverse events (Pronovost et al. 2002; Pronovost, Wu and Sexton 2004). Simulator studies measuring ICU team performance during critical event scenarios have also identified some of the specific communication errors that commonly occur (Lighthall et al. 2003). Examples include team members failing to communicate their care priorities to one another, physicians overloading nurses with requests, a lack of leadership resulting in ineffective use of time and personnel, and a lack of communication on the initiation of new therapies.

Team Communication and Patient Outcomes

Investigations examining communication in the ICU have also shown better communication to be associated with positive patient-related outcomes. Units with higher levels of collaboration between nurses and physicians during patient-transfer decisions have reported lower rates of risk-adjusted mortalities (Baggs et al. 1999). Shortell and colleagues (1992) conducted structured interviews with nurses and doctors in US intensive care units in order to develop a tool for measuring organizational aspects, including communication and leadership. A comparison of interview data from ICU staff members at high and low performing units revealed that the highest performing ICUs reported accurate and open communication between nurses and doctors, flexible leadership patterns with clear goals, and a more collaborative approach to problem solving with the expertise of all team members being utilised. Later studies using the measurement tool revealed, in a survey of 42 ICUs, that the quality of interdisciplinary collaboration was to be associated with ICU performance outcomes, with timely, accurate, and open communication being a major facilitator of well-coordinated patient care (Shortell et al. 1994; Zimmerman et al. 1993). In summary, research investigating the relationship between communication and quality of care in the ICU has shown communication failures as commonly causing errors, and good communication as being associated with positive patient outcomes.

Team Inputs and Team Communication

Having established a relationship between effective team communication and patient outcomes, research within the ICU has attempted to identify the factors that lead to effective communication between team members. As shown in Figure 8.1, a number of team inputs are thought important for group processes; in particular one of the structural factors, the issue of status differences within groups, has been studied in some depth due to its considerable influence on ICU team communication.

Status Differences and Communication

Healthcare teams tend to be quite hierarchical in nature, with senior doctors usually having a higher status than other healthcare professionals. This tends to result in large power distance, where team members who perceive themselves as being of a lower status (for example, nurses and junior doctors) feel as if they have less influence upon team functioning (Hofstede 2003). Group research has shown that group members of a higher status voice their thoughts and opinions more often than those of a lower status (Islam and Zyphur 2005), and individuals of a lower group status are less likely to (a) contribute to group tasks (Berger et al. 1985), (b) play a central role in decision making (Driskell and Salas 1992), or (c) display speaking-up behaviors (Edmondson 2003). Group status has been a topic of particular interest for aviation communication, as research has shown unassertive junior team members (for example, co-pilots) do not speak up effectively in the presence of highly authoritative captains, even when they know the captain is performing unsafely (Foushee and Helmreich 1988). Similarly, lower status individuals in medical teams (for example, residents relative to senior physicians) have reported feeling unable to speak up when recognising potential patient safety lapses due to their perceptions of lower status (Blatt et al. 2006).

In one of the first major studies of ICU status differences and team member interactions, Donchin and colleagues (1995) found an association between patterns of Israeli nurse and doctor communications and occurrences of critical incidences. They observed verbal communication between caregivers in 9 per cent of all activities conducted in the ICU, with most communications being between nurses or between doctors. However, although nurse with doctor communications were found to occur in just 2 per cent of all activities performed in the unit, these were associated with over a third of errors. It was concluded that this might be due to the informal and infrequent communications between nurses and doctors, alongside misperceptions and misunderstandings regarding the information communicated between them. Donchin et al. (1995) reasoned that due to the close proximity to patients, nurses function as an active liaison between physicians and patients, helping to avoid confusion and to bridge information gaps, and thus nurses should be more formally involved in information exchanges during physician activities (for example, the physician rounds). Having a clear two-way flow of information between ICU nurses and doctors is important for ensuring that their knowledge and perspectives can be combined to develop a complete, coherent and up-to-date knowledge base of patient status amongst team members.

Research that we have recently conducted in the UK intensive care environment has studied the degree to which ICU team members of different hierarchical status (for example, nurses and doctors, trainee doctors and senior doctors) have different perceptions of their communications together. According to research on effective team communication, team members should agree on the communication behaviors (for example, speaking up) that are required of themselves and of others (Edmondson 2003). If junior team members believe they cannot communicate openly, this can result in information critical to patient care not being shared, and can reduce the likelihood of concerns being expressed or of guidance being asked for aspects of patient treatment. A survey was conducted with 400 staff (with a 47 per cent response rate) in four Scottish ICUs (Reader et al. 2007). The survey tool used to study perceptions of ICU team members was the "Interdisciplinary Collaboration" self-report questionnaire developed by Shortell et al. (1994). This measure was selected due to it being psychometrically well validated, and the range of questions focusing on communication between interdisciplinary groups (that is, between nurses and doctors), and within interdisciplinary groups (that is, between trainee and senior doctors) in the ICU. Although a range of scales were incorporated in the study, only data from the communication scales are shown in Table 8.1 and discussed here.

Table 8.1 Scales used in ICU communication survey

- **Communication openness between nurses and doctors**—the extent to which ICU nurses and doctors can speak openly with one another without fear of negative repercussions or misunderstanding
- **Communication openness within groups**—the extent to which ICU team members within a group (e.g. between doctors) can speak openly with one another without fear of negative repercussions or misunderstanding
- **Communication accuracy between nurses and doctors**—the degree to which nurses and doctors believe that information conveyed to one another is accurate
- **Communication accuracy within groups**—the degree to which ICU team members within a group (e.g. between senior and trainee nurses) believe information conveyed to one another is accurate
- **Shift communication between groups**—the extent to which ICU nurses and doctors feel between-shift communication with one another is effective
- **Shift communication within groups**—the extent to which ICU team members within a group (e.g. doctors) feel between-shift communication with one another is effective
- **Unit communication timeliness**—the degree to which information about patient care is promptly relayed to relevant caregivers
- **Satisfaction with nurse and doctor communication**—overall satisfaction with the quality of nurse and doctor communication
- **Satisfaction with communication within groups**—overall satisfaction with the quality of between-group (e.g. between nurses) communication

The study showed ICU team members in general to have positive perceptions of their communication with one another, with the majority of the sample reporting being satisfied with communication in their units. Comparisons of the UK sample with the US sample used in the original study revealed relatively little difference between response patterns in the two countries. In particular, perceptions were positive for open communication within professional groups (for example, between nurses) and the timelines of communication between ICU caregivers. However, there were some less favorable results, with just over half of the sample having positive perceptions of the accuracy of communication between members of the same professional group (for example, between doctors). Perceptions regarding the quality of communications between caregivers across shifts were also less positive, indicating some dissatisfaction with shift handovers.

Additionally, for the majority of questions, doctors had more positive perceptions of communication compared to nurses. Specifically, the perceptions of doctors regarding communication openness between nurses and doctors were significantly more positive than the perceptions of nurses. Most doctors (and especially senior doctors) reported perceptions that were classified as very positive (indicating relatively little need for improvement), as compared to just over a third of nurses. This indicated that nurses and doctors (and especially senior doctors) had quite different perceptions of their communications openness together. Divergent perceptions due to seniority were also found relating to communication openness between doctors. The majority of senior doctors reported very positive perceptions of communication openness between doctors, as compared to around just half of trainee doctors. Thus a quite noticeable trend was found, with junior ICU staff being less likely than senior ICU staff to report positive perceptions of communication openness. Interestingly, ICU team members who reported open communication in the ICU also reported having a better understanding of their patient care duties. Furthermore, the quality of senior physician leadership (for example, making clear the behaviors required of ICU staff, emphasizing standards) in the unit was found to be particularly important for encouraging open communication in the ICU. This is consistent with research from other domains, which emphasizes the importance of leadership in developing high-performing teams within a range of industries (Bass et al. 2003; Flin and Yule 2004; Zohar 2002).

The degree to which a team has a steep hierarchical structure can depend on a number of factors, including the distribution of knowledge and expertise relative to a task (LePine and Van Dyne 2001), situational factors, personality of individuals within a group (Fournier, Moskowitz and Zuroff 2002), organizational culture (Edmondson 1999), and perceptions of procedural justice and fairness (Hunton, Hall and Price 1998). Within healthcare, changing the structure of teams in order to develop the ability of junior and senior team members to communicate well together is seen as one of the key ways through which teamwork can be enhanced (Leonard, Graham and Bonacum 2004). Attitudinal studies have shown that ICU caregivers would wish to reduce the hierarchical nature of their teams, with 94 per cent of ICU staff advocating a flat hierarchy in the units (Sexton, Thomas and Helmreich 2000). Furthermore, ICU nurses and doctors tend to be in agreement that junior team members should be able to question senior members, that decision making should include team member input, and that (as is practiced in aviation) team discussions which focus on threats and errors before and after team activities can be an important part of safety and teamwork (Helmreich and Wilhelm 1991). Despite this, nurses still report finding it difficult to speak up, with fewer nurses than doctors feeling that disagreements in the ICU are properly resolved, that input from nurses about patient care is well received, and that teamwork between nurses and physicians is well coordinated (Thomas, Sexton and Helmreich 2003).

Status, Communication and Decision Making

The team processes featured in Figure 8.1 are theorized to be highly interdependent (for example, communication and decision making), as well as being considerably influenced by input factors. The team-based decision-making processes involved in diagnosing patients and developing patient treatment plans constitute a core activity in providing critical care medicine. Experimental research investigating communication and group decision making has shown that in teams with rigid hierarchies, the distribution and sharing of knowledge amongst all team members is associated with decision-making accuracy (Hollenbeck et al. 1995). Additionally, minority dissent in teams with a high level of cohesion and participation has been shown to lead to more creative decisions (De Dreu and West 2001). Furthermore, real-life research during trauma resuscitation has shown the decision-making process (that is, autocratic or democratic) to depend on the severity of patient injuries and team experience, with physicians showing a more directive leadership style when patient trauma is more severe or the trauma team is less experienced (Yun, Faraj and Sims 2005).

Within intensive care, studies have compared the effect of task difficulty upon team communication and decision-making processes. Patel and Arocha (2001) studied the communication patterns of ICU teams during decision making in medical and surgical units. A distinction was found between the decision-making process in the medical ICU (where it is necessary for teams to identify and diagnose the condition of patients and to make decisions about the application of suitable treatments) and the surgical ICU (where teams manage the post-operative, and thus better understood, conditions of patients). In both environments, decisions were made through the use of information collected by all team members, with data being communicated and filtered (to distill the most salient points) from one level of the ICU hierarchy to the next. An analysis of audiotape transcripts from the rounds revealed communication processes in the surgical ICU to be more "democratic," with decisions being made after team discussions which involved contributions from ICU team members of all levels. In contrast, communication in the medical ICU appeared to be more linear, with senior doctors making all of the major decisions, and with nurses communicating after performing information-gathering tasks. This finding indicated that the team communication processes leading up to decision making were partly dependent on the severity and transparency of patient conditions.

A number of studies have attempted to improve communication and decision making in the ICU through implementing communication protocols or encouraging a change in the communication culture. In the US, daily goals sheets have been introduced during the ICU round in order to improve task clarity and team communication (Pronovost et al. 2003). The ICU round is a team-oriented decision-making activity that involves the reviewing of patients, the sharing of information, the formation of treatment plans, and the development of a shared mental model amongst team members for issues of patient care and teamwork. The daily goals sheets formalized the rounds process, and required all team members to participate in the setting of patient care goals and the recording of patient-related information. The implementation of daily goals sheets resulted in a considerable increase in the number of ICU team members who reported understanding their patient care duties, alongside associated reductions in average patient lengths of stay. Both resident doctors and ICU nurses reported that the form clarified work goals and improved communication. In particular, nurses reported that the daily goals form helped them to feel they were an active part of the patient care team. Attempts have also been made to redesign and formalize the ICU rounds process in order to make rounds shorter and more concise; to ensure that short- and long-term patient care plans and problems lists were more explicit and accessible; to ensure that all decision makers were present during rounds; and to generate an atmosphere where all team members showed professional and respectful behavior in a relaxed team-based environment (Dodek and Raboud 2003). This has been found to improve interdisciplinary communication, with large increases being found in the numbers of ICU staff reporting a better understanding of patient care plans as well as higher levels of satisfaction with the process and outcome of ICU rounds.

Our research conducted in a Scottish ICU has examined communication during the ICU physician rounds (Reader et al. 2007). Data were gathered during ICU rounds regarding individual team member anticipations for how the most critically ill patients would progress over the proceeding 48 hours (that is, whether patients would deteriorate, remain on ventilation, or be discharged from the unit), and perceptions of individual involvement during the patient care decision-making process. Physicians and senior nurses used handheld computers to individually record their judgments after the review of 105 patients during 35 ICU rounds. Observational data were also collected by the first author during each physician round in order to measure the contributions of ICU team members to patient care discussions. The preliminary analysis has shown that the degree to which senior and trainee doctors formed a shared understanding for whether patients would deteriorate in condition or would be discharged was associated with the involvement of trainee doctors in the ICU rounds decision-making process. The reported involvement of trainee doctors was associated with the number of verbal contributions made during patient discussions. Furthermore, the analysis found that nurses reported feeling highly uninvolved in the patient review process. The observations of communications during the physician rounds revealed nurses to demonstrate far less communication behaviors than doctors, with their contributions often only being made in response to requests for information.

Interruptions During Team Communication

Research investigating safety in aviation has shown that interruptions to pilots in the cockpit are frequently causal factors in the occurrence of aviation incidents (Turner and Huntley 1991). Communication research in acute clinical environments has shown caregivers to frequently use interruptive communication strategies as a way of requesting or transmitting information to one another (Coiera and Tombs 1998). However, the costs of interruptions can be a loss of attention, forgetfulness, and ultimately error (Reason 2000), and interruptive behavior is particularly disruptive during tasks such as shift handovers, patient reviews, and surgery (Healey, Sevdalis and Vincent 2006; Laxmisan et al. forthcoming). A review of the multidisciplinary rounds processes has reported that interruptions on non-related issues (for example, non-urgent information requests for another patient) are often identified as a barrier to communication during rounds (Gurses and Xiao 2006). Investigations of interruptions during ICU physician rounds have shown a large proportion of the communication during the round to be of an interruptive nature (Alvarez and Coiera 2005). Physicians have been found to interrupt other caregivers roughly twice as often as nurses, with senior doctors interrupting more than junior doctors. This effect may be due to the senior doctors' leadership role in coordinating patient care, and also traditional hierarchical structures within medical teams. However, further research is required to examine how team members cope with interruptions during their routine work, and what effect interruptions have upon safety in the ICU.

Patterns of Communication in ICU Teams

Although team research in intensive care has often looked at specific issues (for example, team structure), ethnographic and interview studies have researched the general patterns of communication that occur in ICU teams during routine tasks. Such grounded theory research (the generation of theory from data) can be informative for understanding the nature and culture of communication.

Ethnographic studies of ICU team communication in Canada have identified a number of "catalysts" that result in ICU team members communicating in a collaborative or conflicting manner (Hawryluck et al. 2002). These "catalysts" include whether the team has a shared perception of who was in the decision-making role during a specific scenario; whether there is time to share perceptions of goals and values between team members and trainees; whether team members work together to reach an understanding on patient conditions; and whether there are demanding time constraints on the delivery of patient care. Similarly, in a US study, observations of physicians and nurses caring for patients in four ICUs have identified various communication strategies (Patterson et al. 2006). These include nurses listening to rounds in order to hear the development of patient care plans, nurses cross-checking physician-generated patient care plans, physicians and nurses providing "heads-up" alerts to each other about pertinent information outside of the rounds, and nurses and physicians speaking privately about care plans after the rounds. Although such ethnographic style studies are useful for understanding how teams function, there remains a gap between analyzing how teams function together and the resultant effect upon team performance.

Albolino, Cook and O'Connor (2007) have studied "collective sensemaking" in ICU teams. They found a variety of communication strategies were used for the team to develop a shared sense of the intensive care environment. In particular the physician round was identified as a key process for sensemaking, with the cases of individual patients being presented to the team, explicit care plans being developed, and summaries being used to recap the discussion and highlight the core duties of team members. Structured interviews have also been used to study the causes underlying the breakdown of shared understanding or "common ground" within the critical care team (McHugh et al. 2005). These include factors such as nurses feeling unable to share valuable information with doctors due to their different professional background and hierarchical position; the work in the ICU being conducted by small or sub-teams which do not necessarily communicate information to the larger ICU team; and the difficulties of ensuring good continuity of care and communication of information between different shifts. Finally, implementing multidisciplinary work-shift evaluations have been indicated to improve reported communication in ICUs (Sluiter et al. 2005). Through team members of a particular shift meeting up regularly to have open discussions on patient care issues, critical incidents, and teamwork, staff reported higher levels of satisfaction and improvement of communication in the unit.

Summary and Conclusions

Studies investigating communication in the ICU have provided a substantial insight into the specific communication practices of intensive care teams. Using the framework described in Figure 8.1, it can be seen that team processes such as the quality of communication and cooperation amongst team members lead to positive outcomes in terms of safety, quality of care, and job satisfaction. Furthermore, the process of ICU team communication is determined by a variety of team-related inputs. These include factors such as group communication norms, the roles and status of team members, expertise required for performing a task, use of protocols for structuring communication, team communication strategies, interruptions, and group reflections on teamwork. Thus, the structure of the team and the roles and status of individual team members appear to be issues particularly important for determining the communication behaviors of ICU team members. Similarly to other healthcare domains, status differences between ICU team members result in team members of different roles and professional groups perceiving communication quite differently. The applied psychology literature has demonstrated that the behavioral norms of a team are important for ensuring high-quality team communication and coordination, and ultimately team performance and safety. Healthcare research has shown that team leadership is particularly important in developing a culture of open communication, with it being essential to create a safe atmosphere where team members feel they can speak up should they have any safety concerns or issues with the quality of care provided to patients (Burke et al. 2004; Leonard, Graham and Bonacum 2004). This atmosphere can be created through team leadership that advocates a flat hierarchy in which junior team member input is welcomed, that shows a willingness to listen to the concerns and ideas of junior team members, that recognizes human limitations and fallibility, and that clearly states expected interaction patterns amongst team members (Nembhard and Edmondson 2006; Sexton, Thomas and Helmreich 2000). For example, in the ICU, senior doctors might wish to encourage trainee members to contribute to the patient care plan decision-making process through asking trainee staff whether they have any alternative suggestions, concerns, or general thoughts on the patient care plans that have been outlined. Also important for developing open communication amongst teams is the implementation of structured communication protocols (for example, communication checklists) that support communication across hierarchical boundaries (Fletcher et al. 2003; Lingard et al. 2005; Pronovost et al. 2003), and team-based training that encourages assertiveness, interdisciplinary communication, and a shared perception of teamwork (Undre et al. 2006).

In conclusion, a considerable amount of research has focused on how ICU team members communicate, the effect on safety and performance, and the factors that influence their communication practices. As with aviation and other high-risk domains, good communication in the ICU is essential for maintaining safety and high levels of performance. Patient safety researchers have argued that through understanding the factors that lead to effective teamwork and communication in settings such as the ICU, team training methods similar to those adopted in aviation can be used to improve teamwork within intensive care (Rall and Gaba 2004). Research in other areas of healthcare—for example, anaesthesia—has led to the development of tools for improving and assessing communication in the operating room. Whilst communication research in the ICU has contributed to the understanding of the various factors that can affect and improve team communication, further research is required to understand the specific communication skills and behaviors that lead to successful and safe performance in the ICU. Although these will doubtless hold to the principles of team communication research developed in aviation and aerospace, there remains considerable scope for conducting research to identify the specific communication skills and behaviors associated with high levels of performance in the ICU.

References

Albolino, S., Cook, R. and O'Connor, M. (2007), 'Sensemaking, Safety, and Cooperative Work in the Intensive Care Unit', *Cognition, Technology and Work* 9:3, 131–7.

Alvarez, G. and Coiera, E. (2005), 'Interruptive Communication Patterns in the Intensive Care Unit Ward Round', *International Journal of Medical Informatics* 74:10, 791–6.

Baggs, J.G., Schmitt, M.H., Mushlin, A.I., Mitchell, P.H., Eldrege, D.H. and Oakes, D. (1999), 'Association Between Nurse–Physician Collaboration and Patient Outcomes in Three Intensive Care Units', *Critical Care Medicine* 27:9, 1991–8.

Bass, B., Avolio, B., Jung, D. and Berson, Y. (2003), 'Predicting Unit Performance by Assessing Transformational and Transactional Leadership', *Journal of Applied Psychology* 88:2, 207–18.

Berger, J., Fisek, M., Norman, R. and Wagner, D. (1985), 'Formation of Reward Expectations in Status Situations', in J. Berger and M. Zelditch (eds), *Status, Rewards, and Influence* (San Francisco: Jossey-Bass) 215–61.

Blatt, R., Christianson, M., Sutcliffe, K. and Rosenthal, M. (2006), 'A Sensemaking Lens on Reliability', *Journal of Organizational Behavior* 27:7, 897–917.

Bowers, C., Jentsch, F., Salas, E. and Braun, C. (1998), 'Analyzing Communication Sequences for Team Training Needs Assessment', *Human Factors* 40:4, 672–9.

Burke, C.S., Salas, E., Wilson-Donnelly, K. and Priest, H. (2004), 'How to Turn a Team of Experts into an Expert Medical Team: Guidance from the Aviation and Military Communities', *Quality and Safety in Healthcare* 13:Suppl. 1, i96–i104.

CAA (2006), *Crew Resource Management (CRM) Training. Guidance for Flight Crew, CRM Instructors (CRMIs) and CRM Instructor-examiners (CRMIEs)* (London: Civil Aviation Authority).

Carson, S., Stocking, C., Podsadecki, T., Christenson, J., Pohlman, A., MacRae, S., Jordan, J., Humphrey, H., Siegler, M. and Hall, J. (1996), 'Effects of Organizational Change in the Medical Intensive Care Unit of a Teaching Hospital: A Comparison of "Open" and "Closed" Formats', *Journal of the American Medical Association* 276:4, 322–8.

Coiera, E. and Tombs, V. (1998), 'Communication Behaviours in a Hospital Setting: An Observational Study', *British Medical Journal* 316:7132, 673–6.

Cullen (1990), *Report of the Official Inquiry into the Piper Alpha Disaster* (London: HMSO).

De Dreu, C.K.W. and West, M.A. (2001), 'Minority Dissent and Team Innovation: The Importance of Participation in Decision Making', *Journal of Applied Psychology* 86:6, 1191–1201.

de Leval, M., Carthey, J., Wright, D., Farewell, V. and Reason, J. (2000), 'Human Factors and Cardiac Surgery: A Multicenter Study', *The Journal of Thoracic and Cardiovascular Surgery* 119:4, 661–70.

Dodek, P.M. and Raboud, J. (2003), 'Explicit Approach to Rounds in an ICU Improves Communication and Satisfaction of Providers', *Intensive Care Medicine* 29:9, 1584–8.

Donchin, Y., Gopher, D., Olin, M., Badihi, Y., Biesky, M., Sprung, C.L., Pizov, R. and Cotev, S. (1995), 'A Look into the Nature and Causes of Human Errors in the Intensive Care Unit', *Critical Care Medicine* 23:2, 294–300.

Driskell, J. and Salas, E. (1992), 'Collective Behavior and Team Performance', *Human Factors* 34:3, 277–88.

Edmondson, A.C. (1999), 'Psychological Safety and Learning Behaviour in Work Teams', *Administrative Science Quarterly* 44:2, 350–83.

Edmondson, A.C. (2003), 'Speaking Up in the Operating Room: How Team Leaders Promote Learning in Interdisciplinary Action Teams', *Journal of Management Studies* 40:6, 1419–52.

Firth-Cozens, J. (2004), 'Why Communication Fails in the Operating Room', *Quality and Safety in Health Care* 13:5, 327.

Fletcher, G., Flin, R., McGeorge, P., Glavin, R., Maran, N. and Patey, R. (2003), 'Anaethesists' Non-Technical Skills (ANTS): Evaluation of a Behavioural Marker System', *British Journal of Anaesthesia* 90:5, 580–88.

Fletcher, G., Flin, R., McGeorge, P., Glavin, R., Maran, N. and Patey, R. (2004), 'Rating Non-technical Skills: Developing a Behavioural Marker System for Use in Anaesthesia', *Cognition, Technology and Work* 6:3, 165–71.

Flin, R., O'Connor, P. and Crichton, M. (forthcoming), *Safety at the Sharp End: A Guide to Non-technical Skills* (Aldershot, UK: Ashgate Publishing).

Flin, R. and Yule, S. (2004), 'Leadership for Safety: Industrial Experience', *Quality and Safety in Healthcare* 13:Suppl. II, 45–51.

Fournier, M.A., Moskowitz, D.S. and Zuroff, D.C. (2002), 'Social Rank Strategies in Hierarchical Relationships', *Journal of Personality and Social Psychology* 83:2, 425–33.

Foushee, H.C. and Helmreich, R.L. (1988), 'Group Interaction and Flight Crew Performance', in E. Weiner and J. Nagel (eds), *Human Factors in Aviation* (San Diego: Academic Press) 189–227.

Gaba, D. (1989), 'Human Error in Anaesthetic Mishaps', *International Anesthesiology Clinics* 27:3, 137–47.

Gaba, D.M., Fish, K.J. and Howard, S.K. (1994), *Crisis Management in Anaesthesiology* (Philadelphia: Churchill Livingston).

Gurses, A. and Xiao, Y. (2006), 'A Systematic Review of the Literature on Multidisciplinary Rounds to Design Information Technology', *Journal of the American Medical Informatics Association* 13:3, 267–76.

Hackman, J.R. (1990), *Groups That Work (and Those That Don't)* (San Francisco: Jossey-Bass).

Halpern, N., Pastores, S. and Greenstein, R. (2004), 'Critical Care Medicine in the United States 1985–2000: An Analysis of Bed Numbers, Use, and Costs', *Critical Care Medicine* 32:6, 1254–9.

Hawryluck, L.A., Espin, S.L., Garwood, K.C., Evans, C.A. and Lingard, L.A. (2002), 'Pulling Together and Pushing Apart: Tides of Tension in the ICU Team', *Academic Medicine* 77:10 Suppl., S73–6.

Healey, A., Sevdalis, N. and Vincent, C. (2006), 'Measuring Intra-operative Interference from Distraction and Interruption Observed in the Operating Theatre', *Ergonomics* 49:5–6, 589–604.

Helmreich, R. and Wilhelm, J. (1991), 'Outcomes of Crew Resource Management Training', *International Journal of Aviation Psychology* 1:4, 287–300.

Hofstede, G. (2003), *Culture's Consequences: Comparing Values, Behaviors, Institutions and Organizations across Nations* (Newbury Park, CA: Sage Publications).

Hollenbeck, J.R., Ilgen, D.R., Sego, D.J., Hedlund, J., Major, D. and Phillips, J. (1995), 'Multilevel Theory of Team Decision Making: Decision Performance in Teams Incorporating Distributed Expertise', *Journal of Applied Psychology* 80:2, 292–316.

Hunton, J.E., Hall, T.W. and Price, K.H. (1998), 'The Value of Voice in Participative Decision Making', *Journal of Applied Psychology* 83:5, 788–97.

Islam, G. and Zyphur, M.J. (2005), 'Power, Voice, and Hierarchy: Exploring the Antecedents of Speaking Up in Groups', *Group Dynamics: Theory, Research, and Practice* 9:2, 93–103.

Jentsch, F., Barnett, J., Bowers, C.A. and Salas, E. (1999), 'Who is Flying this Plane Anyway? What Mishaps Tell Us About Crew Member Role Assignment and Aircrew Situation Awareness', *Human Factors* 41:1, 1–14.

Kanki, B. and Palmer, M. (1993), 'Communication and Crew Resource Management', in E.L. Weiner, B.G. Kanki and R.L. Helmreich (eds), *Cockpit Resource Management* (San Diego: Academic Press) 99–136.

Kanki, B. and Smith, G. (2001), 'Training Aviation Communication Skills', in E. Salas, C. Bowers and E. Edens (eds), *Improving Teamwork in Organizations: Applications of Research Management Training* (Mahwah, New Jersey: LEA).

Kent, R. and McGrath, J. (1969), 'Task and Group Characteristics as Factors Influencing Group Perceptions', *Journal of Experimental Social Psychology* 5:4, 429–40.

Laxmisan, A., Hakimzada, F., Sayan, O.R., Green, R.A., Zhang, J. and Patel, V.L. (forthcoming), 'The Multitasking Clinician: Decision-making and Cognitive Demand During and After Team Handoffs in Emergency Care', *International Journal of Medical Informatics*.

Leonard, M., Graham, S. and Bonacum, D. (2004), 'The Human Factor: The Critical Importance of Effective Teamwork and Communication in Providing Safe Care', *Quality and Safety in Healthcare* 13:Suppl. 1, i85–90.

LePine, J.A. and Van Dyne, L. (2001), 'Voice and Cooperative Behavior as Contrasting Forms of Contextual Performance: Evidence of Differential Relationships with Big Five Personality Characteristics and Cognitive Ability', *Journal of Applied Psychology* 86:2, 326–36.

Lighthall, G.K., Barr, J., Howard, S.K., Gellar, E.E., Sowb, Y., Bertacini, E. and Gaba, D. (2003), 'Use of a Fully Simulated Intensive Care Unit Environment for Critical Event Management Training for Internal Medicine Residents', *Critical Care Medicine* 31:10, 2437–43.

Lingard, L.A., Espin, S.L., Rubin, H.R., Whyte, S., Colmenares, M., Baker, G.R., Doran, D., Grober, E., Orser, B., Bohnen, J. and Reznick, R. (2005), 'Getting Teams to Talk: Development and Pilot Implementation of a Checklist to Promote Interprofessional Communication in the OR', *Quality and Safety in Healthcare* 14:5, 340–46.

McGrath, J. (1984), *Groups Interaction and Performance* (New Jersey: Prentice-Hall).

McHugh, A.P., Crandall, B., Miller, T.E. and Mills, J.A. (2005), 'Cognition in Critical Care: An Exploratory Study', in J.M.C. Schraagen (ed.), *Proceedings of the Seventh International NDM Conference* (Amsterdam).

Moskowitz, D.S., Suh, E.J. and Desaulniers, J. (1994), 'Situational Influences on Gender Differences in Agency and Communion', *Journal of Personality and Social Psychology* 66:4, 753–61.

Nembhard, I. and Edmondson, A. (2006), 'Making it Safe: The Effects of Leader Inclusiveness and Professional Status on Psychological Safety and Improvement

Efforts in Health Care Teams', *Journal of Organizational Behavior* 27:7, 941–66.

O'Connor, P., Flin, R. and Fletcher, G. (2002), 'Methods Used to Evaluate the Effectiveness of Flight Crew CRM Training in the UK Aviation Industry', *Human Factors and Aerospace Safety* 2:3, 235–56.

Orasanu, J. (1990), *Shared Mental Models and Crew Performance*, Technical Report No. 46 (Princeton, NJ: Princeton University).

Patel, V.L. and Arocha, J.F. (2001), 'The Nature of Constraints on Collaborative Decision Making in Health Care Settings', in E. Salas and G. Klein (eds), *Linking Expertise and Naturalistic Decision Making* (New Jersey: Lawrence Erlbaum Associates) 383–405.

Patterson, E., Hofer, T., Brungs, S., Saint, S. and Render, M. (2006), 'Structured Interdisciplinary Communication Strategies in Four ICUs: An Observational Study', *Proceedings of the Human Factors and Ergonomics Society 50th Annual Meeting* (Santa Monica, CA: HFES).

Pronovost, P.J., Berenholtz, S.M., Dorman, T., Lipsett, P.A., Simmonds, T. and Haraden, C. (2003), 'Improving Communications in the ICU Using Daily Goals', *Journal of Critical Care* 18:2, 71–5.

Pronovost, P.J., Wu, A., Dorman, T. and Morlock, L. (2002), 'Building Safety into ICU Care', *Journal of Critical Care* 17:2, 78–85.

Pronovost, P.J., Wu, A.W. and Sexton, J.B. (2004), 'Acute Decompensation After Removing a Central Line: Practical Approaches to Increasing Safety in the Intensive Care Unit', *Annals of Internal Medicine* 140:12, 1025–33.

Rall, M. and Gaba, D. (2004), 'Human Performance and Patient Safety', in D.R. Miller (ed.), *Anesthesia*, 6th edition (Philadelphia: Churchill Livingstone) 3073–3103.

Reader, T., Flin, R., Lauche, K. and Cuthbertson, B. (2006), 'Non-technical Skills in the Intensive Care Unit', *British Journal of Anaesthesia* 96:5, 551–9.

Reader, T., Flin, R., Mearns, K. and Cuthbertson, B. (2007), 'Interdisciplinary Communication in the Intensive Care Unit', *British Journal of Anaesthesia* 98:3, 347–52.

Reason, J. (2000), 'Human Error: Models and Management', *British Medical Journal* 320:7237, 768–70.

Salas, E., Dickinson, T.L., Converse, S.A. and Tannenbaum, S.I. (1992), 'Towards an Understanding of Team Performance and Training', in R. Swezey and E. Salas (eds), *Teams: Their Training and Performance* (Norwood, NJ: Ablex Publishing).

Salas, E., Weaver, J. and Cannon-Bowers, J. (2002), 'Command and Control Teams: Principles for Training and Assessment', in R. Flin and K. Arbuthnot (eds), *Incident Command: Tales from the Hot Seat* (Aldershot, UK: Ashgate Publishing) 239–57.

Schaefer, H. and Helmreich, R. (1994), 'The Importance of Human Factors in the Operating Room', *Anesthesiology* 80:2, 479–82.

Sexton, J.B., Thomas, E.J. and Helmreich, R.L. (2000), 'Error, Stress and Teamwork in Medicine and Aviation: Cross Sectional Surveys', *British Medical Journal* 320:7237, 745–9.

Shortell, S.M., Zimmerman, J.E., Gillies, R.R., Duffy, J., Devers, K.J., Rousseau, D.M. and Knaus, W.A. (1992), 'Continuously Improving Patient Care: Practical Lessons and an Assessment Tool from the National ICU Study', *Quality Review Bulletin* 18:5, 150–55.

Shortell, S.M., Zimmerman, J.E., Rousseau, D.M., Gillies, R.R., Wagner, D.P., Draper, E.A., Knaus, W.A. and Duffy, J. (1994), 'The Performance of Intensive Care Units: Does Good Management Make a Difference?', *Medical Care* 32:5, 508–25.

Sluiter, J., Bos, A., Tol, D., Calff, M., Krijnen, M. and Frings-Dresen, M. (2005), 'Is Staff Well-being and Communication Enhanced by Multidisciplinary Work Shift Evaluations', *Intensive Care Medicine* 31:10, 1409–14.

Steers, M. (1988), *Introduction to Organizational Behaviour*, Scott, Foreman Series in Management and Organizations (New York: Harper Collins).

Steiner, I. (1972), *Group Processes and Productivity* (New York: Academic Press).

Thomas, E.J., Sexton, J.B. and Helmreich, R.L. (2003), 'Discrepant Attitudes About Teamwork Among Critical Care Nurses and Physicians', *Critical Care Medicine* 31:3, 956–9.

Turner, J.W. and Huntley Jr, M.S. (1991), *The Use and Design of Flight Crew Checklists and Manuals*, Technical Report No. FAOE2-A0180 (Washington, DC: Department of Transportation).

Undre, S., Sevdalis, N., Healey, A., Darzi, S. and Vincent, C. (2006), 'Teamwork in the Operating Theatre: Cohesion or Confusion?', *Journal of Evaluation in Clinical Practice* 12:2, 182–9.

Unsworth, K. and West, M. (2000), 'Teams: The Challenges of Cooperative Work', in N. Chanel (ed.), *Introduction to Work and Organizational Psychology* (Cornwall, UK: Blackwell) 327–46.

Wright, D., Mackenzie, M., Buchan, I., Cairns, C. and Price, L. (1991), 'Critical Incidents in the Intensive Therapy Unit', *Lancet* 338:8768, 676–81.

Yun, S., Faraj, S. and Sims, H.P.J. (2005), 'Contingent Leadership and Effectiveness of Trauma Resuscitation Teams', *Journal of Applied Psychology* 90:6, 1288–96.

Zimmerman, J.E., Shortell, S.M., Rousseau, D.M., Duffy, J., Gillies, D.M., Knaus, W.A., Devers, K.J., Wagner, D.P. and Draper, E.A. (1993), 'Improving Intensive Care: Observations Based on Organizational Case Studies in Nine Intensive Care Units: A Prospective, Multicenter Study', *Critical Care Medicine* 21:10, 1443–51.

Zohar, D. (2002), 'Modifying Supervisory Practices to Improve Subunit Safety: A Leadership-based Intervention Model', *Journal of Applied Psychology* 87:1, 156–63.

Chapter 9

Between Shifts:
Healthcare Communication in the PICU

Christopher P. Nemeth, Julie Kowalsky, Marianne Brandwijk, Madelyn Kahana, P. Allan Klock and Richard I. Cook

The coordination of acute care clinical work, authority, and responsibility are critical to patient care, particularly in the intensive care unit (ICU). Transitions between shifts in the ICU, which typically occur twice a day, create potential gaps in the continuity of care (Cook, Render and Woods 2000). Practitioners necessarily rely on distributed cognition (Hutchins 1995) to prevent the formation of gaps during transfers between departments or during work-cycle shift changes. Clinicians manage transitions between shifts using verbal hand-offs, or "sign outs," to coordinate clinical work, authority, and responsibility. The complexity of medical interventions as well as complexity, uncertainty, and rapid changes in patient condition make effective sign outs both essential and difficult.

Our ongoing research into the coordination of clinical work across shift boundaries examines the nature of scheduled exchanges of authority and responsibility (Woods 1993) in order to improve clinician ability to perform sign outs and to improve the continuity of patient care. This chapter presents the early results of an ongoing study of coordination and hand-offs across a group of fellows in a pediatric intensive care unit (PICU).

Background

ICUs are hospital units that are equipped and staffed to provide specialized care for the most critically ill patients. Pediatric intensive care treats children, although patient ages in the unit can range from newborn to early twenties. Typical conditions requiring treatment in the PICU include congenital abnormalities, traumatic injuries, and illnesses such as asthma and epilepsy. Patients' conditions are fragile, unstable, and can deteriorate rapidly. It is common for these patients to need intravenous (IV) medications or ventilator-assisted breathing to support life. The PICU at the research site has a capacity of thirteen patients, with five isolation beds and two open bays with four beds each. The PICU has a 1:1 nurse-to-patient ratio to care for those who suffer from severe, acute conditions. The Step Down Unit (SDU) provides intermediate level care for up to twenty patients. The SDU is located near the PICU but does not directly adjoin it. Ten of the rooms are private, while the two open bays have four or six beds. The SDU has a ratio of one nurse for every three patients, who typically suffer from a chronic illness.

Attending physicians and nurses routinely staff the PICU at private hospitals. Because of its role as an educational institution, PICU staff in teaching hospitals also includes residents (physicians who have finished medical school but are learning a specialty such as pediatrics) and fellows (physicians who have completed residency and are performing additional training that may include graduate research). Their role as new physicians and the span of their training period (four to six years) makes the study of resident and fellow work in the PICU particularly productive.

US hospitals reduced resident work hours to a maximum of 80 per week (ACGME 2002) in response to patient safety recommendations in the 1999 Institute of Medicine report (IOM 2000). While the intention was to reduce fatigue among resident physicians, one of the mandate's effects was to increase the need for residents from other units to replace, or "cross cover," residents who had reached their hourly maximum. The increased frequency of patient care turnovers that resulted made effective sign outs more crucial to patient care in teaching hospitals.

The severity of patients' conditions in ICUs requires a practitioner to be present in the unit at all times. Hand-offs are necessary in an ICU because the length of a patient's stay often exceeds the amount of time one individual can offer. Each hand-off conveys complex information about extremely ill patients and that information may be misrepresented, forgotten, misunderstood, or misreported. Hand-offs in hospitals are routinely performed between peers. Nurses hand-off to nurses, residents to residents, fellows to fellows, and physicians to physicians. The complexity, uncertainty, unpredictability, and the dynamic nature of disease and therapy put a premium on the caregivers' ability to make their communications about patients effective. The complex nature of interventions and the possibility of rapid deterioration in patient conditions make communication between caregivers essential in order to ensure continuous, efficient, and effective patient care. The safety of PICU patients relies on the quality of care and the speed with which it is administered, and any breakdown in communication directly affects patients' health.

The nature of what occurs during sign-out conversations can be understood through the work of H.P. Grice (1913–88). Grice's writings on the philosophy of language in the 1970s and 1980s changed the debate over the nature of meaning from linguistic representation to mental representation. His "Cooperative Principle" (Grice 1975, 45–6) describes general features of conversation that participants are expected to observe: "Make your conversational contribution such as is required, at the stage at which it occurs, by the accepted purpose or direction of the talk exchange in which you are engaged." Those who engage in conversation and who follow four categories, or maxims, would produce results that reflect the Cooperative Principle:

- *Quantity*: Make your contribution as informative as is required (for the current purposes of the exchange). Do not make your contribution more informative than is required.
- *Quality*: Do not say what you believe to be false. Do not say that for which you lack evidence.
- *Relation*: Be relevant.

- *Manner*: Avoid obscurity of expression. Avoid ambiguity. Be brief (avoid unnecessary prolixity). Be orderly.

We sought to determine whether sign out conversations reflect Grice's maxims, and to accurately describe sign out content and form.

Methods

The project employed three methods to conduct research: direct observation, process tracing, and conversation analysis.

Direct Observation

Hand-off data were collected through direct observation and audio recording during regular operations in the PICU. On the same day, the researcher (MB) also completed a unit floor plan diagram to identify patient location, condition, and level of demand for care. The team developed three measures (ventilation, cardiac condition, and the number of IV pumps) to estimate care demand, which is the level of work effort that caregivers devote to a patient based on the patient's medical condition. Each measure was assigned a relative weight based on its estimated contribution to clinician work load. Ventilation was allocated ten points; cardiac, five; and each IV pump, one. The sum of all three represented a patient's care demand. For example, a cardiac patient with ten IV pumps would have a care demand of 15, while a patient on a ventilator with three IV pumps would have a demand of 13.

Our research analyzed between-shift hand-offs that were conducted among five intensivist fellows over six weeks in the PICU of a major urban teaching hospital. After obtaining informed consent according to institutional review board requirements, we observed 12 unit-level exchanges as the fellows handed off the 13-bed PICU and 20-bed SDU. Exchanges were conducted between an off-going and on-coming fellow during the morning (7:30 am) or afternoon (4:30 pm) shift change. One of the authors (MB) participated in the exchanges as part of the routine clinical rotation and made audio recordings of each discussion which were then transcribed. We used two methods to analyze the hand-off data: process tracing (Woods 1993) and conversation analysis (Drew and Heritage 1992).

Process Tracing

Two of the authors (MB and CN) reviewed audio recordings of each exchange while seated at a workstation that was equipped with an audio cassette player, microphones, and a video camera pointed down at the desk surface. They played the recording of each hand-off, discussed what occurred during the exchange, and moved a token across a floor plan diagram of the PICU to indicate where the fellows were located in the unit. The sessions traced the process of unit-level review between the off-going and on-coming fellow. The process enabled MB to provide context, identify expectations, and describe physical position and gestures that occurred during the exchanges. This enabled CN to pose naïve questions that elicited further reflection and identified traits that occurred across the series of hand-offs. Videotapes of the analyses captured the original sign-off audio, the commentary about the exchange, and the image of the floor plan with token.

Conversation Analysis

Process tracing could not determine how the structure and use of language changed during the hand-offs and how that occurred. That detailed level of analysis is only available through conversation analysis. Conversation analysis (CA) is used to develop a detailed, coded transcription from which aspects of conversation such as turns at talk and patterns of conversation style can emerge. An episode of conversation is transcribed to discover, describe, and analyze the "*structures*, the *machinery*, the *organized practices*, the *formal procedures*, the ways in which order is produced" (ten Have 1999, 41). CA avoids concerns that are associated with other qualitative studies such as imprecise intuition and recollection, selective attention, and biased experimental design. Like interaction analysis, CA "exposes the practical reasoning activities of participants themselves in a way which avoids them having to remember, justify or even know what they did" (Frohlich 1993). Furthermore, the audio recording that the method includes allows for repeated review of a particular event exactly as it occurred. This reproducibility enhances observations, permits collaboration with colleagues using first-hand data, and shares the authentic data with the public so that analytic claims may be evaluated and the data may be applied in comparative studies. CA has been used in healthcare research to better understand the doctor–patient relationship by examining patient counseling, and the use of medical records (Drew and Heritage 1992; Heath and Luff 2000).

Another member of the research group (JK) observed hand-offs to become familiar with their nature and the PICU context, viewed videotapes of the process tracing analyses, then performed conversation analysis on eight of the twelve exchanges using Computerized Language Analysis (CLAN) software. CLAN is designed to analyze data that has been transcribed in the format of the Child Language Data Exchange System (CHILDES). CLAN can be used to perform frequency counts, word searches, co-occurrence analyses, Mean Length of Utterance (MLU) counts, interactional analyses, text changes, and morphosyntactic analysis (to reveal an ordered, dynamic relation between one linguistic form and another).

The hand-off audio recordings were digitized by connecting the field cassette recorder to a Dell personal computer and using the Sound Recorder utility program to convert analog recordings to digital files. Initial review of transcripts accounted for the content, speaker, and length of each exchange. The CLAN software's voiceprint display (Figure 9.1) made it possible to specify the timing of conversational elements during each exchange to the level of fractions of a second, revealing utterance duration, overlaps, and pauses. Results of the analysis could then be represented in the form of annotated transcripts and diagrams such as timelines.

H: first hour I was here she was having seizures every five (to ten)
    minutes And so we reloaded her withten of Phenobarb again (1.0)
    Otherwise everything has been [the same]
R: [Okay   ]
H: [And since that load   ]
R: [Did you have to go up o]n the Propofol?
H: No
R: [Okay]
H: [She d]idn't

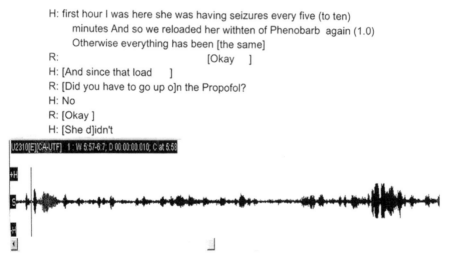

Figure 9.1 CLAN software voiceprint display

Results

We anticipated that communications among practitioners would adhere to Grice's maxims of quantity, quality, relation, and manner. Work-cycle characteristics place a high premium on efficient communications between practitioners, and we found that clinicians do meet this need through communications with characteristics that reflect Grice's maxims. Figures 9.2 through 9.5 depict selected portions of the hand-offs in which one of the maxims apply. Complete transcripts of hand-offs are available in Kowalsky (2004).

Figure 9.2 illustrates the maxim of quantity, by showing a conversation of length and density that depends on patient population size and acuity. The exchange provides as much information as needed in a context (but not more). It uses compact reference to manage quantity. The off-going fellow nods and points in the direction of a patient and says "Fine" three times in a row. Instead of a routine review of vital signs that is fixed in content and duration, this exchange varies from extended monologue summaries to casual interchanges.

Figure 9.3 depicts a fluid, dynamic exchange that is subject to distraction and interruptions. Rather than a seamless transfer of quantitative information such as vital signs, the hand-off's success depends on the on-coming physician's confidence in quality and completeness of information: whether the truth about the patient is being presented. The hand-off fluctuates on the aptitude of, and confidence in, the off-going and on-coming physician. By attending to the quality of the hand-off, the fellows protect truth through high sensitivity to the patient context.

In Figure 9.4, the fellows discuss the entire unit while remaining at the nurse's station in the center of the PICU. The fellows also discuss one patient while standing at another's bed, and discuss patients in other departments while standing in PICU. These are gestures that are used to refer to information that matters, but can be conveyed most efficiently through references to patients who are elsewhere on the unit and the facility. Instead of a series of discussions about each patient at each patient's bedside, this hand-off uses gestures to convey information in order to be relevant to the patient care context.

```
J: urine output has steadily dropped to like really minimal.It's grossly
bloody. He's got grossly bloody secretions from his endotracheal tube as well.
Uhmm, he's on amp gent and flagyl The gent I held
M: I am gonna go because they're gonna talk
J: Yeah, he's got a level ordered for later today
M: ok, he's a full court press
M: ok, anything else major? this is ??
```

```
[standing at the nurses station]
J: no, I. got reintubated this morning at about 6.30.
(Nods/ points in the direction of the patient)L. is fine.
(Nods/ points in the direction of the patient)Fine.
(Nods/ points in the direction of the patient)Fine.
(Nods/ points in the direction of the patient) Had some climbing pCO2's we
played with the vent, she's better
M: ok; who's that?
J: and then, J. came down here,
M: oh ok
J: she had a pCO2 of  greater than 105
M: ok thanks
J: there is 2 kids in step down [pause] by the way.  There is a two year old
that got beat up
M: correct
J: (Nods/ points in the direction of the patient)Liver lac.
(Nods/ points in the direction of the patient)Stable.
M: thanks J.
J: high LFT's, two thousands.
M: great, great way to
```

(margin label, rotated:) Five critical patients

**Figure 9.2 Hand-off complies with quantity maxim of Grice's
Cooperative Principle**

```
H: Just keep coming down to like 20 on her rate. Uhmm (pause) this is the
same settings that she's been on forever so I don't know the difference
except that she's just totally out  so that she's not fighting at all or
not making any motion against the vent
***
Overhead page by RN "Who has the new shedule?"
H: [making a non verbal gesture]
R: [Laughs]
***
MK: This is easy. It's going to be easy. The little trauma
H: yes
MK: can go down. cause she looks really good. This one??
H: yes
MK: and [pause] he could go down.
H: ok
MK: and T. could go down. Now I am not going [unintelligible] to move
anybody till I [unintelligible] the traumas, because once I see the
traumas then we'll know
H: right, right
MK: but [short pause] we got play
*****
```

(margin label, rotated:) Announcement, Attending, interrupt

**Figure 9.3 Hand-off complies with quality maxim of Grice's
Cooperative Principle**

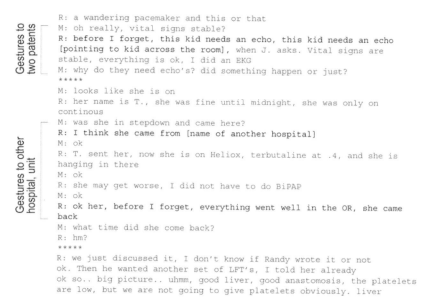

**Figure 9.4 Hand-off complies with relation maxim of Grice's
        Cooperative Principle**

In Figure 9.5, a negotiated discussion occurs in which control is shared, maintained, and invited by cues. For example, the on-coming physician controls closure over each portion of the dialog through incremental acceptance. Instead of the off-going shift providing a fixed information brief for the on-coming shift, the hand-off uses stylized protocols and expressions to maximize accuracy and to avoid ambiguity.

We expected that the greatest amount of attention (expressed in the length of time that care providers spent discussing an individual's condition) would be paid to patients who required the greatest amount of care. If this was true, patients who were ventilator-dependent, required cardiac care, or required multiple intravenous medications would receive the greatest amount of attention. However, as Figure 9.6 shows, correlations between discussion time and care demand were not significant. In the scatter plot, the patient population in the PICU and SDU during the time the data were collected is represented according to their care demand and discussion time. Note that the fellows do not favor discussion of the most demanding patients in their hand-offs. The average discussion time for any patient (excluding patients with discussion time equal to 0 seconds) is 36.5 seconds.

J: Yep
M: So and the only access we have is a small peripheral IV in her foot
J: last time [unintelligible] vagal nerve stimulator
M: right so you have uh
J: yep
M: just so you know. Uhm .. The ECMO patient you know, she was put back
on ECMO, uhm or he was put back on ECMO
J: 2.30 Saturday morning
M: Yeah, something like that. Doing ok, uhmm, really no significant
problems. Lactate had been rising a little bit to like 2.7 but
stabilizing there. The only thing was that uhmm platelets uhmm they are
accepting lower platelet counts of 50,000 but we've had to transfuse a
couple times for platelets like 11 or 14,000
J: ok
M: uhmm... the other thing is there was a little bit of swelling on the
uhmm
J: right leg
M: right inguinal area, no, in the inguinal area moving toward the
buttocks, over the day. Lisa noticed that. We just .. We put a pressure
dressing on, and we kept an eye on it. The pulses are ok, so we're just
gonna watch
J: ok, uhmm...... alright, what is the gram negativ
M: uhm it is S. and uhmm yeah
J: where
M: everywhere, every single.. uhmm line
J: surprise surprise
M: it's not good, according to A. once it's in the circuit, it's in the
circuit; not good. C., he's basicly the same; he's low grade fever, like
38.5 so I did culture him. Uhmm he...he's gonna get a trach at the
bedside this afternoon if they get consent and I heard he is going for
CT this morning but I just heard that from the nurse but I have not
heard
J: ok
M: anything about that.
J: He never went last week because
M: ok so maybe that is why
J: he just needs a follow-up to see what his ventricles look like
M: ok, uhmm, L., uhmm, she is doing just fine. She is diuresing quite
aggressively and obviously needing Potassium supplements
J: ok
M: I think both of these can be cut back. She is otherwise doing ok. She
she starts to through PVC's uhmm when her uhmm Potassium goes down
J: less than 2.7
M: Yeah, I think are we giving it now? [talking to RN]
RN: no I just sent some , I'll check them in a minute
M: ok
RN:[unintelligible]
M: ok
J: 2.7 is her number to start throwing PVC's
M: she she is .....like she needs a higher level than some of the other
kids. C. is C., not really anything new.
J: extubated, though
M: extubated,she is doing good, uhmm, ... started Captopril, I think
the Milrinone is off, and uhmm, I think they're gonna do a Echo today,so
J: [unintelligible] M: [unintelligible] as far as I know
J: she looks comfortable
M: she looks comfortable [unintelligible] J:[unintelligible] main stem
M: she is not very awake or interactive, so, I mean part of it is , I'm
sure, weaning sedation but I would have .. I would have liked to see her
a little more awake in between. This little one was extubated uhm like
early yesteday, not, uhmm early yesteday morning or the day before

On-coming fellow provides incremental closure, co-constructs shared cognition

**Figure 9.5 Hand-off complies with manner maxim of Grice's
        Cooperative Principle**

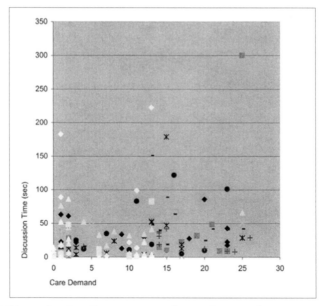

Figure 9.6 Discussion length versus care demand per patient
Copyright © 2007 Cognitive Technologies Laboratory. Reprinted by permission.

Further analysis of the transcripts revealed that it is *uncertainty* about patient condition that influences hand-off content and form. Sign outs are primarily used to account for what is known and not known about a patient's condition, and how both are likely to play out through the oncoming shift.

Hand-off analysis also showed that clinicians vary the content, form, and structure (strategy) of their hand-offs as a way to cope with the demands of their uncertain, complex work setting.

Content

The proportion of time that is spent on patients, compared to other content, varies among the hand-offs. Some hand-offs are almost exclusively patient-related. Others incorporate considerable discussion of topics other than patient condition. The percentage of a hand-off that is spent on discussion of individual patients ranges from nearly all of it (97 per cent) to just over half of it (56 per cent). Our conversation analysis found six additional types of hand-off content: introduction, walking, interruption, unit resources, patient population, and socializing. Table 9.1 shows six other categories that we identified, followed by a definition and an example from the data.

Table 9.1 Hand-off content

Topic	Characteristic	Example
Patient	Information related to the condition of a particular patient.	H: So this little guy came back from (.) the (0.8) OR and he had uhm just evidence of clinical coarc essentially so he was taken back to the operating room again at ten thirty with D1 to (0.5) uhm (1.3) there was significant gradient like I guess twenty millimeters of mercury difference so he was taken back to the OR. Came back on ECMO and have been doing that ever since
Introduction	Hand-offs may begin with an announcement that it is time to start or a confirmation that everyone is ready to proceed.	J: Okay Are you ready? M: Yep I am[a]
Walking	The fellows may walk to each bed where they discuss the patient.	(relatively long pauses of silence, or inaudible talk of people the fellows pass)

Interruption	An event or person interrupts the hand-off with a question or comment unrelated to the hand-off.	H: What
		N: You know what that neurology resident's name is
		R: (D3)
		H: (D3) (the fellow?)
		?: ((??))
		H: Yeah
		N: Oh she's a fellow
		H: Yeah
		N: Already good I'll have this (for you (tomorrow))
		H: (He thinks)
		   you stole the grey chart
		   : (0.7)
		?: She stole the gray chart
		M: ((Laugh))

Socializing	Teasing, joking, or talking about topics unrelated to patients and often pertaining to their personal lives such as parties, sports, sleep.	A: Oh yeah I'd love to come next Sunday J: Next Saturday the eleventh A: A week from Saturday Okay M: A (girls' night) R: ((There) all girls) (.) party? J: All girls' party

Unit resources	Discussion of bed availability, patients that can be transferred to another unit (from the main unit to step down or from step down to the floor), and new admittances that will soon be arriving in the unit from the emergency room, operating room, or an outside hospital.	H: So what (.) the only reason why I'm saying all of this is that just right before I went and got a shower we got a call that there's two pediatric traumas One is ap- Both from Indiana One is apparently a head, one is apparently a pelvis (0.7) So they were gonna have to sit in the ER for a while but if he can move (0.6) this would be the other one also that she was saying could potentially move So you have beds to put the traumas both up here : (1.1) R: (she can move to stepdown) H: (And then in step down) you'll have one RSV patient left that was on the CPAP that ((??)) R: (right) She's still on the CPAP H: She's still on the CPAP looking good R: O(kay) H: (The) other one can go out to the floor (serv)ice R: (Okay)[b]
Patient population	Talk about the unit at a general level (overall status, rounds, and responsibilities) including individual or multiple patients who were previously on the unit, have since returned home, or passed away.	R: And everybody else (.) they're okay? H: Yeah D6 D6 was not (here more than ??) M: uh R: Yeah Busy busy H: It was just busy[c]
Conclusion	Hand-off may end with the on-coming fellow signaling that all of the information has been understood and there are no further questions, or the off-going fellow may inquire if the hand-off may end.	*R: Good* *: (2.1)* *R: Alrighty* *: (1.8)* *R: Thank you (.) H[d]*

Notes:
[i] Hand-off #2 Lines 10–11
[ii] Hand-off #1 Lines 311–24
[iii] Hand-off #1 Lines 426–430
[iv] Hand-off #1 Lines 443–7

Form

Subjects employed three forms of talk, shown in Table 9.2: two types of soliloquies and one type of colloquy. Table 9.2 includes the forms, a definition, and example of each.

Table 9.2 Hand-off form

Form	Definition	Example
Soliloquy (type 1)	Unidirectional occurrence of talk in which one person does all of the speaking.	*R: Uh P62 okay P62 is six years old (0.6) uhm (0.6) an: d he was in this (.) apartment fire (0.6) He: (.)aparently arrest- was down for fifteeen minutes (.) in the field (0.5) and when he got to South Shore Hospital he was down uh He got Epi in the field and then he came back (0.7) And I don't know what he got at South Shore they didn't tell us (0.5) No no medications Okay so (.) alright (0.8) Uh:m (1.1) his carboxyhemoglobin outside was thirty-two percent (1.6) Uhm (.) when he got here (1.2) uh (.) we got an a- axillary art line He has a triple lumen central line in his groin (0.6) He had one episode of his blood pressure going down to the thirties but that was a cuff pressure before we got all the lines in He got about two hundred cc's of volume (1.1) uh: His first blood gas here showed a carboxyhemoglobin of four (0.5) and a methemoglobin of one point four which is normal We ordered thiosulfate anyway and we decided to give it anyway (0.7) uh: (0.6) These are his vent settings (.) uh PRVC two twenty (.) and a hundred percent FiO2 His PaO2 was good (.) Five eighty-eight (0.8) uh:m (1.3) So the plan o(kay)* *J: (What was) his initial pH [i]*
Soliloquy (type 2)	Monologue but has the additional feature of verbal acknowledgement of understanding.	*R: So we're working up endocrine (.) extensively and genetic and (.) everything (0.5) So (1.0) he needed like D fifteen to maintain his glucose (0.7) So what we did is uh you know obviously we were worried about like growth hormone and things (like that) and because growth hormone is episodic* *J: (umhm)* *R: (We wanted) to challenge him* *J: (Sure)* *R: So the moment we stopped like decreased his glucose infusion for an hour his glucose* *went down to twenty-four* *M: Oh wow*

| Colloquy | Reciprocal transfer of information involving two or more persons. | R: *So they're gonna do a Ross: (0.9)*
J: *They (are)*
M: *(They) are*
R: *Yeah*
: *(0.7)*
?: *They're gonna what*
M: *(But) that's*
J: *Do a (Ross)*
R: *(Ross)*
M: *How do they feel the LV is Is the*
         (LV working better   )
J: *(Do we know (anything for sure) though)*
R: *On pressors it (was pe)rfect ((for this much))*
M: *(yeah)   (oh great)*
   And you ((don't) give him (??) so that's good)
R: *((what happens on Epi) so   )*
: *(0.6)*
M: *But still we're (a lot   )*
J: *(We're doing) another ECHO today*
R: *Yeah*
M: *Okay[ii]* |

Notes:
[i] Hand-off #9 Lines 14–32
[ii] Hand-off #9 Lines 292–313

In a *soliloquy*, one person does all of the speaking, as in a monologue. A *colloquy* is a reciprocal transfer of information involving two or more persons, as in a dialogue. Colloquy includes question–answer series, testing–confirmation series, exchange of ideas, and problem-solving. The forms demonstrate the same variable, emotion-laden, dynamic, and complex traits as the work domain that they are used to manage (Conant and Ashby 1970). Figures 9.7 and 9.8 show timelines for two of the exchanges, representing their content and form. In each of the diagrams, the column at left is a timeline for a single hand-off. Discussion about patients is indicated by a black field. Discussion about other topics is shown on a white field. The number and types of topics displays the diversity of hand-off content. Hand-off form, or conversation style, is represented by four columns on the right. Each of the columns from left to right denotes a specific conversation type: soliloquy, soliloquy with interjections, colloquy. The fourth allows for occasions in which language in the audio recording was inaudible. Using this approach, both the hand-off content and form of discourse can be determined at any point during the hand-offs.

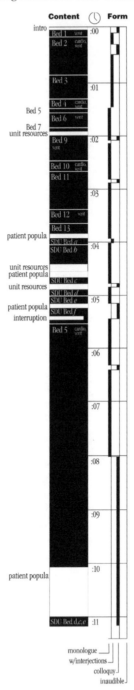

Figure 9.7 Hand-off content and form – Saturday am
Copyright © 2007 Cognitive Technologies Laboratory. Reprinted by permission.

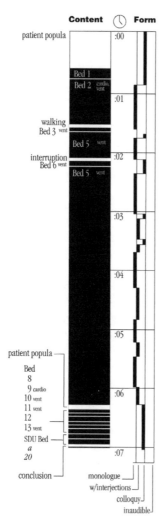

Figure 9.8 Hand-off content and form – Wednesday am
Copyright © 2007 Cognitive Technologies Laboratory. Reprinted by permission.

Strategies and Patterns

In this study, hand-off length ranged from six minutes to 25 minutes and 40 seconds. What accounts for that spread? Aspects of the work setting such as limited time, the onset of general rounds, or a critically ill patient impose different constraints on the clinicians. Clinicians respond by employing different strategies to organize the structure of their hand-offs. In some cases, efficiency is paramount. In others, objectives may involve the discussion of every patient, the solution of a problem concerning a particular patient, unit resources, or development of rapport with peers. The structures of hand-offs are as diverse as the varied constraints on hand-offs.

The analysis discovered three kinds of hand-off strategies. The first strategy (example 1) is the form of a hand-off that is generally expected. Strategies 2 and 3 develop from adaptations to the usual hand-off strategy as a way to deal with pressure from external constraints.

Strategy Example 1: Bed to bed, make sure all is said. The Friday hand-off in Figure 9.7 depicts the presumed, or canonical, form of a hand-off. It is the geographic strategy, in which the fellows start their patient discussion at Bed One. They then proceed around the unit in a precise order, methodically moving from bed to bed. Each patient is discussed in turn as the fellows stand at the bedside of that patient. The fellows can see the next bed and anticipate what is to follow. The progress of the hand-off can be determined by their physical location in the unit. By knowing what has been completed and what lies ahead, the hand-off pace can be altered as needed. The geographic hand-off strategy is best suited to circumstances in which time is available. Most hand-offs belong to this category.

Strategy Example 2: Save the sick, do the others quick. The imminent start of unit rounds is an example of a constraint that leads to selection of this "do the others quick" strategy, shown in the Saturday timeline in Figure 9.7. The fellows change shift at 7:30 am. Daily, at 8:00 am, the attendings, fellows, residents, surgeon and cardiologist, charge nurse, social worker, and nurse at the bedside of the patient gather to conduct rounds. These rounds involve a parade through the unit to each bedside where the resident presents the patient, the patient is evaluated, and the plan is identified. The fellows' sign out needs to be completed before rounds begin. This hand-off has a rigid time constraint of which the fellows are aware before the hand-off begins. Using this strategy, the fellows can focus on what they consider to be the most important issue(s) to discuss. They also know that other events that are scheduled for later in the day will provide additional information beyond the sign out.

Strategy Example 3: New demand, change the plan. In the Wednesday hand-off in Figure 9.8, the fellows begin with the geographic strategy. They proceed from bed to bed until they reach the fifth patient. An obstacle arises that threatens to interrupt or truncate the hand-off and puts orderly completion of the task in jeopardy: unit rounds are beginning early. As the fellows talk, they also watch the crowd gathering across the room in anticipation of starting rounds. The geographic hand-off strategy they are using will no longer suffice. Both fellows are aware that the most critical information must be transmitted immediately and concisely. In this case, the most critical patient is in Bed Five, so discussion continues until time nearly runs out. The remaining seconds are spent on concise statements about several other patients with one or two significant details.

Discussion

Hand-offs are not reports, but are instead conversations. Expertise in hand-off communications depends on the ability to choose what to include and what to leave out, to prioritize relevant information, and to transfer insights. Effective communication depends as much on what is left out as on what is included.

Clinicians use variations of monologue and dialogue to transfer information at a high level. Both forms demonstrate the same variable, emotion-laden, dynamic, and complex traits as the work domain that they are used to manage (Conant and Ashby 1970). We find that sign outs account for both what is known and what is not known about a patient's condition, and are used to assess expectations for the oncoming shift. The fresh perspective of the on-coming individual can increase the likelihood that misperceptions due to fixation bias will be detected (Patterson et al. 2004; Wears et al. 2003). Uncertainty about patient condition influences hand-off content and form. Clinicians change the amount of time that they allocate to hand-offs based on other aspects of workload, such as rounds or procedures. Clinicians apportion time to discuss individual patients according to the perceived severity and stability of each patient's condition.

Why are hand-offs like this? Acute healthcare is similar to other complex high stakes technical work. Patient care responsibility and authority are transferred using communication strategies that are tailored to support the distribution of cognition across time and space. Practitioners necessarily distribute cognition in order to prevent gap formation during work-cycle shift changes. These processes are reminiscent of the hand-offs in combat information centers in US Navy ships (Klein 2000).

Acute healthcare hand-off language follows Grice's four maxims for a number of reasons. The ICU and its patients are complex. It is impossible to fully describe everything that is relevant. While there are specific details that matter, they vary from patient to patient and from time to time. Circumstances change so rapidly that the content of a hand-off will be stale within a short time. The ICU and its patients are beset by uncertainty, and hand-offs include information about the nature and scope of the uncertainty. Clinicians use language in certain ways in order to manage work domain complexity. Patient progress is not a direct course of improvement, is complex, and is unpredictable. As a result, clinician hand-offs are complex and flexible in their structure, focus on what is uncertain, are necessarily variable in their content, and take multiple forms. Patterson, Roth and Render (2005) found wide variability in healthcare hand-off strategies, media, and order across and within wards, over both time and individuals. In their study of patient hand-offs by ED physicians, Matthews et al. (2002) also reported a variety of communications patterns, and lack of a "controlled" turnover process.

Even though they affect patient care quality and continuity, sign-outs are not taught, but are instead learned on the job. Findings from this study and further analyses can be used to develop training in hand-offs for junior clinicians such as nurses and residents, as Philibert and Leach (2005) contend. Formulaic "canned" approaches to handling sign-outs are a poor match to deal with the uncertainty and complexity of the critical care environment. Clinicians create hand-offs that are unique in content and form in order to manage PICU circumstances. Attempts to improve continuity of care must reflect this.

The study was subject to two limitations. As an exploratory project, lack of funding limited the study's scope to one site and a period of six weeks, and one of the authors (MB) served as both subject and analyst. One limitation of conversation analysis is that "transcriptions ... are always and necessarily selective" in terms of the "sensitivity and precision" of interactional details (ten Have 1999, 78).

Conclusion

Our research has shown that pediatric ICU fellow hand-off content varies, but exchanges conform to Grice's maxims by demonstrating high context sensitivity, compact reference, gestures, and stylized expressions. The conventional view considers hand-offs to be data-focused, simply structured, uniform in content, and singular in form. By contrast, our data show that hand-offs focus on what is uncertain, are complex and flexible in their structure, necessarily variable in their content, and take multiple forms. This is because patient progress is not a direct course of improvement, but is instead complex and unpredictable. Relevant, efficient hand-offs significantly affect the ability of clinicians to provide care at the unit level, within and between departments, and across specialties. Improvement of their ability to perform this vital task through training promises to benefit both care providers and patients alike.

Acknowledgements

Dr Nemeth's work is supported by a grant (LM007947) from the Agency for Healthcare Research and Quality. Dr Cook's work is supported by a grant (HS11816) from the Agency for Healthcare Research and Quality.

References

Accreditation Council for Graduate Medical Education (ACGME) (2002), *Report of the ACGME Work Group on Resident Duty Hours*, Chicago, 11 June.

Brandwijk, M., Nemeth, C., O'Connor, M., Kahana, M. and Cook, R. (2003), 'Distributing Cognition: ICU Handoffs Conform to Grice's Maxims', paper presented at the *Proceedings of the Society for Critical Care Medicine National Conference*, January, San Antonio, TX.

Conant, R.C. and Ashby, W.R. (1970), 'Every Good Regulator of a System Must Be Model of That System', *International Journal of Systems Science* 1:2, 89–97.

Cook, R.I., Render, M. and Woods, D.D. (2000), 'Gaps in the Continuity of Care and Progress on Patient Safety', *British Medical Journal* 320:7237, 791–4.

Drew, P. and Heritage, J. (1992), *Talk at Work* (New York: Cambridge University Press) 3–100, 331–58.

Frohlich, D.M. (1993), 'Adding Interaction Analysis to the User Research Portfolio. Rethinking Theoretical Frameworks for Human Computer Interaction', *InterCHI '93* (Amsterdam: Association for Computing Machinery).

Grice, H.P. (1975), 'Logic and Conversation', in P. Cole and J.L. Morgan (eds), *Syntax and Semantics: Speech Acts*, Volume 3 (New York: Academic Press) 41–58.

Heath, C. and Luff, P. (2000), *Technology in Action* (New York: Cambridge University Press) 1–60, 217–51.

Hutchins, E. (1995), *Cognition in the Wild* (Cambridge, MA: MIT Press).

Institute of Medicine (IOM) (2000), Kohn, L., Corrigan, J. and Donaldson, M. (eds), *To Err is Human* (Washington, DC: National Academies Press).

Klein, G. (2000), *Sources of Power* (Cambridge, MA: The MIT Press).

Kowalsky, J. (2004, August), *PICU Hand-Offs: Characterizing the Technical Work Context of Intensive Care Units*, Report available from the Cognitive Technologies Laboratory, University of Chicago, 5841 S. Maryland Avenue, MC4028, Chicago, IL 60637.

Kowalsky, J., Nemeth, C., Brandwijk, M. and Cook, R.I. (2005, January), 'Understanding Sign Outs: Conversation Analysis Reveals ICU Handoff Content and Form', *Critical Care Medicine* 32:12, A29.

MacWhinney, B. (2000), *The CHILDRES Project: Tools for Analyzing Talk*, 3rd edition (Mahwah, NJ: Lawrence Erlbaum Associates).

Matthews, A.L., Harvey, C.M., Schuster, R.J. and Durso, F.T. (2002), 'Emergency Physician to Admitting Physician Handovers: An Exploratory Study', *Proceedings of the Human Factors and Ergonomics Society 46th Annual Meeting* (Santa Monica, CA: HFES).

Nemeth, C. (2004), *Human Factors Methods for Design* (New York: Taylor and Francis/CRC Press).

Patterson, E., Roth, E. and Render, M. (2005), 'Handoffs During Nursing Shift Changes in Acute Care', *Proceedings of the Human Factors and Ergonomics Society 49th Annual Meeting* (Santa Monica, CA: HFES) 1057–61.

Patterson, E., Roth, E., Woods, D., Chow, R. and Gomes, J.O. (2004), 'Handoff Strategies in Settings with High Consequences for Failure: Lessons for Health Care Operations', *International Journal for Quality in Health Care* 16:2, 125–32.

Philibert, I. and Leach, D.C. (2005), 'Reframing Continuity of Care for this Century', *Quality Safety in Healthcare* 14:6, 394–6.

ten Have, P. (1999), *Doing Conversation Analysis: A Practical Guide* (London: Sage Publications).

Wears, R.L., Perry, S.J., Shapiro, M., Beach, C. and Behara, R. (2003), 'Shift Changes Among Emergency Physicians: Best of Times, Worst of Times', *Proceedings of the Human Factors and Ergonomics Society 47th Annual Meeting* (Santa Monica, CA: HFES) 1420–23.

Woods, D.D. (1993), 'Process Tracing Methods for the Study of Cognition Outside of the Experimental Psychology Laboratory', in G. Klein, J. Orasanu and R. Calderwood (eds), *Decision Making in Action: Models and Methods* (Norwood, NJ: Ablex Publishing Corporation) 228–51.

Chapter 10

Collaborative Cross-checking

Jeffrey P. Brown

Background

Cross-checking has been described as the ability of individuals or groups to assess the validity or accuracy of others' assumptions or actions (Patterson et al. 2007). Thus, cross-checking may provide opportunity to detect, reveal, and intervene in erroneous actions or inactions before they cause harm (Carthey, de Leval and Reason 2001; Klein 2006; Klein et al. 2005b; Patterson, Render and Ebright 2002; Patterson et al. 2007; Uhlig et al. 2001). It is also a means by which the consequences of errors or anomalies may be detected and mitigated (Helmreich 2000; Klein et al. 2005b; Mudge 1998; Woods 2005).

The potential of cross-checking to enhance problem detection is perhaps greatest in the context of interdisciplinary teamwork. Teams comprised of individuals with varied backgrounds and perspectives may have a greater chance of avoiding or detecting problems, relative to individuals or more homogenous teams (Helmreich 2000; Klein 2006; Leape et al. 1999; Weick 2001; Woods, O'Brien and Hanes 1987). Yet, it is rare to observe cross-checking as an element of interdisciplinary teamwork in clinical settings. When cross-checking is observed in clinical settings, it is most often seen as a facet of an individual's practice, or as a required cross-check for a high-risk procedure, such as blood transfusion (Kosnik, Brown and Maund 2007). The focus of this chapter will be on cross-checking as an elemental team process, rather than as a routinized or required monitoring task.

A Definition of Collaboration

The term "collaborative cross-checking" implies a compact among personnel to aid one another in avoiding misstep. This compact is fulfilled through both verbal and non-verbal communication and, accordingly, I have selected the following definition of collaboration from Kinnaman and Bleich (2004: 311) for the purposes of this chapter:

> Collaboration is a communication process that fosters innovation and advanced problem solving among people who are of different disciplines, organizational ranks, or institutional settings; band together for advanced problem solving; discern innovative solutions without regard to discipline, rank, or institutional affiliation; and enact change based on a higher standard of care or organizational outcomes.

The process of collaboration requires mutual respect, differing but complementary competencies, a distributed balance of power between the parties, and evidence of satisfying teamwork that results in change.

In this light, the term "collaboration" embraces the greater promise of team-based practice, and collaborative cross-checking may be seen as an elemental team process; an outgrowth of conditions for effective teamwork enacted through communication. In settings where there is high consequence for failure, such as flightdeck operations and air traffic control, collaborative cross-checking may be observed as part of the fabric of teamwork. It is a practice integral to problem detection, analysis, and resolution that is woven into interaction among team members (Hollnagel, Woods and Leveson 2006; Mudge 1998; Patankar and Taylor 1999). Let us consider how the current context of hospital-based care may foster or deter collaborative cross-checking and other team processes.

The Context for Collaborative Cross-checking in Hospital-based Care

Research has shown that information gathering and analysis by health professionals is primarily mediated through conversation (Coiera 2000). This suggests that effective individual performance, while important, is insufficient for successful navigation of patient needs. Health professionals must continually align and adjust their assessments and actions with members of other disciplines to guide safe and effective patient care. Yet, hospitals were not conceived to support interdisciplinary clinical practice. Instead, they were conceived and organized to support the practice of affiliated physicians with facilities, technologies, and support personnel such as nurses, therapists, and pharmacists (Ludmerer 1999; Merry and Brown 2001; Brown 2005b; Sharpe and Faden 1998).

The Organizational Roots of Hospitals

In the early twentieth century, hospitals were organized to support a hospital–physician relationship in which: (a) physicians received the privilege of admitting and caring for their patients in a given hospital, and (b) hospitals received revenue from patients admitted by affiliated physicians through the provision of beds, supplies, and care from nurses (Merry and Brown 2001; Sharpe and Faden 1998). Then, as now, hospital administrators were accountable for the financial viability of the hospital and for the provision of facilities, technologies, and patient care resources to support the practice of affiliated physicians. Medical staff members (physicians), in turn, were accountable for the quality of medical care. Medical staff responsibilities such as credentialing and peer review were overseen by medical staff executive committees. Hospital responsibilities were fulfilled under the auspices of hospital chief executives. Both reported to the same board of trustees. Beneath the layers of regulatory, organizational, and managerial complexity that have accreted over the last century, this conceptual and structural divide between medical and hospital functions and processes remains intact. Conceived to support the independent practice of physicians, the organizational and governance structures of hospitals sustain a clinical context in which physician autonomy frequently trumps close attention to the management of role interrelationships and interdependencies among care providers (Lawrence 2002; Merry 2005; Starr 1982). This is evident in role-based hierarchy found within and across disciplines (Rafferty, Ball and Aiken 2001), but the authority gradient is especially steep in interaction between physician and non-physician healthcare providers.

The Effect of Role Hierarchy on Team Processes

The role relationship between medical and non-medical personnel manifests fundamentally as follows: (a) physicians assess patients and write patient care orders in the patients' medical records, and (b) the disciplines tasked by those orders fulfill them. As new patient care roles have been created over the years, hospitals have established clinical departments such as physical therapy, dietetics, and social work, among others, which deploy their members to clinical units to fulfill their tasks as ordered by physicians. Nurses, therapists, social workers, and other clinical professionals may be observed on virtually any US hospital ward reviewing physician orders, independently gathering information from patients (much of it redundant), developing a plan of care specific to their professional function, and then entering these plans into the patient's medical record. The medical record is the traditional mechanism for coordinating patient care activities among health professionals; a function for which it has become increasingly ill-suited in the face of rising social and technological complexity. Stale or ambiguous data entry, informational gaps, and changes in patient status necessitate frequent interaction with members of other disciplines to provide or seek alternative perspectives, make sense of changes, or otherwise clarify information. These purposes are pursued through phone calls, paging, and random interactions in hallways, cafeterias, and other locations. There are few, if any, "designed-in" opportunities in workflow for interdisciplinary sensemaking, planning, and provision of care. The end result of this approach to managing role interrelationship and patient care interdependencies is fragmentation of effort that may create or exacerbate problems as much as resolve them (Brown 2005b; Patterson, Render and Ebright 2002; Tucker and Edmondson 2003; Rafferty, Ball and Aiken 2001; Sutcliffe, Lewton and Rosenthal 2004).

But Most Hospitals Assign Clinical Care to Teams, Right?

It is common to hear from clinical and administrative health professionals that care is provided by teams or interdisciplinary teams in hospital settings. Yet, as noted above, observation of clinical work in hospitals often reveals members of various disciplines fulfilling patient care tasks independently rather than in concert, even when in the same physical space at the same time. The following quote is from a unit secretary, whose role is clerical rather than clinical:

> Yesterday, a consulting cardiologist came to my intensive care unit and examined a patient. He then came to the nursing station where I sit, directly across from the patient's room, to talk with the patient's nurse. Meanwhile, the patient's surgeon showed up and went into

her room. After examining her he went over to the computer, put in an order, then left. I do not know if he saw the cardiologist, but the cardiologist had not seen him. A little while later, the surgeon's order was discovered by the cardiologist and I could tell from his facial expression that he thought it was not appropriate. He asked me to track down the surgeon and the two of them ended up playing phone tag for the better part of two hours before they finally spoke and agreed on what to do. I do not know if there was any bad effect on the patient from this delay, but I have sometimes seen patients get really sick before stuff like this gets sorted out. I have tried to make sure people do not miss talking to each other, but this is not always appreciated and I am not always right about thinking they might need to check in with each other. I do not want to be viewed as meddling outside of my role, but sometimes I just get really concerned.

And the following observation from an operating room illustrates that poorly coordinated task fulfillment can lead to unchecked actions capable of placing patients at immediate risk of injury.

A five-year-old boy had experienced a laryngeal spasm while under anesthesia. This was managed successfully, but after the surgical procedure had been completed the Certified Registered Nurse Anesthetist (CRNA) decided to monitor the boy in the operating room (OR) a bit longer than usual, to ensure that he was truly stable before being transferred to the Post Anesthesia Care Unit (PACU). Meanwhile, other nursing personnel began cleaning the OR and prepping equipment for the next case. In the course of fulfilling these tasks, one of the nurses disconnected the electrical power to monitoring equipment that was still attached to the boy. The CRNA expressed alarm, then noted what had happened and requested that it be re-connected.

While the event described above was not deemed consequential by anyone involved, it illustrates the potential for more serious consequences resulting from coordination and cross-checking deficits. These may arise when personnel do not consider how their activities and actions might impact the overall situation in which they are embedded. Explicit communication practices, such as announcing an intended change in equipment configuration, are commonly used by flight crewmembers to invite cross-check and preclude misstep. Such communication practices are not yet exercised as a professional standard in healthcare. Another factor contributing to the event described above is production pressure, which exacerbated the tendency for task-myopia in this busy operating room. The nurse who had prematurely disconnected the monitoring equipment later explained:

We have to turn those rooms around, quick. We have cases waiting and we're accountable for efficient throughput. If cases get backed up it hurts the hospital's bottom line and surgeons get upset because it hurts their bottom line, too. We are very concerned with patient safety here, I just hadn't thought about the impact of what I was doing on anyone else.

What we are held to account for strongly influences what we attend to (Woods 2004). Being held to account for individual fulfillment of tasks, rather than the performance of tasks in close coordination with other care providers, remains a powerful source of fragmentation and patient harm (Brown 2005b; Patterson, Render and Ebright 2002). Although the extent varies with the social dynamics of any given unit or organization, the fulfillment of clinical tasks in contemporary hospital-based care is more an individual activity than truly team-based (Dominguez et al. 2005; Gittell et al. 2000; Lawrence 2002). And while many clinical units have "check-ins" on patient needs and care plans called "interdisciplinary" or "multidisciplinary rounds", these vary greatly in terms of participation and rigor. The following illustrative quote is from a social worker:

> One type of rounds at my hospital is called "interdisciplinary discharge rounds". Even though called interdisciplinary, these rounds in fact do not include the patient, family members, or physicians—or even a quorum of the disciplines that may have had a "hands-on" role in the care of the patient who is going to be discharged. Hospitals are very busy and while members of each discipline are expected to go to discharge rounds, they are not accountable for attendance; they are accountable for fulfilling their assigned tasks with patients, which is pretty time-pressured. So, what actually happens is that you often only have a nurse, a social worker, and maybe a member of another discipline who actually attend. This is a problem because we might have eight or ten patients admitted in the morning and by noon they are to be transferred or discharged and no one person, or even two or three members of different disciplines, can put together the whole picture—a bunch of people in other disciplines may have interacted with the patient, including attending physicians and maybe a consultant, and they may not have had a chance to enter their notes in the patient's medical record. Even if you have notes from members of other disciplines who are not in attendance, these often require clarification and you have to track down that person (if they are still on shift) which often happens later, after discharge. For example, you can look at the physical therapy notes but they are all in the code-talk of physical therapy. And even though discharge may be recommended by the attending physician and other disciplines, you might have no indication in the notes that the physician who wrote prescriptions for the patient realizes that the patient has no prescription drug insurance and will be unable to afford the drugs prescribed. And the physical and occupational therapists who are recommending discharge may not be aware that the patient lives on the third floor of an apartment building with no elevator and there is nobody to help him up and down the stairs. Discharge rounds are driven by pressure to get the patient out of the hospital with very little consideration of what happens to that patient upon discharge. Consequently, we commonly have patients discharged this week return the next because their overall situation is never coherently examined. Because of this incoherence in discharge planning we are probably a bigger reason than anyone realizes for the existence of so many "frequent flyers". These are patients who are regularly admitted to the hospital, over and again. We do not assemble all of the minds necessary to do discharge rounding well, and we do not have the organizational structure and incentives to do so. Each discipline is held accountable for their productivity and/or billable time—which equates to a focus on fulfilling their assigned tasks independently with patients. Consequently, no matter how much we may want to, we never fully understand how our role fits into the overall process of care experienced by the patient.

Although some health professionals cite experience with exemplary team-based practice in hospitals, the conditions for poor quality care described above remain all too common and are fundamentally "hard-wired" into the social architecture and governance structure of hospitals. These conditions have arisen because the social and technological complexity of contemporary healthcare is overwhelming the century-old model of hospital organization and management that was conceived to support the independent practices of physicians (Merry and Crago 2001; Merry 2005; Sharpe and Faden 1998; Starr 1982). Although the current picture may seem bleak, the good news is that clinical environments are rich in diverse intellectual resources which, if harnessed through team processes, may yield significant improvements in the safety and quality of care (Lawrence 2002; Leonard, Graham and Bonacum 2004; Uhlig et al. 2001 and 2002).

The Importance of Harnessing Intellectual Variety in Clinical Care

The ability to detect and diagnose problems or anomalies, and adapt activity to avert failure, has been discussed by numerous researchers as instrumental to safety and reliability (Hollnagel, Woods and Leveson et al. 2006; Klein 2006; Rasmussen 1982; Reason 1997; Roberts and Bea 2001). There is increasing consensus that team processes may enhance this adaptive capability (Lawrence 2002; Patterson et al. 2007; Uhlig et al. 2001; Weick, Sutcliffe and Obstfeld 1999). Teams comprised of members with diverse expertise and perspectives may be especially capable of problem detection, analysis, and resolution (Bolman 1980; Klein 2006; Sarter and Alexander 2000; Woods, O'Brien and Hanes 1987). Per Karl Weick (2001):

> When technical systems have more variety than a single individual can comprehend, one of the few ways humans can match this variety is by networks and teams of divergent individuals ... Whether team members differ in occupational specialties, past experience, gender, conceptual skills, or personality may be less important than the fact that they do differ and look for different things when they size up a problem. If people look for different things, when their observations are pooled they collectively see more than any one of them alone would see.

Weick also points out that as team members become more alike, or homogenous, their collective observations are less distinguishable from their individual observations, and they are likely to gain little advantage in understanding a problem collectively rather than individually.

Ashby's Law of Requisite Variety asserts that the greater the variety of actions available to a control system, the greater the variety of perturbations it may compensate for (Heylighen 1992). The application of Ashby's Law to human systems (Zeleny 1986) suggests that promoting variety and diversity of perspective through interdisciplinary teamwork may increase the likelihood of problem detection and resolution. Harnessing the intellectual variety represented by the many disciplines that care for patients requires flattening of hierarchy and creating a context in which clinical personnel feel safe to express concern, inquire, or advocate for another perspective, without fear of repercussion.

Psychological Safety and Trust

Although change is coming (Baker et al. 2005; Greiner and Knebel 2003), the processes of training and education for physicians and members of other health professions continue to instill a theory of practice that is centered in professional autonomy and independent role-based task fulfillment, not teamwork (Helmreich and Merritt 1998; Brown 2005a and 2005b; O'Connell and Pascoe 2004). This orientation is coupled with a deep and abiding sense of individual accountability and responsibility for the welfare of patients. While desirable and admirable, this sense of responsibility remains rooted in the view that errors are de facto evidence of incompetence, if not moral failure (Brown 2005a). To identify a possible problem, ask clarifying questions, or seek more information may be perceived and treated as a challenge to another's competence, or evidence of one's own incompetence. Inter-professional and intra-professional shaming continues to dampen the willingness of physicians, nurses, and other personnel to ask questions or voice concerns with any but their most trusted colleagues (Coiera 2000; Fuedtner, Christakis and Christakis 1994; Hafferty and Franks 1994; Hicks et al. 2001; Manderino and Berkey 1997; Thomas 2003). The following quote from an intensive care nurse provides some insight into psychosocial barriers to collaborative cross-checking:

> It is difficult for any healthcare professional to speak up and question what other care providers are doing, or what they might not have done. If you really know the other person and trust them, then it becomes possible. But, it is especially hard to do this with a physician—to suggest that something might not be right—that they could have missed something. And it is *really* not okay to do this with any care provider in front of a patient or members of a family because you do not want to give the impression that you and others do not know what you are doing.

The development of an environment in which team processes such as cross-checking may thrive requires freedom from concern about being shamed or censured as a consequence of engaging in inquiry and advocacy (Argyris and Schon 1974; Bolman 1980; Edmondson 2003; Helmreich 2000). Moreover, personnel must trust that there will be no later reprisal for speaking up. Edmondson (1999 and 2002) used the term "psychological safety" to describe the extent to which people view their work environment as enabling them to engage in the interpersonal risk of pointing out their own mistakes, voicing a concern, or speaking up to intervene in another's erroneous action or inaction. In psychologically safe environments people believe that they will not be rebuked for identifying a problem, asking assistance, or seeking additional information.

Common Ground

Psychological safety is necessary for the development of "common ground": the shared beliefs, values, and assumptions among team members that serve interpredictability and support a climate in which team members may develop the norm of assisting each other in avoiding or mitigating missteps (Klein 2006; Klein et al. 2005a; Sexton 2004). Ultimately, the achievement and maintenance of common ground is pursued through dialogue. Inquiry and discourse enable the development of a team's tacit if not explicit compact to cross-monitor and cross-check (Edmondson 2003; Helmreich 2000; Klein et al. 2005a).

Developing a collaborative social context characterized by psychological safety and common ground requires time, space, and dialogue. In hospital-based care, opportunities for the development of psychological safety and the emergence of common ground have largely been eclipsed as an unintended consequence of organizational efforts to increase efficiency and productivity.

The Impact of Productivity and Efficiency Pressure on Collaboration

The United States healthcare system is under intense and escalating societal pressure to provide healthcare that is accessible, equitable, safe, reliable, and cost effective (Kohn, Corrigan and Donaldson 2000; Corrigan et al. 2001; Sandroni and Sandy 2003). This pressure comes at a time when the number of hospital beds has declined across the United States and patients admitted to hospitals are sicker than in the past, and remain in hospitals longer (Aiken et al. 2002; Locker et al. 2005). Coupled with personnel shortages in key patient care roles such as nursing, hospitals are increasingly operating near the limits of their capacity (JCAHO 2004). Moreover, declining reimbursements for patient care services have compelled cost-cutting and efficiency actions that have further narrowed human and material capacity, eroding the ability of hospitals to cope with situational increases in demand (Cook and Rasmussen 2005; Holtom and O'Neill 2004). The following quote from a nurse illustrates how a focus on financial/productivity goals may limit the ability of personnel to engage in collaborative processes, and conceal process problems and inefficiencies:

> An effort was made by one of our physicians, a hospitalist, to bring together members of all disciplines to round on patients at the same time. This was achieved just once, after substantial negotiation with managers of the various clinical departments involved. Physical therapy and occupational therapy professionals, for example, are accountable for their billable time. Rounding as a member of a team is not an activity for which they can bill. After immense effort the hospitalist succeeded and we had one day where we all rounded at the same time at each patient's bedside. He asked us to each share our thoughts on the patient's care needs from our professional perspective, aloud. Even though it was awkward and everybody was looking at each other askance, some interesting things came up that we didn't expect. When one of the nurses mentioned that the patient was to be taken for a radiological procedure later in the morning the social worker revealed that the patient already had that procedure the day before. The patient said he knew he was going to have a radiological procedure that day, but hadn't realized it would have been an unnecessary repeat. It turns out that we had some kind of problem with our computer system that sometimes led to patients being collected and transported for radiological procedures more than once. Usually, the error was recognized in radiology and the patient sent back—often after the patient insisted that they had already had the procedure. Two other people spoke up and said that this had happened with other patients before, but at the time they thought it was just a fluke and had never mentioned it. It made me and others wonder how many things like this go on that we never make visible because we don't get together as a team with all the disciplines to talk about the whole process of care. We only came together as a team that one time; the hospitalist couldn't make it routine given the many different department managers he had to win over. And he couldn't find a way to pay for the time of some of the disciplines so that they could be there. But it was a really rich experience—from that one time I learned things about what members of the other disciplines thought was important to note about patients that I had been unaware of. I suspect that there are lots of expensive inefficiencies that operate in our organization that

are invisible because our drive for efficiency and billable time prevents us from coming together as a team and identifying them.

The above quote illustrates not only endemic challenges to team-based practice in contemporary healthcare settings but, ironically, how efforts to increase efficiency often render inefficiencies invisible. Through interdisciplinary discourse regarding patients' needs and plans of care, clinical process problems and other patient care issues may be revealed—whether they have roots only in the clinical setting or across multiple functional areas of the hospital. Finally, this quote also suggests that learning about how one's role fits into the larger processes of patient care does not occur automatically. Lave and Wenger (1991) have described the importance of participation in collaborative decision-making processes as a vehicle for knowledge acquisition. In other industries, such as aviation, there has been substantial exploration of how to structure communication and interaction to limit error and promote learning (Bolman 1980; Helmreich 2000; Mudge 1998; Patankar and Taylor 1999).

Cultivating Collaborative Practice: A Tale of Doing and Undoing

There follows the story of a multidisciplinary group of care providers that utilized lessons from aviation and other industries to become a high performing interdisciplinary team.[1] Through collaboration they cultivated psychological safety, trust, and common ground. Collaborative cross-checking and other team processes emerged and prospered for over three years. During that time the quality and safety of patient care provided by the team, while already highly rated against national benchmarks, improved significantly and the team was recognized in the United States for its innovative approach to clinical teamwork (Uhlig et al. 2002).

The story of the team, eventually known as the Cardiac Surgery Care Team, reveals how they created time and space for collaboration and how collaborative cross-checking and other team processes may serve the improvement of patient care. Yet, despite their success, the team was ultimately disbanded in the face of powerful cultural push-back. Their experience underscores the difficulty of sizing up both medical staff and hospital readiness for change and the challenges faced by change agents in navigating the development of new organizational forms in healthcare. A high performing clinical team, it turns out, may upset not only traditional role hierarchy, but contemporary approaches to hospital administrative control.

In late 1999, health professionals caring for open heart surgery patients at a mid-sized community hospital began re-thinking care processes for their patients. The provision of care for open heart surgery patients is socially and technically complex. Surgeons, therapists, nurses, pharmacists, social workers, and other disciplines must coordinate their assessments and therapeutic actions with one another and with patients and families. The traditional approach to patient care, discussed earlier in this chapter, is characterized predominantly by independent interactions with the patient by members of each discipline who enter their notes and plans in the patient's

---

1 This story has been shared previously in a discussion of the ethical import of the team's decision-making process in Brown (2005b).

care record. For the past 100 years, the patient's medical record has been cast as the primary coordination medium for role-based task fulfillment in hospital care. Notwithstanding this expectation of the medical record, numerous issues compel care providers to coordinate directly with other health professionals. Because there is little or no designed-in opportunity in clinical work for interdisciplinary collaboration, this is accomplished through phone calls, paging, and interactions on the clinical floor and elsewhere. Care provided in this traditional manner is vulnerable to oversights and inappropriate or conflicting actions based on ambiguous information, stale or mistaken understandings of patients' situation, and/or uncertainty about the overall plan of care. Moreover, the "coordination cost" of this traditional approach to care is often high and stressful (Klein 2006); care providers must expend significant time and effort throughout any given shift to locate other health professionals in order to close informational gaps, correct flawed concepts, and otherwise ensure that patients' needs are understood and met. Knowledge of these inefficient conditions, coupled with a desire to restore opportunity for meaningful interrelationship with patients and families, led the Cardiac Surgery Care Team to engage in dialogue about change in practice.

The Beginnings

Members of each discipline providing care for open heart surgery patients met outside of work to learn about each other's roles and responsibilities. Through dialogue the existence of shared beliefs and values with respect to patient care became apparent and common ground began to develop. There was also opportunity to test assumptions and gain clarity about roles and responsibilities across disciplines. The group discovered that upwards of 80 per cent of the information each discipline collected from patients during their rounds process was the same; only around 20 per cent was discipline-specific. (Patient rounds are conducted to assess the patient's situation and needs, and to plan care.) The reason patients so often said "don't you people *ever* talk to each other" became very apparent. As redundancies became visible, it was also clear that the fragmentation of effort across disciplines was a leading source of the wear and tear associated with having to routinely track each other down to ensure that the plan of care, and coordination of care, was as it should be. In response to these and related insights, the group stated that they wanted to become a "true team". They would embark on this journey by convening all disciplines that worked interdependently in caring for open heart surgery patients at the same time on rounds. Patients and family members would be integral members, and the team would meet at their patients' bedsides.

While the inclusion of patients and family members as central team participants during rounds may seem a mundane expectation from a patient's viewpoint, it is not as common as one might expect. While there are many variations across care units, such as emergency departments, medical-surgery units, or intensive care, rounds will not necessarily:

- significantly involve the patient or their family member(s), if at all;
- be conducted at the bedside;

- involve more than one health professional or more than one discipline, for example, nurses may round alone and medical residents may round in groups.

When rounds do occur with more than one care provider at the bedside, communication will likely be directed to a senior clinician, rather than the patient, for example, a patient's nurse will report patient care information to a charge nurse or physician, or a resident physician will report to an attending physician (Dominguez et al. 2005). Reporting of information is hierarchical, from lesser rank and authority to higher rank and authority. Moreover, information will be couched in medical jargon, rendering discourse literally and figuratively over the head of the patient. These and other traditional approaches to rounding often leave families and patients with a high degree of uncertainty and anxiety about what will happen next, both during the hospitalization and following discharge from the hospital. It was common for the Cardiac Surgery Care Team, for example, to receive many post-discharge phone calls from patients and family members attempting to clarify the plan for recuperation. The Cardiac Surgery Care Team hoped to preclude this uncertainty and anxiety by including patients and families in daily care planning, beginning on the first day of post-surgical experience in the hospital. To facilitate meaningful involvement of the patient and family, each discipline would communicate their assessment and care recommendations to the patient in lay language, rather than to the surgeon in medical jargon. Team members agreed to monitor one another and to speak up to clarify meaning if any of them lapsed into jargon when addressing the patient and family. By having each discipline explicitly communicating their understanding of the patient's situation and needs, and engaging in dialogue as a team to revise and improve understanding, they would develop a plan of care that represented their best collective judgment. Cross-monitoring and cross-checking, to avoid missteps in care, would be enhanced by: (a) the collaborative development of a shared understanding of the patient's situation and the plan of care, and (b) knowledge of other team members' routine and non-routine roles and responsibilities in fulfilling the patient's plan of care. The team also agreed that any deviations from intended care would be identified during rounds for later review. The purpose of reviewing deviations from intended care was not to cast blame, but to understand the implications of a deviation for quality of care (positive or negative) and to investigate systemic origins and support process improvement. A separate meeting called "System Rounds" would be conducted outside of the clinical context each week for this purpose.

The decision to conduct rounds together posed scheduling challenges, because departments generally do not coordinate staff schedules with other departments. Instead, schedules are optimized to meet departmental needs rather than serve interdisciplinary or cross-functional processes. And, in some instances, team members had to negotiate their participation with their supervisors because collaborative rounding was not "billable time". They needed to justify participation in rounds as a non-revenue event, or participate on their own time if their schedule permitted.[2] And underlying all challenges to conducting collaborative rounds was the countercultural flavor of the entire idea. Especially from the point of view of physicians, the notion of collaborative decision making may be received as an affront to a deeply engrained belief in the responsibility of the physician to independently assess the patient and write patient care orders. Seen from this perspective, allowing other disciplines a significant say in care decisions could be viewed as abdicating control and professional responsibility for the patient. From the point of view of administrators, who might chance by the unit and see the team gathered around a patient, it could seem like people were wasting valuable time when they should be working.[3]

Getting Underway

Despite various obstacles, the Cardiac Surgery Care Team launched their collaborative rounding process in the fall of 1999. As previously noted, team membership was determined by identifying all roles that work interdependently to care for open heart surgery patients along the entire care path—into, through, and out of the hospital. Hence, in addition to the patient and family member(s), the full team could include the unit nurse, physician assistant, nurse practitioner, social worker, surgeon, spiritual care counselor, home care/visiting nurse coordinator, pharmacist, physical and occupational therapists, respiratory care therapist, dietitian, diabetic educator, office manager, cardiac rehabilitation specialist, and utilization review coordinator.

To guide their development as a team at the bedside, the group looked for an approach to team communication and decision making. Much has been learned in aviation about how to structure communication and interaction to limit error, develop common ground, and to provide feedback on systemic problems so that they may be corrected (Helmreich 2000; Mudge 1998; Patankar and Taylor 1999). These team-based decision-making and management methodologies differ from traditional team-based management training in that they are expressly designed to improve the safety of high-risk/high-consequence activities. Mudge (1998) and Patankar and Taylor (1999) described a communication protocol for flight crew decision making called the Concept Alignment Process (CAP). This crew decision-making methodology influenced the process of communication for the Cardiac Surgery Care Team. The description below is an adaptation of Patankar and Taylor's description of CAP that reflects its application by the Cardiac Surgery Care Team:

> The CAP is a simple "structured communication" protocol with a specific strategy, structure, and process. The strategy addresses risk management by focusing on team decision-making. In so doing, it is acknowledged that safety should be equated to risk

---

2 With the exception of the surgeon and a few others, team members had patient care responsibilities scheduled on other units and floors where collaborative practice was not in play.

3 In reality, although not occurring at the same time, each discipline engaged in traditional rounds would see the same patient independently for a similar period of time, then spend significant time chasing down information from other caregivers in an effort to test understandings, correct misunderstandings, and sort out the whole plan of care.

management and the responsibility for such risk management is shared by all the stake-holders, including patients and families. Thus, it provides patients, families, physicians, nurses, therapists, social workers and other disciplines with a standard decision-making process to effect better communication, workload management, situation awareness, cross-monitoring, cross-checking, etc. The "structure" is the requirement for briefings among all disciplines that work interdependently to care for patients. CAP provides a way of ensuring that all parties are acting on the same concept. If not, it provides a way of resolving ambiguous and/or conflicting viewpoints among the communicating parties.

The basis of the Concept Alignment Process is a simple communication protocol that desensitizes rank and provides means for all the individuals to share information. At the heart of this protocol is the concept. A concept is defined as an idea, remark, or an observation that is stated by one person and is either affirmed or challenged by co-workers. If a difference between the points of view is stated, it is the team's responsibility to seek validation for that concept from an independent third source. If one concept can be validated and one cannot, the validated concept shall become the working concept. If both can be validated, the choice of which becomes the working concept is up to the primary authority. If neither concept can be validated, the most conservative of the two is chosen. Once a working concept is agreed upon, it shall be further scrutinized using a predefined judgment process. Often in this process, the team members discover underlying causes of discrepancies in the concepts and recommend appropriate changes. Changes have been made in operating policies and procedures, care protocols and other documentation and practices as a direct result of this process.

The Cardiac Surgery Care Team named their approach to structured communication the "Collaborative Communication Cycle". The term "collaborative" as used by the team is consistent with the definition of collaboration shared at the beginning of this chapter. The following description of the structure and process of the Collaborative Communication Cycle and its application in patient care is taken from Brown (2005b):

> The Collaborative Communication Cycle is a team briefing and debriefing process that begins when team members assemble with family members around the patient's bed. This generally took the form of a circle, of which the patient is a part. Conceptually, the needs of the patient are at the center of this circle, to be defined and addressed by all team members, including the patient and the patient's family member(s). To desensitize rank and promote open communication, the surgeon participated in the process as a team member. Facilitation of the assessment and decision-making process was provided by the nurse practitioner or physician assistant, and, at times, other disciplines. Although the surgeon had final decision-making power, in most instances team process rather than individual choice was used to make a shared assessment and determine a plan of action.

> The goal of the communication process was to ensure that a complete, shared concept of the patient's situation and needs was obtained by harnessing the knowledge and information resources of all team members. From this shared concept, a care strategy would be developed which represented the team's best collective response to their shared concept of patient situation and needs. An integral element of the communication process was a debriefing that enabled identification of any variation between intended care and actual care received by the patient.

Deviations from intention were recorded during rounds, to enable subsequent analysis of human, technical or organizational factors—either to intervene in potentially unsafe conditions, or to evaluate and disseminate a serendipitous discovery of practice improvements. Given the cultural expectation in traditional health care of error-free performance, generally the word "error" is stress provoking. To emphasize that most errors are actually context and system events, team members, including patients and families, were asked to identify any "G.L.I.T.C.H.es" in care since the last briefing. G.L.I.T.C.H. is an acronym for Gathering Little Insights That Can Help. Building sufficient trust to share G.L.I.T.C.H.es was a fragile process that took time, and was attended by initial ups and downs in the willingness of providers to discuss such deviations openly.[4] The leadership of the surgeon was instrumental in building this trust. A willingness to disclose and discuss his glitches and to discuss the glitches of others in a non-punitive manner, focused on learning, set the climate and tone of the process and proved essential to the practice being normalized. This simple debriefing mechanism catalyzed a robust reporting process, eliciting important information daily with respect to the functioning of the clinical unit, and of deleterious or beneficial side effects of "upstream" organizational decision-making. Through this mechanism, the Cardiac Care Team became a learning sub-system, capable of driving organizational learning.

During the patient's first experience of collaborative care, post-surgery, the briefing leader advised the patient and her or his family that each team member would introduce himself or herself. They were also advised that they should interrupt anytime they need clarification, or additional information. The concept of a glitch was also introduced. Patients and family members quickly adapted to the process. During the first day following surgery they might have listened more than participate, but by the second day they were more involved, and by day three they were actively engaged and had questions or concerns to be addressed. Process components of the "collaborative communication cycle" included the following:

- The briefing leader recapitulated the previous day's plan of care.
- The briefing leader stated his/her concept of the patient's current status and asked the patient and his/her family how they are doing and if they have any concerns. Following their response and interaction, a re-statement of the patient's needs, wants, and situation as then understood was offered to the whole team.
- Beginning with the patient and family, each team member then contributed additional information or insight. Clarifying information was provided or requested from other team members as needed. From these insights, shared decisions were made about actions such as new medications, different therapies, etc. In this way, a care plan based on a shared concept of patient situation and needs was crafted collectively by all team members. Any unusual or special roles were explicitly stated and acknowledged. Further, contingency plans and tolerances were explicitly stated to assist team members in monitoring and noting if the patient's condition deviated from expectations, allowing early intervention to prevent or mitigate harm to the patient.
- Patients, family members, and providers were asked to identify any glitches associated with the execution of the previous day's plan. All glitches were recorded in the "Glitch

---

4 An example glitch (Uhlig et al. 2002): "A single, one-time dose of furosemide (Lasix; Aventis Pharmaceuticals, Bridgewater, NJ) was ordered following surgery. The order was misinterpreted and recorded as a daily dose. During the collaborative rounds process on the following day, this glitch was identified and corrected before an additional dose was administered."

Book." Some were addressed immediately, and the others addressed in a separate weekly team meeting known as "system rounds" designed for discussion of system issues.

- Throughout the communication process, a team member wrote down the emerging plan. When the team completed formulating the plan, this team member then read back the "plan of care"—the strategy that has been developed to address the needs of the patient over the next twenty-four hours (barring need for adaptation based on evolving experience). This provided a final opportunity to correct any misunderstandings, and elicit any latent insights that might yield an adjustment to the plan. Should there be revisions at this point a final summary would be made, incorporating these changes.

The entire process took about twelve minutes, longer when a patient was more acutely ill. Team members departed with a common concept of the patient's situation and care plan, including contingency plans and tolerances for their execution. Even though changes in patient situation might occur that are not addressed by specified contingencies, the practice of contingency planning was also intended to encourage vigilance for any change in patient status or situation as care providers went about their independent work following rounds.

An important feature of the collaborative rounds process was how it served the development of overlapping role and task knowledge among team members. Disciplines that might not previously have been capable of recognizing an error in medication processes, for example, now knew the normal utilization of medications for open heart surgery patients, and of specific adjustments for each patient. On one occasion during rounds the spiritual care coordinator articulated that a patient's slow recovery might be due to an oversight—a medication that was supposed to have been discontinued was still being administered. As a function of participating in interdisciplinary rounds she had developed sufficient knowledge of a medication side effect to cross-check the medication process, detecting a G.L.I.T.C.H. that hadn't been detected by the pharmacy or by members of other clinical disciplines. Through an open and explicit process of communicating, team members learned enough about each other's roles and tasks to more effectively cross-monitor and cross-check the entire process of patient care to which they each contributed. This is an essential capability for intervening early to avoid misstep and to improve the chance of noticing and mitigating harm from a misstep that has already occurred. Another apparent benefit, for novice care providers who accompanied senior mentors, was the ability to note the patient symptoms or information that were significant to the experts that they were shadowing. This may assist novices in advancing their judgment processes by making important facets of expert decision-making visible—to witness thought and proposed action uncoupled and discussed for pros and cons. Learning early about potential pitfalls in decision-making, based on the expert's process of judging and deciding, may help new practitioners avoid potentially harmful cognitive errors as they gain hands-on experience (Croskerry 2003a and 2003b; Lave and Wenger 1991).

Results

Fundamentally, the Cardiac Care Team altered the context of care, from one that revolved around the tasks and the independent actions of physicians and other clinicians, to one where the focus was on collaboration and the development of a collective understanding of patient needs and a strategy of care that harnessed the knowledge and skill resources of the entire interdisciplinary team. Following are some of the context-changing purposes and functions at the core of the Collaborative Communication Cycle:

- Achieve alignment among care providers, patients, and patients' families regarding the patient's situation and plan of care. All care providers, including family, and patients were included as team members in this alignment process, with a clear voice in decision-making. Rather than the traditional approach to "reporting", wherein a subset of professional disciplines will communicate with each other, literally and figuratively "over the head" of the patient, each discipline would address his/her thoughts and recommendations to the patient, using accessible language. Medical jargon would be translated into lay language; conversation was directed toward the patient instead of toward other practitioners.
- Establish a philosophical foundation for communicating and collaborating characterized by respect, relationship, inclusion and self-care. Rather than a narrow diagnostic and treatment discourse, focused on the patient's disease, the patient would be affirmed as a whole person and their progress in healing and adjusting to their altered health status would be noted and acknowledged.[5] The team recognized that while they may view open heart surgery as routine, for patients the experience is a frightening and difficult life adjustment. They would do their best to provide a healing and caring relationship that would help alleviate the anxiety of patients as they recovered from the stressful experience of open heart surgery and began to adapt to this significant interruption in their life routine.
- Create a psychologically safe communication environment. To serve the foregoing purposes, the team needed to establish an environment in which patients, patients' family members, and all clinical disciplines would feel free to voice information and share alternative perspectives—even if the information or perspective conflicted with the views of the traditional authority, i.e., surgeon. By developing an environment in which information flows freely, the intellectual resources of the entire team may be harnessed to achieve the best possible understanding of the patient's situation and the best possible care strategy. As trust in the interpersonal safety of the communication process grew so did a sense of joint accountability for the entire process of care to which each individual contributed.
- By establishing trust and common ground, team members also established an information-rich decision-making environment. This strengthened the team's chances of avoiding errors due to informational deficiencies that were rife in the traditional approach to rounds. Further, a sense of joint accountability for the entire process of care allowed team members to cross-monitor and cross-check—to speak up in order to identify and trap an error before it could cause harm to the patient. The team was also more likely to detect and mitigate an error that had already affected the patient before the consequences became critical.
- By deliberately and routinely harvesting information about deviation from intentions in the fulfillment of care processes (a.k.a., glitches or errors) the team became a source of continual intelligence on error-provoking conditions and hazards. They also identified practice improvements associated with such deviations. If coupled with a

---

5 In other words, while the patient's disease or diseases would continue to be treated in a manner consistent with the best medical technology and techniques available, the psychological focus of patient and provider interaction was on the patient's wellness and productive adaptation rather than a narrow discourse centered on the status of a diseased organ.

robust analysis and intervention process, the team had the potential to act as an engine for continual learning and improvement—at unit and organizational levels.

Patient Care Outcomes

- The cardiac surgery program at this hospital participated in a collaborative database called the Northern New England Cardiovascular Disease Study Group (NNE). This is a voluntary consortium that includes all open heart surgery programs in northern New England, USA. The NNE tracks the clinical outcomes of its members, using risk models and observed mortality for all open heart surgery patients in the region. Prior to implementation of collaborative rounding, operative mortality for the Cardiac Care Team's patients was consistent with that predicted by NNE data, one of the best benchmarks in the United States for open heart surgery. Following implementation of the collaborative rounds process, observed mortality of the Cardiac Care Team's patients began to decline significantly from expected rates, relative to the NNE (Uhlig et al. 2002). Within two years of beginning the collaborative rounding process, operative mortality for the Cardiac Care Team's patients was less than half of that expected based on NNE prediction.
- Patient satisfaction was tracked using a survey managed by Press Ganey Associates. Following implementation of the collaborative rounds process, the cardiac surgery program consistently achieved ratings that were in the 97th to 99th percentile, relative to national figures, across the USA. Patients and families expressed how important it was to have the team convene each day, and to listen and interact over questions and concerns. They were less anxious because they were not chasing after caregivers to find out what was happening with their loved ones. One family member stated (Uhlig et al. 2002):

"We were comforted as we watched this team gathered around my husband's bed, discussing his care together. We were empowered as we realized that our personal [patient] knowledge, our observations, and our questions were important to all those making the care decisions. We felt positive because we were involved and had no doubt that this medical team was informed, involved, and working together to provide my husband with the very best care possible."

- Staff also expressed increased satisfaction with the collaborative rounds process, relative to traditional rounds (Uhlig et al. 2002).
- In recognition of the safety and quality improvements brought about by the Collaborative Communication Cycle, the Joint Commission and the National Quality Forum awarded the team one of the first John M. Eisenberg Patient Safety Awards for System Innovation in 2002. This national recognition is given to a handful of individuals and organizations each year.

It should be noted that the foregoing improvements were achieved without additional human or materiel resources. The improvements were accomplished by altering patterns of practice, including communication and interaction. Of particular interest with respect to patient safety is the fact that operative mortality decreased significantly from expected through NNE following implementation of the Collaborative Communication Cycle in post-surgical care. This decline in operative mortality suggests that a significant number of deaths attributed to surgical processes may in fact be linked to problems in post-surgical care management. And, the team's outcomes suggest that many of these deaths might be prevented through the use of structured communication to guide interdisciplinary teaming.

Although the glitch harvesting process captured rich information for the improvement of system functionality, these data were not meaningfully incorporated in the organization's process improvement program. Changes and improvements were made if within the purview of team members, or if team members were successful in efforts to resolve problems with members of other units of the hospital. Fundamentally, the G.L.I.T.C.H. harvesting process was never properly assessed as a tool for identification, analysis and intervention in latent failure conditions.

Consistent with the description of the Concept Alignment Process (CAP), the Collaborative Communication Cycle: (a) desensitized rank; (b) evaluated all of the concepts being presented by team members in the analysis, mitigating the influence of personal bias on the decision process; (c) required the users to continuously evaluate their chosen path of action in the light of any new information that may have become available over time; and (d) required the users to actively attempt to identify the root causes that may have led to the presentation of multiple concepts or of invalid concepts so that systemic errors might be eliminated prior to further compromises to safety. In addition to establishing a shared concept of each patient's situation, structured communication methodologies may guide decision makers in blending rule-based and risk-based responses to patient care situations (Reason 1997). This assists providers in adapting formal and tacit clinical protocols based on unique patient needs. Further, under conditions of high uncertainty, structured communication guides knowledge-based problem solving, to help care providers arrive at the best possible risk-based assessment and response when no protocol/rule is known to apply.

Despite both measured and perceived benefits to patients and providers, and national recognition for the hospital, the Collaborative Practice Model developed by the Cardiac Surgery Care Team was ultimately suspended. The reasons are complex, and reflect how good people in clinical and administrative roles may clash when change challenges deeply held beliefs and assumptions.

Some Reflections on the Undoing of the Cardiac Surgery Care Team

The development of a high performing Cardiac Surgery Care Team was a frontline initiative led by health professionals who, by nationally accepted measures, were already providing excellent care when they began developing as a team. Despite already doing well, they wanted to do even better for their patients. They succeeded in large measure due to the passion for improvement embodied by all team members and the committed involvement of patients and their families in the decision processes of care. Also of critical importance was the willingness of a heart surgeon to learn to exercise his authority in a new way—one that enabled the expertise of other disciplines to be brought to bear proactively in developing a plan of care. While the surgeon retained final authority for the care of the patient, he visibly demonstrated that it was not only safe but expected that members of each discipline share their professional assessment of each patient's situation and care needs—even if they contradicted his view. He participated as a team member, rather than as the team facilitator, to demonstrate that he was committed to collaboration. Patients began to see each team member as a credible participant in their care whose word they could trust—because the surgeon clearly did.[6] The care plan represented a response to the pooled "best" understanding of the patient's needs by the team, which included patient and family perspectives.

Despite the benefits, the existence of a high performing team amidst organizational structures and processes designed to support autonomous task performance ultimately contributed to its demise. One issue arose as the team sought to report quality improvement opportunities for action within the hospital. Quality improvement initiatives in US hospitals are commonly conceived at "upper" management levels and implemented by middle level managers. Quality improvement coordinators deploy a plan, conduct education or training, and then measure for desired outcomes. The Cardiac Surgery Care Team presented an unusual situation—they had set the goal to become a high performing team and began self-educating, training, and developing this capability in-situ, without an organizational mandate. As their "Glitch" harvesting began to surface opportunities for process and other improvements, at both clinical and organizational levels, the team sought to collaborate with personnel managing the organization's variance reporting program. The issues and opportunities surfaced by the team did not fit neatly into the existing reporting scheme and the response by variance reporting personnel, understandably, was to attempt to educate the Cardiac Surgery Care Team on what was acceptable to report. The opportunity to develop new analysis strategies, to harness the rich source of intelligence on system improvement opportunities, was neither recognized nor tapped.

Reaction to the collaborative rounding model on the medical side of the hospital ranged from curiosity to ardent dislike. For some, the practice of team decision making ran against the grain of a deeply held theory of practice that is centered in professional autonomy. Ironically, physicians, nurses, and other clinical personnel visited from around the US (attracted by Press Ganey scores or other performance data) to observe the collaborative rounding process. Some subsequently implemented similar practice in their home organizations (Brown et al. 2006; Dominguez et al. 2005).

Ultimately, there was medical and administrative rejection of the practice of collaborative rounding. It was as if the team was a foreign protein being rejected by the body of the organization. A movement arose to stop the practice of collaborative rounding which, by late 2003, succeeded. The surgeon who had been instrumental to the success of the collaborative rounding model subsequently joined another organization to continue research and support for collaborative practice and the practice of collaborative rounding. Remaining surgeons did not subscribe to collaborative rounding in the care of their patients and the practice withered.

---

6 Team members expressed that, prior to collaborative rounding, patients had been more likely to question their veracity and insist on having validation of their word from the surgeon.

Summary

If an organization's processes and procedures are not adapted iteratively to support the implementation and development of collaborative practice, it will likely be perceived as a source of turbulence and disruption to those who remain engaged in the status quo. Without the committed support of senior medical and administrative leaders, who anticipate significant organizational change as an implication of cultivating team processes, it is difficult to sustain a meaningful frontline teamwork initiative in hospital settings. Moreover, a clinical team that develops the practice of routinely identifying quality and safety improvement opportunities may be perceived as upending traditional "top to bottom" approaches to quality and safety improvement in hospitals. This may be disquieting to managerial personnel at all levels of the organization.

Among other prospective concerns, flattening of frontline role hierarchy will invariably be a red flag to some members of medical staff, and even to members of other disciplines, such as nursing. All of the foregoing may be among the reasons why research findings on the effect and merit of collaborative cross-checking have been somewhat mixed in the healthcare literature (Patterson et al. 2007). Regardless, experiences such as that of the Cardiac Surgery Care Team speak to the potential for significantly improved care as a function of collaborative practice. The reframing of hospital organization and management to support team-based practice will require passion and persistence by health professionals in clinical and administrative roles. The following quote from the spouse of a cardiac surgery patient who suffered serious complication provides a compelling reason to rise to this challenge:

> Everyone knows that things can and do go wrong, and that mistakes can and do happen in every part of life. When patient and family know that a team is working together to prevent mistakes, and reacting quickly to adapt care to correct any glitches as quickly as possible, they also know that they are getting the best possible care humans can provide. Anger comes when families feel helpless to stem or correct unfortunate situations, and it escalates when they feel others do not care. When patient and family are part of a team who cares, problems become a time to "roll up one's sleeves" and help. And when the solution may protect someone else [other patients] it's a positive outcome amidst the angst.

References

Aiken, L.H., Clarke, S.P., Sloane, D.M., Sochalski, J. and Silber, J.H. (2002), 'Hospital Nurse Staffing and Patient Mortality, Nurse Burnout, and Job Dissatisfaction', *Journal of the American Medical Association* 288:16, 1987–93.

Argyris, C. and Schon, D.A. (1974), *Theory in Practice: Improving Professional Effectiveness* (San Francisco: Jossey-Bass).

Baker, D., Salas, E., King, H., Battles, J. and Barach, P. (2005), 'The Role of Teamwork in the Professional Education of Physicians: Current Status and Assessment Recommendations', *Joint Commission Journal on Quality and Safety* 31:4, 185–202.

Bolman, L.G. (1980), 'Aviation Accidents and the Theory of the Situation', in G.E. Cooper (ed.), *Resource Management on the Flight Deck* (National Aeronautics and Space Administration: Ames Research Center).

Brown, J.P. (2005a), 'Ethical Responsibilities of Educators, Regulators and Professional Organizations in Healthcare', in M. Patankar, J.P. Brown and M.D. Treadwell (eds), S*afety Ethics. Cases from Aviation, Healthcare, and Occupational and Environmental Health* (Aldershot, UK: Ashgate Publishing).

Brown, J.P. (2005b), 'Key Themes in Healthcare Safety Dilemmas', in M. Patankar, J.P. Brown and M.D. Treadwell (eds), S*afety Ethics. Cases from Aviation, Healthcare, and Occupational and Environmental Health* (Aldershot, UK: Ashgate Publishing).

Brown, J., Dominguez, C., Zipperer, L. and Stahl, G. (2006), 'Multidisciplinary Perspectives on Collaborative Rounds', *Proceedings of the Human Factors and Ergonomics Society 50th Annual Meeting* (Santa Monica, CA: HFES).

Carthey, J., de Leval, M.R. and Reason, J.T. (2001), 'Institutional Resilience in Healthcare Systems', *Quality in Health Care* 10:1, 29–32.

Coiera, E. (2000), 'When Conversation is Better than Computation', *Journal of the American Medical Informatics Association* 7:3, 277–86.

Cook, R. and Rasmussen, J. (2005), 'Going Solid: A Model of System Dynamics and Consequences for Patient Safety', *Quality and Safety in Healthcare* 14:2, 130–34.

Corrigan, J., Donaldson, M., Kohn, L., Maguire, S. and Pike, K. (eds) (2001), *Crossing the Quality Chasm: A New Health System for the 21st Century* (Washington, DC: National Academies Press).

Croskerry, P. (2003a), 'The Importance of Cognitive Errors in Diagnosis and Strategies to Minimize Them', *Academic Medicine* 78:8, 775–80.

Croskerry, P. (2003b), 'Cognitive Forcing Strategies in Clinical Decision-making', *Annals of Emergency Medicine* 41:1, 110–20.

Dominguez, C., Uhlig, P., Brown, J., Gurevich, O., Shumar, W., Stahl, G., Zemel, A. and Zipperer, L. (2005), 'Studying and Supporting Collaborative Care Processes', *Proceedings of the Human Factors and Ergonomics Society 49th Annual Meeting* (Santa Monica, CA: HFES).

Edmondson, A. (1999), 'Psychological Safety and Learning Behavior in Work Teams', *Administrative Science Quarterly* 44:2, 350–83.

Edmondson, A. (2002), 'The Local and Variegated Nature of Learning in Organizations: A Group Level Perspective', *Organization Science* 13:2, 128–46.

Edmondson, A. (2003), 'Managing the Risk of Learning: Psychological Safety in Work Teams', in M. West, D. Tjosvol and K. Smith (eds), *International Handbook of Organizational Teamwork and Cooperative Working* (New York: Wiley Publishing).

Fuedtner, C., Christakis, D.A. and Christakis, N.A. (1994), 'Do Clinical Clerks Suffer Ethical Erosion? Students' Perceptions of their Ethical Environment and Personal Development', *Academic Medicine* 69:8, 670–79.

Gittell, J., Fairfield, K., Bierbaum, B., Head, W., Jackson, R., Kelly, M., Laskin, R., Lipson, S., Siliski, J., Thornhill, T. and Zuckerman, J. (2000), 'Impact of Relational Coordination on Quality of Care, Postoperative Pain and Functioning, and Length of Stay: A Nine-Hospital Study of Surgical Patients', *Medical Care* 38:8, 807–19.

Greiner, A. and Knebel, E. (eds) (2003), *Health Professions Education: A Bridge to Quality* (Washington, DC: The National Academies Press).

Hafferty, F. and Franks, R. (1994), 'The Hidden Curriculum, Ethics Teaching, and the Structure of Medical Education', *Academic Medicine* 69:11, 861–71.

Helmreich, R. (2000), 'On Error Management: Lessons Learned from Aviation', *British Medical Journal* 320:7237, 781–5.

Helmreich, R. and Merritt, A. (1998), *Culture at Work in Aviation and Medicine: National, Organizational, and Professional Influences* (Aldershot, UK: Ashgate Publishing).

Heylighen G. (1992), 'Principles of Systems and Cybernetics: An Evolutionary Perspective', in R. Trappl (ed.), *Cybernetics and Systems Research '92: Proceeds of the Eleventh European Meeting on Cybernetics and Systems Research* (Singapore: World Scientific) 3–10.

Hicks, L., Lin, Y., Robertson, D., Robinson, D. and Woodrow, S. (2001), 'Understanding the Clinical Dilemmas that Shape Medical Students' Ethical Development: Questionnaire Survey and Focus Group Study', *British Medical Journal* 322:7288, 709–10.

Hollnagel, E., Woods D.D. and Leveson, N. (eds) (2006), *Resilience Engineering: Concepts and Precepts* (Aldershot, UK: Ashgate Publishing).

Holtom, B.C. and O'Neill, B.S. (2004), 'Job Embeddedness: A Theoretical Foundation for Developing a Comprehensive Nurse Retention Plan', *Journal of Nursing Administration* 34:5, 216–27.

JCAHO (2004), *Managing Patient Flow* (Oakbrook Terrace, Illinois: Joint Commission on Accreditation of Healthcare Organizations).

Kinnaman, M. and Bleich, M. (2004), 'Collaboration: Aligning Resources to Create and Sustain Partnerships', *Journal of Professional Nursing* 20:5, 310–22.

Klein, G. (2006), 'The Strengths and Limitations of Teams for Detecting Problems', *Cognition, Technology and Work* 8:4, 227–36.

Klein, G., Feltovich, P.J., Bradshaw, J.M. and Woods D.D. (2005a), 'Common Ground and Coordination in Joint Activity', in W.B. Rouse and K.R. Boff (eds), *Organizational Simulation* (New York: John Wiley and Sons Inc).

Klein, G., Pliske, R., Crandal, B. and Woods, D. (2005b), 'Problem Detection', *Cognition, Technology and Work* 7:1, 14–28.

Kohn, L., Corrigan, J. and Donaldson, M. (eds) (2000), *To Err is Human. Building a Safer Health System* (Washington, DC: National Academies Press).

Kosnik, L., Brown, J. and Maund, T. (2007), 'Learning from the Aviation Industry', *Nursing Management* 38:1, 25–30.

Lave, J. and Wenger, E. (1991), *Situated Learning: Legitimate Peripheral Participation* (New York: Cambridge University Press).

Lawrence, D. (2002), *From Chaos to Care: The Promise of Team-based Medicine* (Cambridge, MA: Perseus Publishing).

Leape, L., Cullen, D.J., Clapp, M.D., Burdick, E., Demonaco, H.J., Erickson, J.I. and Bates, D.W. (1999), 'Pharmacist Participation on Physician Rounds and Adverse

Drug Events in the Intensive Care Unit', *Journal of the American Medical Association* 282:3, 267–70.

Leonard, M., Graham, S. and Bonacum, D. (2004), 'The Human Factor: The Critical Importance of Effective Teamwork and Communication in Providing Safe Care', *Quality and Safety in Healthcare* 3:Suppl., i85–90.

Locker, T., Mason, S. Wardrop, J. and Walters, S. (2005), 'Targets and Moving Goal Posts: Changes in Waiting Times in a UK Emergency Department', *Journal of Emergency Medicine* 22:10, 710–14.

Ludmerer, K.M. (1999), *Time to Heal: American Medical Education from the Turn of the Century to Era of Managed Care* (New York: Oxford University Press).

Manderino, M. and Berkey, N. (1997), 'Verbal Abuse of Staff Nurses by Physicians', *Journal of Professional Nursing* 13:1, 48–55.

Merry, M. (2005), *Hospital-Medical Staff Culture Clash: Is it Inevitable or Preventable?* (Rensselaer, NY: Health Trustees of New York State).

Merry, M. and Brown, J. (2001), 'From a Culture of Safety to a Culture of Excellence: Quality Science, Human Factors, and the Future of Healthcare Quality', *Journal of Innovative Management* 7:2, 29–46.

Merry, M. and Crago, M. (2001), 'The Past, Present and Future of Health Care Quality', *Physician Executive* 27:5, 30–35.

Miller, A. and Xiao, Y. (2007), 'Multi-level Strategies to Achieve Resilience for an Organisation Operating at Capacity: A Case Study at a Trauma Centre', *Cognition, Technology and Work* 9:2, 51–66.

Mudge, G. (1998), 'Airline Safety: Can We Break the Old CRM Paradigm?', *Transportation Law Journal* 25:2, 231–43.

O'Connell, M. and Pascoe, J. (2004), 'Undergraduate Medical Education for the 21st Century: Leadership and Teamwork', *Family Medicine* 36:Suppl., S51–6.

Patankar, M. and Taylor, J. (1999), *Corporate Aviation on the Leading Edge: Systemic Implementation of Macro-Human Factors in Aviation Maintenance*, SAE Technical Paper 1999-01-1596.

Patterson, E., Render, M. and Ebright, P. (2002), 'Repeating Human Performance Themes in Five Health Care Adverse Events', *Proceedings of the Human Factors and Ergonomics Society 46th Annual Meeting* (Santa Monica, California: HFES).

Patterson, E.S., Woods, D.D., Cook, R.I. and Render, M.L. (2007), 'Collaborative Cross-Checking to Enhance Resilience', *Cognition, Technology and Work* 9:3, 155–62.

Rafferty, A., Ball, J. and Aiken, L. (2001), 'Are Teamwork and Professional Autonomy Compatible, and Do They Result in Improved Hospital Care?', *Quality in Health Care* 10:Suppl. II, ii32–7.

Rasmussen, J. (1982), 'Human Errors: A Taxonomy for Describing Human Malfunction in Industrial Installations', *Journal of Occupational Accidents* 4:2–4, 311–33.

Reason, J. (1997), *Three Levels of Performance in Managing the Risk of Organizational Accidents* (Brookfield, VT: Ashgate Publishing Company) 68.

Roberts, K. and Bea, R. (2001), 'When Systems Fail: From the Titanic to the Estonia', *Organizational Dynamics* 29:3 179–91.

Sandroni, S. and Sandy, L. (2003), 'Homeostasis without Reserve: the Risk of Health System Collapse', *New England Journal of Medicine* 348:14, 1410.

Sarter, N. and Alexander, H. (2000), 'Error Types and Related Error Detection Mechanisms in the Aviation Domain: An Analysis of Aviation Safety Reporting System Incident Reports', *International Journal of Aviation Psychology* 10:2, 189–206.

Sexton, J.B. (ed.) (2004), *The Better the Team, The Safer the World. Golden Rules of Group Interaction in High Risk Environments: Evidence Based Suggestions for Improving Performance* (Ladenburg, Germany: Gottlieb Daimler and Karl Benz Foundation, Rüschlikon, Switzerland: Swiss Re Centre for Global Dialogue).

Sharpe, V. and Faden, A. (1998), *Medical Harm: Historical, Conceptual, and Ethical Dimensions of Iatrogenic Illness* (Cambridge: Cambridge University Press).

Starr, P. (1982), *The Social Transformation of Medicine: The Rise of a Sovereign Profession and the Making of a Vast Industry* (New York: Basic Books).

Sutcliffe, K., Lewton, E. and Rosenthal, M. (2004), 'Communication Failures: An Insidious Contributor to Medical Mishaps', *Academic Medicine* 79:2, 186–94.

Thomas, S. (2003), 'Horizontal Hostility: Nurses Against Themselves: How to Resolve This Threat to Retention', *American Journal of Nursing* 103:10, 87–8, 90–91.

Tucker, A. and Edmondson, A. (2003), 'Why Hospitals Don't Learn from Failure: Organizational and Psychological Dynamics that Inhibit System Change', *California Management Review* 45:2, 55–72.

Uhlig, P., Brown, J., Nason, A., Camelio, A. and Kendall, E. (2002), 'System Innovation: Concord Hospital', *Journal on Quality Improvement* 28:12, 666–72.

Uhlig, P., Haan, C.K., Nason, A.K., Niemann, P.L., Camelio, A. and Brown, J. (2001), 'Improving Patient Care Through the Application of Theory and Practice from the Aviation Safety Community', *Proceedings of the 11th International Symposium on Aviation Psychology* (Columbus, Ohio: The Ohio State University).

Weick, K. (2001), *Making Sense of the Organization* (Malden, MA: Blackwell Publishing) Chapter 14, 333.

Weick, K., Sutcliffe, K. and Obstfeld, D. (1999), 'Organizing for High Reliability: Processes of Collective Mindfulness', in B.W. Staw and L.L. Cummings (eds), *Research in Organizational Behavior*, Volume 21 (Greenwich, CT: JAI Press) 81–123.

Woods, D.D. (2004), 'Conflicts Between Learning and Accountability in Patient Safety', *De Paul Law Review* 54, 485–502.

Woods, D.D. (2005), 'Creating Foresight: Lessons for Enhancing Resilience from Columbia', in W.H. Starbuck and M. Farjoun (eds), *Organization at the Limit: Lessons from the Columbia Disaster* (Malden, MA: Blackwell Publishing) 289–308.

Woods, D.D., O'Brien, J. and Hanes, L.F. (1987), 'Human Factors Challenges in Process Control: The Case of Nuclear Power Plants', in G. Salvendy (ed.), *Handbook of Human Factors and Ergonomics* (New York: Wiley).

Zeleny, M. (1986), 'The Law of Requisite Variety: Is it Applicable to Human Systems?', *Human Systems Management* 6:4, 269–71.

Chapter 11

Maintaining Common Ground: An Analysis of Cooperative Communication in the Operating Room

Leila Johannesen

Practitioners engaged in managing a dynamic process, such as operating room staff performing a surgery, must maintain a common situation assessment. An observational study of anesthesiologists and operating room staff, focused on the nature of their communications, provides some insights into how they do this. Information exchanges among team members in the operating room are typically brief, relying on different types of contexts. Team member communications throughout the operation help to facilitate relatively quick diagnoses that may be needed during critical situations. By applying an analytical perspective from cognitive psychology and, in particular, the concept of maintaining the common ground, we offer some insights into the nature of effective team situation assessment.

Introduction

Certain fields of practice involve the management and control of complex dynamic systems. These include flightdeck operations in commercial aviation, control of space systems, chemical or nuclear process control, and anesthetic management during surgery. These domains have demands of complexity and time pressure, as well as high consequences of failure. In these situations, fault diagnosis typically occurs while the monitored process is on-line and in conjunction with maintaining system integrity. Some other characteristics of these domains include: the need to form interpretations of the situation before all the data are available; the need to continuously update these interpretations as data comes in or is changed; and the need to act based on these interpretations in order to prevent possible dire consequences (Woods 1994).

Building a common situation assessment among team members is particularly important in these domains because of the time pressure and potential serious consequences. How do they support one another's situation assessment and how do they engage in fault diagnosis when there is a problem? In particular, what are their communications to each other like—what do they say and how do they say it? A useful framework for understanding the nature of communication is the notion of the "common ground"—the set of beliefs and presuppositions that each participant assumes are held by both, that is, what they take to be their mutual knowledge and mutual beliefs (Stalnaker 1978; Clark and Schaefer 1989). How common ground is built up, its role and functions was originally studied in the domain of conversation. But all coordinative activity requires moment to moment updating of the common ground (Clark and Brennan 1991).

Maintaining common ground about the state of problem solving and about the state of the monitored process requires knowing about the relevant activities of other team members, because their activities may impact the process. This is important in order to be able to manage the process effectively—because knowing what to do depends in part on knowing what has been done, what is expected and what is planned for. It is also clearly important for diagnosis (in order to know what may be the cause(s) of an anomaly). Furthermore, team members also need to be grounded about relevant assessments of others, because these can potentially affect expectations and plans.

This chapter describes research to understand how teams, who are engaged in managing some dynamic process, support one another's situation assessment and how they engage in fault diagnosis when there is a problem. This was done by conducting an observational study of anesthesiologists as they manage a patient's physiological process during an operation. An observational study allows one to study behavior in varied situations and under the actual constraints faced by practitioners.

The practitioners were recruited by a practitioner-researcher who asked them if they would agree to being videotaped during an operation for a study he was conducting on physician–automation interaction and expertise in anesthesiology. They were not told that this was a study of communication or explanation until after the study.

I begin by providing some general background on what anesthesiologists do pertaining to the goals of the research.

General Goals and Activities of Anesthesiologists

The anesthesiologist's main goals during an operation are to maintain the health and safety of the patient and to create appropriate surgical conditions. From the anesthesiologist's point of view, the operation is divided into the following basic phases: pre-induction, induction, maintenance, emergence, and recovery. Pre-induction involves preparation of the patient for anesthesia, which includes establishing intravenous access, placement of the patient on the operating table, placement of the monitoring sensors for the electrocardiogram, blood pressure, pulse oximetry, and so on. During induction, the patient is put to sleep, intubated and artificially ventilated. The beginning of a case, before the surgeon makes an incision, is a busy period for the anesthesiologists; they must undertake several activities such as attaching the equipment that monitors the patient's vital signs, placing catheters in the patient (for delivery of drugs and fluids and for monitoring critical parameters), getting drugs ready, administering drugs to the patient, and intubating the patient.

In some settings, especially teaching hospitals, more than one practitioner is involved in many of these tasks. During the maintenance phase of the operation, drugs and fluids are administered to keep the patient anesthetized for the duration of the operation and to maintain normal physiological functions (for example, intravenous fluid to replace blood loss). During the emergence phase, when the surgical procedure is finished, the administration of drugs is discontinued and the patient is awakened and extubated.

The major functions and signs that anesthesiologists must monitor are: depth of anesthesia, circulatory function, blood loss, respiratory function, respiratory and anesthetic gases, renal function, neuromuscular function, body temperature, and other system functions depending on the type of surgery or the health of the patient (for example, blood sugar, electrolytes, hemoglobin). Clinical means (for example, inspection, palpation, auscultation) as well as several instruments are used to provide indications of these functions and signs. Several devices and monitors are used to measure vital signs. Data from many of these measurements are available on an integrated computerized display (which we refer to in the text as the vital signs monitor). While some of these data are continuously available (for example, the heart rate), others are available at intervals (cuff blood pressure), and still others require some explicit activity by the practitioner (for example, cardiac output). Also, not all data is immediately available. For example, an arterial blood gas sample requires analysis in a remote lab and ten minutes may elapse between drawing the sample and receiving the results.

Management actions, such as administering drugs, blood, or fluids, are taken on the process depending on its state and past history. Many drugs, each with specific actions, side effects and contraindications, are available to the anesthesiologist. Some types of drug that are typically used during the maintenance phase of the operations observed are: inhalation anesthetics (for maintaining unconsciousness), narcotic analgesics, muscle relaxants, hypotensive agents, vasopressors, and vasodilators. For more on the cognitive activities of anesthesiologists, see Cook, Woods and McDonald (1991) and Xiao (1994).

Practitioner Roles and Relationships

The operations I observed were done at a large teaching hospital and involved at least two anesthesiologists: an attending anesthesiologist (or simply "attending") and one or two residents. The attending is a senior member of the anesthesiology staff, who holds a faculty position. In all cases, the attendings observed here were board-certified. The attending is responsible for overseeing several operations concurrently. He or she is always present during the induction phase of the operation, and typically returns periodically throughout the case. The attending adapts his schedule of visits depending on expectations about how the case will go and on assessments of the resident's competence to handle the case alone; for a relatively routine case, he may only be present during induction.

The resident, an anesthesiologist gaining practical experience for four years after medical school, is present throughout the case, and in general manages the case. He is typically a senior resident (in his third or fourth year of residency). The operations with two residents had a senior resident and a junior resident (usually in his second year).

The attending is the more experienced, generally more knowledgeable, team member. He or she oversees the process and the resident, setting the general strategy and specifying certain actions and or decision choices. The resident defers to the attending in these decisions. Both attending and resident monitor and take actions on the process, but the resident is present during the whole operation, while the attending is present only some of the time (since he supervises other cases as well). When he returns to the operation, he needs to update his situation assessment (for example, determine what events have occurred, how certain vital signs are proceeding); the resident will typically assist him in this process.

In the operations involving a senior and a junior resident, the relationship between them was similar to that of an attending and resident, in the sense that the senior resident directs strategy while the junior resident typically defers to the senior resident's decisions.

Present in this domain are general issues of coordination and communication among team members managing some process and having different areas and levels of expertise. The attending and resident(s) must communicate and coordinate with one another, as well as with other personnel, such as surgeons and nurses who have different tasks, and who have the same high-level goal of preserving the integrity of the physiological process, although their lower level goals may be quite different.

The Observational Study

Research Questions

The main guiding questions for this study were: How do team members support each others' situation assessment? How do they communicate about interpretations and assessments? How do they provide explanations for their assessments? How do team members keep informed about the relevant actions of others? How do they engage in diagnostic behavior?

Data and Analysis

I observed and transcribed ten neurosurgery operations from videotapes. The neurosurgeries involved one of the following: clipping of a cerebral aneurysm, removal of a brain tumor, or a laminectomy.

The data sources relied on in the analysis were: (1) verbal communications made by the anesthesiologists and those directed to them by others, or those that may have been overheard by them; (2) actions taken by the anesthesiologists, such as: looking at the monitor, any interactions with the machines, any adjustments to drugs or objects, any samples taken (and how taken), or drugs given; (3) actions taken by other personnel when interacting with the anesthesiologists; (4) behavior of the dynamic process as indicated by the patient record kept during the operation, and as displayed by the various monitors and machines, and a record of vital signs.

Three cameras were placed in the operating room so as to capture these data sources. One camera was focused on the various anesthesia machines and displays. Another focused on the area at the head of the operating table and in front of the machines, where the anesthesiologists spend most of their time. Finally, another camera focused on the patient, which captured close-up actions taken on the patient.

Transcription

The guiding questions drive the episodes selected for analysis, as well as the transcription process to some extent. The videotapes were transcribed in two passes. The first pass consisted of transcribing all verbalizations made by the anesthesiologists and verbalizations made by other team members to the anesthesiologists. The only verbalizations omitted were those that were obviously social chatting. Also recorded were various activities undertaken by the anesthesiologists, including interactions with the machines, or other equipment, or administration of drugs or other fluids.

The next stage involved reviewing the transcript to identify particular episodes of interest, which are described in the next section. Then I went through the transcripts of the episodes of interest and described them in a general or domain-independent way. I used the general problem-solving concepts, or concepts from the common ground framework, for this generalized interaction description.

Episodes of Interest

In general I focused on situations in which team members talked about their activities, interpretations, and assessments of the process. I was particularly interested in the following kinds of episodes.

Management and Diagnosis   These are situations in which team members are engaged in managing the process and/or diagnosing faults in the process. Monitoring and management occur continually. Of particular interest are episodes in which two or more team members are engaged in managing the process and/or in anomaly detection. The beginning and end points for an episode are not well defined a priori. But, generally speaking, this kind of episode will begin with a focus of attention on some anomaly, and end when an interpretation is arrived at and/or management action is taken, and the topic is dropped, resolved or otherwise attains some closure.

Updates   Update episodes are situations in which a team member (typically the attending) returns to the operation and is informed ("updated") about the state of the process. Particularly interesting are those updates that occur after some critical event (one of which is described in the "Findings" section.)

Assumptions and Limitations

The interactions among practitioners were studied as exemplars of good performance. However, this does not mean that performance is flawless or optimal. But on the whole, I think we can assume that the patterns we see reveal effective team interaction.

Not all of the operations yielded episodes that are discussed in the findings. Some cases were routine and relatively uneventful. Unlike simulator studies where the researcher can design the scenarios to address the questions of interest, field studies provide serendipitous opportunities. The virtue of this is that they offer unique conditions and situations that researchers might not have thought of ahead of time, or could not possibly devise in a simulator study.

The video recording did not capture everything that may have been relevant. In this study, for example, some exchanges among team members may have occurred off-camera, or out of line of sight. Also, not all utterances were captured on tape; some were inaudible, or incomprehensible.

Representations of the Findings

Understanding the information exchanges among team members and how these exchanges support dynamic fault management relies both on understanding the domain particulars (for example, to know why mentioning blood pressure now is informative) and on understanding the context for the episode (that is, what relevant events occurred prior to the episode). Just as an utterance may take on any of several meanings depending on its context, the meaning or significance of many episodes cannot be understood without knowing their context (for example, what occurred previously in the case, what parameters have been of concern, what practitioner expectations are).

The "Findings" section contains transcripts (corresponding to an episode of interest). To assist in the analysis, a domain-independent description is provided alongside the transcript. Episodes that involve diagnosis also contain a third column, indicating phase of problem solving. Some episodes are short and do not contain additional columns beyond the transcript. The conceptual level description of each episode, that is, why the episode is significant for the purposes of the study, is contained within the text.

The utterances in the presented transcripts are not time-stamped (though this data is available from the videotapes) because the dialogues in the episodes typically do not have long pauses between utterances. Where relatively longer pauses are found, these are noted.

An identifying code is used before each episode. The code indicates the case in which the episode occurs and the transcript time, as follows: [case|hour: minutes: seconds].

Below are the codes used in the transcripts.

Key to Transcription Symbols

- Ellipsis indicates missing, inaudible or incomprehensible text
- Ellipsis in parenthesis indicates approximate number of incomprehensible words represented by the dots
- Italics indicates actions

- Words in parenthesis express some uncertainty about the actual words
- R = resident (used in cases where there is only one resident)
- RS = senior resident
- RJ = junior resident
- A = attending
- M = medical student
- S = surgeon
- SA = assistant surgeon
- N = nurse
- P = patient
- v.s. monitor = vital signs monitor, an integrated monitoring system that displays all the patient's vital signs

Findings and Discussion

Anesthesiologists continually monitor and manage the patient's physiological process and diagnose unexpected anomalies. In order to perform the high level goals of management and diagnosis effectively, practitioners in this domain must form expectations about the future, plan courses of action, keep track of what has occurred, and evaluate past management actions and interventions. We observed team members keeping one another "in the loop" to facilitate management and diagnosis of the ongoing process in several ways. They do this by (1) informing others about relevant actions, (2) explaining in the flow of events, and (3) drawing attention to anomalies and parameters of concern.

Unprompted Communications about Actions

We observed several instances of team members telling one another about relevant actions they intend to take, are taking or have taken. Many of these statements are unprompted—that is, they are not responses to questions. These statements can serve several functions.

One function is *informative*—they serve to inform others of a new influence on the process. For example, the attending may administer a stimulant and tell the resident what he has just done. This lets the resident know how to interpret an increased heart rate. It helps him maintain an accurate model of the potential influences on the process, which is necessary for ongoing management as well as for possible future troubleshooting.

A second function served is *validative/corrective*. Telling other team members what one intends to do provides the opportunity for another team member to validate the action or point out evidence suggesting a different course of action. In the first example below, a statement of action is acknowledged and the action is validated:

RJ: I'm gonna turn the nitrous back on now *{RJ is reaching up to the knob.}*
RS: Yeah.
{The junior resident then turns it on.}

In the next example, the statement of suggested action proposed by the senior resident is not validated. Instead the response to the proposed action is that it has already been done. Besides "correcting" the proposed action, the response serves to repair a gap in the senior resident's knowledge of the influences acting on the process.

> *{The senior resident walks in and looks at the vital signs monitor}*
> RS: Why don't we try a little ephedrine on her [Patient]. *{RJ is looking at vital signs monitor}*
> RJ: Yeah, he [attending] just gave some ephedrine.
> RS: Did he? Okay.

Still another function served by some statements about actions or intended actions is *coordinative*. That is, they serve to tell others about an action that can potentially affect the behavior or actions of these other team members. In the following example, the resident cautions nearby team members not to touch a sterile kit he is opening up:

> *{Resident brings a movable stand near the patient and sets a sterile kit on it. Another practitioner stands a couple of feet from the tray and is working on the patient's leg.}*
> R: Okay, I'm gonna be opening up a kit here so just watch your elbows.

Information Through Noticing

Clearly not every action taken or about to be taken that impacts the monitored process needs to be verbally stated. Much information about the state of the process and management can be picked up by being able to overhear and see what other team members are doing. Assessments and plans may also be picked up or inferred in this way. It is not necessary for team members to always direct attention and explicitly provide this information to one another. Some actions taken by team members will be evident from the context and do not need to be mentioned. For example, if the team members have agreed upon a division of labor of some task (for example, intubating the patient), one team member may not need to mention all the subactions that he or she is taking, because everything is proceeding normally. Another example is that anesthesiologists can tell what drugs other team members have given by looking at the anesthesia record, or by seeing what ampoules are empty on the drug cart. All of this information is ultimately valuable in allowing team members to update their situation assessment and expectations of the monitored process.

Some work environments foster "open" interactions, that is, interactions that are observable and understandable by others (Hutchins 1990; Segal 1994). The particular interactions afforded by the task environment and tools affect the nature of grounding. In the domain of ATC operations, Hughes, Randall and Shapiro (1992) point out that the tools used (for example, flight strips) allow for open interactions—they allow all the relevant participants to easily see the state of the system and to see what actions others take on the system. On the other hand, some characteristics of work environments may inhibit the ability to ground. For example, Woods et al.

(1994) point out that multifunction controls and displays used in the cockpit tend to suppress cues about the activities and intent of the other human crew member. This disrupts their ability to maintain a common situation assessment, which can degrade communication and coordination across the crew. In the healthcare domain, insertion of computer technology in the form of electronic patient records might have a similar effect in suppressing cues to activities and intent of other team members.

Team members notice what others are doing, and on relatively rare occasions may observe behavior that they do not understand, that does not fit with their expectations, or that suggests that the other team member could use assistance. They have a sense of how activity should be occurring and are able to pick up on discrepancies in the expected activity—when things seem "unusual." It is generally in such instances that a team member questions another about his activity, as in the example below. Open interactions allow possibilities for individuals to detect actions that may be inappropriate in context and to initiate recovery before outcome failures occur.

[4|0:39:25]
{RS sprays numbing medication into P's mouth, turns to get gloves, turns back, RJ is lifting P's left arm slightly, touching pressure cuff line}
RS: What are you looking for?
RJ: Just to see if that was *{points towards monitor}* correlating with that.[1]
RS: *{looks towards monitor, putting on gloves}* They were correlating yeah, very well. *{looks back to P}* She's just a little anxious with me doing this.

Another source of information for updating the common ground is the "self-talk" of others. Team members occasionally talk aloud when engaged in a task or when trying to figure something out. This may serve a dual purpose. First of all, it may help the practitioner who is talking to "keep track" of things, for example, of required actions or possible alternatives. Second, it is also a mechanism that allows other team members to notice someone's activities, plans or reasoning, and to provide assistance, if necessary. That this is accomplished generally without distracting or demanding attention is important. A common, brief form of self-talk which is found in the transcripts is saying "okay" or "alright" (or sometimes sighing) upon completion of a task or subtask. This can, in some circumstances, assist in coordinating behavior by letting someone else know that a particular stage is finished (see Heath and Luff 1992 for examples in the transportation domain).

Information about the state of the process and of problem solving can also be picked up from the tools that are publicly available to the team members, such as the various displays and the anesthesia record. In order to maintain a common frame of reference, these public tools need to afford information access in a way that is consistent with all team member expectations. Consider a shared artifact like the anesthesia record. It is used by several people, both for recording actions and values

---

1 The blood pressure measurement as indicted by the arterial catheter and that measured by the sphygmomanometer (pressure cuff). A check on the arterial line blood pressure measurement is done initially by seeing if it correlates with the blood pressure cuff measurement. (The arterial line may fail or stop reading because of a blood clot at the tip of the catheter or some technical problem.)

(for example, what drug was given when and how much, or what the blood pressure has been for five-minute intervals throughout the case) as well as for retrieving that information. A representation that is used and modified by team members in different ways can create divergences in the common ground. We observed a situation in which a team member noticed a difference in how another team member was annotating the record and commented on this:

[10|7:56:40]
RS: *{looking at record}* oh, you just drew another gas
RJ: yeah, I just sent
RS: I usually end up putting the next gas, when you go to a new page over here so you can look down
RJ: oh so you can follow it
RS: it's not a big issue, that's what I usually do. No big deal.

Notice how the senior resident justifies how he does it ("so you can look down") and the junior resident restates this justification at a meta-level ("oh so you can follow it").

Explaining In the Flow of Events

Sometimes a statement of an action or an assessment may include an "explanatory tag"—that is, a short justification or rationale. These explanations typically come immediately after the statement of action or assessment, are not in response to any query, and are brief. In the following exchange, the attending tags his assessment with a justification (which in this case is observed evidence).

{A has been talking to the resident about non-case related domain knowledge, and then without pause says:}
A: .... He probably needs some fluid I would think, his urine looks pretty dark.
RS: Yeah, let's give him some of this.

In the next example, the attending takes an action, and as he takes it, states what he is doing and why.

A: I think...should be air and O2 only *{adjusts knob}* he's not liking nitrous very much.

The general tendency to provide unprompted explanations is useful for adding to the mutual knowledge and thereby forestalling future misunderstandings. They also serve another purpose: they can minimize the need for long explanations in the future.

Drawing Attention to Anomalies and Joint Problem Solving

Team members draw one another's attention to and talk about anomalies—parameters that are abnormal for the particular situation. Drawing attention to an anomaly is often the initiating point for a joint problem-solving interaction. The example shown in Figure 11.1 begins with one of the residents calling attention to an anomaly. The interaction then quickly turns to figuring out whether the parameter's value is accurate and taking the appropriate management action.

[10|4:22:38] Dialogue	Generalized Interaction
{RJ looks at vital signs monitor}	
RJ: [R's name]	
RS: Yes?	
RJ: His pressure's now reading 177 *{R2 hits blood pressure button to start cuff measurement}*	Draws attention to anomalous value
RS: They must've just stimulated something.	Suggests explanation
{RJ adjusts anesthetic agent, gets syringe}	Gets ready to take action to counter anomaly (no verbal comment)
RS: Don't give him anything yet, see what the cuff pressure is.[i] It's a lot better waveform than we were having, so I think it's probably true, they stimulated something *{both looking at v.s. monitor}*	Proposes waiting to see results of another parameter value, with explanation
RJ: yeah, his heart rate picked up 5 points *{indicates to monitor}*	Points out corroborating evidence
RS: yeah, you'll see that when they're doing cervical, especially anterior, posterior not so much but the anterior, you'll definitely see, you gotta be looking for vagal stimulation, you got the vagus... you got the carotid (body), you gotta be watching for all those things it's just a real touchy surgery...this is not abnormal at all.	
[...]	
RS: Give him another 50 mics of fentanyl.[ii] I think it's a true pressure	Directs corrective action
{RJ administers the drug}	Takes corrective action

Figure 11.1 Anomalies and joint problem solving

Notes:
[i] Blood pressure is measured by two sensors: from an arm cuff and from the arterial line. The arterial line displays blood pressure continuously as a waveform. The cuff pressure, by contrast, is a discrete value measured intermittently. When an arterial line is present, cuff pressures are measured typically every 15 to 30 minutes.
[ii] A narcotic which blunts the response to stimulation.

In the next example, shown in Figure 11.2, one team member points out the anomaly which leads the other team member to review the management strategy he has taken so far, and mention an idea for another management action. The attending thinks it is a good one and they proceed with it. Note: prior to the dialogue shown here, the patient had lost a lot of blood. The patient's temperature became a parameter of concern early on, as did his urine output.

[1|3:3:40] Dialogue	Generalized Interaction
{Attending and Resident are looking at vital signs monitor}	
A: temperature...	Draws attention to anomalous value
R: I've been turning the room temp up, there's not much more we can do unless we get, they don't have any of those um, one time, they demonstrated a Bear Hugger™ that could be used interop?	
A: yeah,..bring the Bear Hugger™, you know	Recommends corrective action
R: {gets on phone} could we have one interop Bear Hugger™...	Takes corrective action

Figure 11.2 Reviewing a parameter of concern

Joint Assessment of the State of Management

Team members will jointly assess the state of management, that is, they will talk about the effects of interventions, about modifications to the management plan, or make predictions about the results of tests. They also comment upon parameters that are generally important (such as blood pressure) or become important in the particular operation, even though they are not anomalous. We could call these "parameters of concern." For example, hematocrit may be especially important to monitor because the patient has lost a lot of blood. In this way, team members keep one another calibrated in the moment-to-moment interpretation and management of the case.

The following example illustrates this joint assessment of the state of management. Notice how both are involved in assessing the state of management and implicitly agree about the course of action:

[1|3:23:40] Dialogue	Generalized Interaction
R: I'm gonna go ahead and send another gas.[i]	Statement of intended action
A: yeah, let's send another gas and	Confirmation
R: see where we're at. Have a feeling it's[ii] still gonna be low, he's just oozing all over the place[iii]	Prediction with explanation tag
A: I think once we bring the temperature up, we have done all we can do, you know, he's still putting out urine,[iv] I think I see more there.	Evaluation of management plan Drawing attention to parameter of concern
R: Yeah, there is a little more there. I'm gonna empty that in a couple of minutes.	Validation of observation Statement of intended action

Figure 11.3 Joint assessment

Notes:

[i] Blood gas. Sending a blood gas means sending a sample of blood for analysis of: pH, partial pressure of oxygen, partial pressure of carbon dioxide, hematocrit, base excess, sodium, potassium, calcium and glucose.

[ii] Hematocrit.

[iii] A reference to the patient's bleeding.

[iv] Low urine level has been a concern so far in this case.

The following episode shows how the team members keep one another involved in the evaluation of the effects of interventions. When the senior resident returns from his break, the junior resident informs him of new data. The senior resident relates these results to previous interventions in an evaluative statement.

[2|2:15:00] Dialogue	Generalized Interaction
{Senior resident has just returned to the operating room after a short break} RJ: I did another output and it was five four, something like that	Statement of action taken and result
RS: So she likes the dobutamine	Interpretation of result
RJ: Her SVR came down (8 point 2)	Statement of relevant parameter, reference and value
RS: So she likes—that's—we could come back down on the nitro, come down about a half if you want	Suggests management action
{RJ turns it down on infusion device}	Takes management action

Figure 11.4 Joint evaluation of the effects of interventions

Relative Referencing

When updating a team member about an anomaly or a parameter of concern, one notable characteristic is that these are often discussed in a *relative* way, that is, with reference to what the parameter value was earlier. This is useful because it provides an opportunity to validate that team members have mutual knowledge about the situation. Consider the last example in the previous section. The resident stated the value for SVR in both precise ("8 point 2") and relative terms (it "came down."). This patient's SVR had previously been high. Another example is found in this exchange:

A: What was the calcium? *{looks at record on table}*
R: It was down a bit, 1.84
A: I'd give him 500... *{R gets up}*

Queries and Informative Responses

Another characteristic of updating communications, and of communications in general, is that questions are not simply answered with a minimal response, but with relevant elaborations (that is, extra information). Consider the following example:

{Attending returns to room after a break}
A: Something I can help ya with?
RS: Nothing, he's doing okay.
A: Did you get an output recently?
RS: *{turning v.s. knob}* Yeah, 7,9 let's see
A: Really?
RS: yeah, that was a combination of 3 outputs so it's pretty accurate. His index is 3,4. It's still low but I'm just
A: I would just...

Rather than simply answering yes to the question and providing the output value, the resident also provides accuracy information ("it was a combination of 3 outputs so it's pretty accurate") and also provides information about another parameter value (that is, cardiac index) that is related to the cardiac output.

Team members will use the management or process context to provide informative responses. Even though a particular parameter value may be the same in two contexts, we observe that response provided to a question will vary depending on the context. Below is an example of how the response elaboration to the question "what's the blood pressure now?" differs even though the process value is the same. A bit of background is necessary for this example, which is taken from a cerebral aneurysm clipping surgery. Before the clipping, deliberately induced hypotension is generally used in order to minimize the chances for rupture, facilitate placement of the clip and also to reduce blood loss if bleeding occurs. The anesthesiologist, because he is the team member who administers the drugs, must coordinate with the surgeon concerning the start, duration, and degree of hypotension. Right before the clipping, this exchange occurs:

S: What's the blood pressure?
R: Still at 100, I'm giving Nipride right now.

This exchange occurs shortly after the clipping:

S: What's the blood pressure?
R: 100 over 50, back up to normal.

In the first asking instance, the anesthesiologist states the blood pressure value plus a "tag" that informs the surgeon that the value should soon drop to the expected value. After the clipping, when the pressure is to be brought up again, almost the same blood pressure value is stated, along with a tag that, this time, specifies how the value is related to the normal value. This example illustrates that team members provide a more "complete picture" for the information seeker than that which would be provided by simply answering their explicit question. In answering queries about process data, providing an informative response means providing information about factors that will or might affect the value within a certain horizon of the future.

The sophistication in the responses that team members can provide has implications for the nature of the questions that team members need to ask. It means that information seekers do not always need to formulate their questions precisely to get good answers. Team members can respond to open-ended questions. For example, an attending might ask some variant of "What's up?" upon returning to the operating room. An observation statement such as "temperature 35.2, eh?" in a particular context, besides being a comment on the temperature being low, can be interpreted by the resident to mean something like "tell me what you know about this parameter being low." Indeed, even when team members ask specific queries, responders often do not simply answer the explicit question posed to them. They go beyond the question to provide what they deem an informative response. People are sensitive to the intentions and goals that requesters have when asking for information, and they answer accordingly (for example, Pollack, Hirschberg and Webber 1982). Team members readily grasp the context, intuit the intent, and respond to the intention of ill-formed questions. Contrast this to computer systems that generally do not understand the context or the intent, and require precisely formed questions. The lack of this ability makes information seeking from computer systems burdensome, especially in dynamic fault management situations.

Updating the Common Ground when a Team Member Returns

We have already seen some examples of episodes that begin when one team member returns to the flow of events after a break. The attending is the main team member that is typically "in and out" of a particular operation. If things seem to be going normally, the attending may leave and then, when he or she returns to the flow of events, will typically receive an "update" from the resident. In the next example, we look in detail at the nature of one of these update episodes in which a significant event occurs during the attending's absence.

Overview of Episode The episode occurs during the maintenance phase of an operation to clip a cerebral aneurysm. The episode occurs about an hour after induction and before the surgeons have exposed the aneurysm. Initially, the senior resident is the only anesthesiologist present; the attending has been away for about half an hour and the junior resident is on a break. In this episode the senior resident detects an anomaly—bradycardia (very low heart rate). He takes corrective action by administering atropine, a drug that raises the heart rate. The junior resident returns from the break. The senior resident has the attending paged. He mentions the event to the surgeons and enquires whether they "might have been doing anything." They answer no. The attending arrives after a few minutes and together they arrive at a diagnosis.

To a practitioner, the bradycardia event is quite dramatic. The pulse rate as indicated by the beeping of the pulse oximeter suddenly slows down. When this occurs in the operation, the resident, who has bent down (apparently to check the urine output or to begin a cardiac output measurement), immediately gets up to look at the monitor. Five seconds later he injects the atropine. See Figure 11.5.

Bradycardia may be expected in certain situations. For example, certain drugs given during maintenance can result in a lower than normal heart rate. Also, a low heart rate indication could be expected in the case of a known artifact with monitoring equipment. However, in this case, bradycardia of such severity is unexpected. Because of its severity, it is critical to treat it immediately, before its consequences begin to propagate. It is also important to understand its etiology because it could be a premonitory event, that is, indicative of a fault that needs to be managed or corrected to prevent the condition from recurring or to prevent other possible disturbances. After investigating the surgeons' actions as a source of the event, the resident pages the attending to help him uncover the cause and also to make the attending aware of a potential premonitory event.

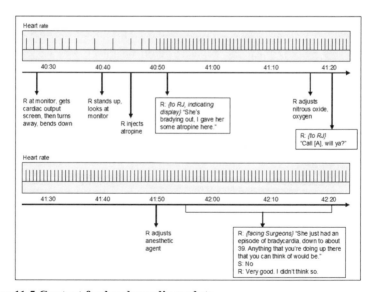

Figure 11.5 Context for bradycardia update

Updating and Joint Problem Solving   Figure 11.6 shows what occurs when the attending arrives. Notice, first of all, that the resident answers the attending's open-ended query with a detailed recounting that is rather like a story, preserving the order of events. Such a recounting would seem to benefit causal analysis. He begins by mentioning a related process event (less severe bradycardia) that occurred before the severe event. He provides information about the dynamics of the antecedent event, of the event itself, and of another relevant parameter (blood pressure).[2] He mentions what action he was taking on the process while the event occurred, the limiting values reached and the corrective action he took and the process response to it. Finally he informs the attending about the state of problem solving, that is, that he has no explanation. He has rejected one hypothesis (that is, "nothing [the surgeons] were doing"), though he does not elaborate. At the end of the initial update, the attending queries him on this point. The resident's response is the same, unelaborated.

At this point, the state of problem solving seems to reach an impasse (that is, when the attending says that he "can't necessarily explain that.") However, the resident continues the problem solving by telling the attending about various management influences on the process (that is, drugs being given). He then tells the attending about the hypotheses he has considered but discarded, and his reasons for doing so.

The attending then lists causes for this kind of event, based on his experience. In reaction to this, the resident seems to re-evaluate the data that fed into his conclusion that it could not have been due to the surgeons. He "revisits" what was occurring during the important time-frame (as pointed out by the attending). By going over in detail what was occurring then, he comes to the conclusion that the surgeons were indeed engaged in an activity that could have given rise to the event.

In this example, the diagnosis process is collaborative. The resident has access to the relevant data by having been present during the event, while the attending has access to more etiological knowledge. Both are essential for the appropriate diagnosis in this case. Notice too that the interaction has a useful property: that of being "robust"—in the sense that an initially discarded hypothesis is reintroduced and taken as the best explanation for the event.

---

2 Severe hypertension may cause bradycardia by a reflex pathway, but the absence of high blood pressure rules out this mechanism.

Transcript	Domain Independent Description	Problem- Solving Phase
A: *{enters room}* Nice and tachycardic [1]	Comment on process	
R: Yeah, well better than nice and bradycardic…		
A: What's going on guys?	Open-ended request for update	
R: *{takes end of printout, seems to show to A}*. She had an episode of just kinda, all of the sudden, bradying down to 50, 52 then came right back up, nothing they were doing, then all of the sudden out of the blue, I was shooting an output and she dropped down to 32, 38 somewhere around there, pressure dropped down to 60 so I gave her .5 of atropine and ah, kicked her up to 6.5; she liked that, but no explanation. This is at 50 millimeters per second, twice the speed.	Mentions: - previous related event, including dynamics and approx. values - discounts hypothesis of other agent's activities as cause - action taken while event occurred - dynamics and approx. values of relevant parameter during event - corrective action taken and process response - has no good candidate explanation Supplements description with artifact preserving data history	Initial update of significant event
A: They weren't in the head doing anything?	Requests information concerning other agents' activities at time of event	Hypothesis building
R: Nothing.	Discounts hypothesis without elaboration	
A: Okay. Well I can't necessarily		
R: The only thing		
A: I can't necessarily explain that	States he has no explanation	
R: Yeah, neither can I. The only thing we're doing right now is just trying to open her up and fill her up *{points to IV tree}*. She's up to a mic per kilo of nitro and then she's still at the 5, started out at 3 and a half of dobutamine and it did absolutely nothing, so I'm up to 5	Provides more information on current and previous actions	Context building
A: Okay		
R: So I don't know if she doesn't like contractility or I can't think of anything else we're doing. The line went in perfectly normal, I can't imagine that she has a pneumo or anything that would be causing tension, her peak area pressures have not changed. Just all of the sudden—boom—out of the blue—her potassium is 3 point 3 and we're getting ready to replace that and we have been hyperventilating but I don't know if low potassium can affect heart rate.	Offers hypothesis but discounts based on his knowledge Offers another hypothesis but discounts based on data Dynamics of event repeated Process variables mentioned, action to be taken mentioned Offers a third hypothesis but voices lack of knowledge	Hypothesis discounting

A: yeah, I don't know, I can't give you cause and effect on that. In my experience it's usually been stimulation of the trachea, it's something traction on the dura	Mentions two causes of significant event based on past experience	Case-based discussion
R: yeah (absolutely)		
A: you know things		
R: yeah, it may have been dura	Remarks that one of these causes may have been cause in this case	
A: ...sort of a reflex, pressure on an eye	Provides another possible cause based on past cases	
R: *{animated}* Actually it was when they were sawing the dura open	Remarks that event occurred during a time when one of the causes mentioned by A could have occurred	Discounted hypothesis reconsidered
A: well that's		
R: putting tension on it		
A: you touch the dura you'll get that	States mechanism	
R: okay		
A: 'cause the dura is ennervated by the fifth I believe, and it somehow makes its way back to the (.) ganglion, same thing that causes oculocardiac reflex	Describes mechanism whereby hypothesized cause leads to the significant event	
R: I'd be willing to bet you're absolutely right	Expresses confidence for hypothesis	Hypothesis acceptance
A: is the same mechanism whereby you get (bradycardial traction) on the dura, so my guess is that's exactly what it was	Continues explanation of mechanism	
R: Okay	Concurs with hypothesis	
A: you know and for future reference, if you suspect this lady's probably not going to mind this experience because she, we don't think she's really significantly sick, we're being a little overly cautious with her, my preference is, if you have a patient that you think has a bad heart and you think they have a vagal problem via traction or an eye...		

Figure 11.6 Updating episode: bradycardia

Notes:
[i] Tachycardia refers to rapid heart rate, while bradycardia refers to a slow heart rate.

Summary

Team members assist one another in maintaining an up-to-date interpretation of the process in several ways. For example, they draw attention to anomalies, events, and parameters of concern and they speak about them relative to expectations. Team members also provide informative responses, that is, with elaborations tailored to the information needs in the current context. Communication among human team members, like conversation in general, reflects a sensitivity to what is informative and relevant to others (Grice 1975). Team members also provide unprompted communication of relevant activities (that is, their influences on the process) and assessments. They talk about strategies and evaluate the effects of past interventions. This articulation of strategies and expectations among team members has been noted in a simulator study of aircraft crews and has been interpreted in a similar way; Orasanu (1990) suggests that these communications help to provide a context in which information takes on meaning, that is, build a shared mental model for the situation.

When the common ground is built up among team members, it will be unusual for team members to ask "why" questions like: "why do you think that?" or "why did you do that?" These questions, which express a need for explanations, indicate a rift in the common ground. Breakdowns in cooperative interaction between pilots and cockpit automation are marked by just these questions (Sarter and Woods 1995). The findings of the study are consistent with those of other studies, particularly work on cockpit resource management, that indicates the importance of continual verbal interaction in keeping team members attentive and informed (Foushee and Manos 1981; Hutchins 1990; Norman 1989).

In general, team members invest heavily in communicating about the state of the monitored process and problem solving. There are several good reasons for them to make this investment in the common ground. One reason is that diagnosis entails disentangling the various potential influences acting on the process, some of which may be due to the interventions of other team members. Hence, it is important for team members to keep one another aware of their interventions on the process.

At another level, an important reason to invest in the common ground is to help keep other team members in a state of readiness so they are able to assist in the management and diagnosis of faults in the process. The same level of effort to keep someone updated is not warranted if they are not true team members. This is reflected in an episode in which an update to a medical student was cut short in order to deal with what was perceived to be a more pressing task.

Another important function of maintaining a common ground is that it allows for more efficient communication during higher tempo periods; less needs to be said because information can be communicated relative to what is already mutually known. This is consistent with Orasanu's (1990) cockpit crew simulator study findings concerning the temporal-sensitive nature of communication; she found that captains in high-performing crews talked less than captains in low-performing crews *when workload was high*; also, the captains of high-performing crews requested slightly less information during abnormal phases of flight, whereas captains of poor-performing crews requested more information during these phases.

Establishing common ground can make the need for retrospective explanations of assessments or actions less necessary. This is useful because such explanations would be resource-consuming at high-tempo, high-criticality times, when concentration needs to be devoted to understanding the process behavior, rather than in mending a problem in a team member's understanding. We observed an episode in which the attending puts off an explanation of his decision until a more opportune time. In this purpose, maintaining common ground is similar to anesthesiologists' preparatory or anticipatory behaviors (Cook, Woods and McDonald 1991; Xiao 1994), that is, a task undertaken at the moment, so that things will be easier later on, when they can be expected to be more busy.

Team Member Capabilities for Supporting Dynamic Management

Based on this study and other research findings discussed, we can summarize some key team member communication capabilities that are needed for effectively supporting dynamic fault management. Team members need to be able to:

- *Provide unprompted communications about actions and assessments.* Communication about relevant assessments and actions serves to build up their common ground, serves to coordinate subsequent team activity and allows for error recovery if needed. Also, this includes explaining or justifying actions where needed, in the flow of events (typically with the use of explanatory tags).
- *Draw attention to anomalies and parameters of concern where appropriate.* This serves to keep other team members in the loop and engages them in joint problem solving.
- *Reference values in a relative way when appropriate.* Rather than simply stating a value, a relative indication may be stated if it would be informative to the context and goals of the team members.
- *Answer questions by going beyond minimal responses.* Team members provide responses that are sensitive to the situation and goals of information seekers. They go beyond a minimal response by providing context-sensitive response elaborations. They can deal with imprecise questions and still provide informative answers.
- *Limit the need for others to search for information.* By providing unprompted information about activities or assessments, directing attention to anomalies and relevant events, context-sensitive elaborations to queries, team members are, in effect, helping one another find the right information at the right time. This is a key ability because cognitive demands increase with the tempo and criticality of operations (Woods 1994). Contrast this to some computer systems with user interfaces that provide a mass of data and force serial access to highly related data (Cook, Woods and Howie 1992).
- *Communicate in various shared contexts.* A salient characteristic of team member communications is their "compactness." By compactness I mean that a phrase, word or gesture is packed with meaning—meaning that would generally not be extractable by a lay person, without extra information or

explanation.[3] Mutual knowledge of various kinds allows for this compactness. This mutual knowledge or mutual potential knowledge can be viewed as different kinds of shared context within which communication occurs. The team members use these different contexts to know what is relevant to say when. These shared contexts of various kinds are simultaneously available.

- One shared context is the *shared domain knowledge*. The team members share domain knowledge about the subject matter and practice of anesthesiology, which allows them to understand for example, what a phrase like "taking a gas" means. It allows one to understand why the attending might say "Let's give him some dobutamine" and how to take this action, or what "Why don't you put the A-line in" means, why it would need to be done, and how to do it.

- Another context is *shared local knowledge*, that is, shared knowledge about how the team, or particular team members, tend to do things that can be done in more than one way. Often there is no one right way to do something, and the department or team may have particular ways of doing them, for example, the default induction drug to use. Also, team members may have different "styles." For example, the data showed attendings varied in their approach to drug dosage or fluid replacement therapy; these variations are stable and are recognized by other team members.

- Another context is the *shared temporal context*. This refers to knowledge about the history of the process, including what interventions were taken, what the evolution of the state of the process has been and of problem solving.

- A fourth context is the *physical context* which consists of both the *task environment* and the *set of available monitored process representations*. Communicating within the context of the same physical environment means that grounding is less costly because the constraints of copresence, visibility, audibility, and cotemporality are present. These constraints allow team members to ground without explicit informing; information is available about what other team members do through peripheral access—being able to see what others do, even though one is not explicitly monitoring for it. The other aspect of the physical context concerns the monitored process views. The transcripts showed that team members often talk about interpretations of the process while looking at displays and pointing. Pointing (deitic reference) makes for compact communication—

---

3 Interestingly, reference can be so compact that it involves neither words nor direct pointing. In one episode observed, a medical student elicits an explanation of the resident by "waving" towards the vital signs display. The resident turns to look at the monitor and states "cause the cuff is up. That's the pulse oximeter." Of all that is on the vital signs display, the resident picks out the flattened pulse oximeter waveform as the reference. From the resident's point of view, the flat waveform is expected because the blood pressure cuff was on the same arm as the pulse oximeter monitor; whenever the cuff inflates it squeezes off blood flow, which leads to a spurious pulse reading. However, it is the atypical item—that which would be anomalous in another context. The reference is understood partly because of the critical role of anomalies in dynamic fault management.

pointing to some item on the display can substitute for a description or an explanation in some situations. A useful representation on a display can provide a wealth of information (for example, trend information), that is conveyed to the viewer by a simple pointing gesture.

- *Communicate without distracting.* The communications of team members are not a break in the flow of activity; in the usual case, it is not necessary for team members to drop what they are currently doing in order to gain information from another team member. Building up the common ground in the flow of events and using the various shared contexts allows for concise communication, and prevents the need for explanations that might distract from the situation.

- *Update a supervisor effectively.* A subordinate team member has to be able to recognize that the situation is in danger of escalating beyond his or her competence, that is, knowing when to call the supervisor. Secondly, the subordinate must be able to provide some kind of reconstruction of the event that emphasizes relevant events, actions, and relationships in order to provide the supervisor with a coherent recounting of the events that led to the present state.

Acknowledgements

I thank David D. Woods and Richard I. Cook for their contributions to the research on which this chapter is based. The research was sponsored by NASA JSC under Grant NAG9-390, whose support I also gratefully acknowledge.

References

Clark, H.H. and Brennan, S.E. (1991), 'Grounding in Communication', in L. Resnick, J. Levine and S. Teasley (eds), *Socially Shared Cognition* (Washington, DC: American Psychological Association).

Clark, H.H. and Schaefer, E.F. (1989), 'Contributing to Discourse', *Cognitive Science* 13:2, 259–94.

Cook, R.I., Woods, D.D. and Howie, M.B. (1992), 'Unintentional Delivery of Vasoactive Drugs with an Electromechanical Infusion Device', *Journal of Cardiothoracic and Vascular Anesthesia* 6:2, 238–44.

Cook, R.I., Woods, D.D. and McDonald, J.S. (1991), 'Human Performance in Anesthesia: A Corpus of Cases', *Cognitive Systems Engineering Lab Technical Report 91-TR-03* (Columbus, OH: The Ohio State University).

Foushee, H.C. and Manos, K.L. (1981), 'Information Transfer within the Cockpit: Problems in Intracockpit Communications', in C.E. Billings and E.S. Cheaney (eds), *Information Transfer Problems in the Aviation System*, NASA Technical Paper 1875 (Moffett Field, CA: NASA Ames Research Center).

Grice, H.P. (1975), 'Logic and Conversation', in P. Cole and J. Morgan (eds), *Syntax and Semantics*, 3 (New York: Academic Press).

Heath, C. and Luff, P. (1992), 'Collaboration and Control: Crisis Management and Multimedia Technology in London Underground Line Control Rooms', *Computer Supported Cooperative Work (CSCW): The Journal of Collaborative Computing* 1:1, 69–94.

Hilton, D. (1990), 'Conversational Processes and Causal Explanation', *Psychological Bulletin* 107:1, 65–81.

Hughes, J., Randall, D. and Shapiro, D. (1992), 'Faltering from Ethnography to Design', *Computer Supported Cooperative Work. Proceedings of the 1992 ACM Conference on Computer-supported Cooperative Work* (New York: ACM Press) 115–22.

Hutchins, E. (1990), 'The Technology of Team Navigation', in J. Galegher, R. Kraut and C. Egido (eds), *Intellectual Teamwork: Social and Technical Bases of Cooperative Work* (Hillsdale, NJ: Erlbaum).

Krauss, R.M. and Fussell, S. (1991), 'Constructing Shared Communicative Environments', in L. Resnick, J. Levine and S. Teasley (eds), *Socially Shared Cognition* (Washington, DC: American Psychological Association).

Mastaglio, T. and Reeves, B. (1990), 'Explanations in Cooperative Problem Solving Systems', *Proceedings of the Twelfth Annual Conference of the Cognitive Science Society* (Mahwah, NJ: Lawrence Erlbaum Associates).

Norman, D. (1989), 'The Problem with Automation: Inappropriate Feedback and Interaction, Not "Over-automation"', presentation at Discussion Meeting on *Human Factors in High-Risk Situations*, The Royal Society, Great Britain, June 28–29.

Orasanu, J.M. (1990), 'Shared Mental Models and Crew Decision Making', *Princeton University Technical Report CSL 46* (October).

Pollack, M., Hirschberg, J. and Webber, B. (1982), 'User Participation in the Reasoning Processes of Expert Systems', *Proc. AAI '82*, 358–61.

Sarter, N. and Woods, D.D. (1995), '"How in the World Did We Get into That Mode?" Mode Error and Awareness in Supervisory Control', *Human Factors* 37:1, 5–19.

Segal, L. (1994), 'Actions Speak Louder than Words: How Pilots use Nonverbal Information for Crew Communications', *Proceedings of the Human Factors and Ergonomics Society 38th Annual Meeting* (Santa Monica, CA: HFES).

Stalnaker, R.C. (1978), 'Assertion', in P. Cole (ed.), *Syntax and Semantics: Pragmatics*, 9 (New York: Academic Press).

Woods, D.D. (1993), 'Process Tracing Methods for the Study of Cognition Outside of the Experimental Laboratory', in G.A. Klein, J. Orasanu and R. Calderwood (eds), *Decision Making in Action: Models and Methods* (New Jersey: Ablex).

Woods, D.D. (1994), 'Cognitive Demands and Activities in Dynamic Fault Management: Abductive Reasoning and Disturbance Management', in N. Stanton (ed.), *Human Factors in Alarm Design* (London: Taylor and Francis) 62–93.

Woods, D.D., Johannesen, L., Cook, R.I. and Sarter, N. (1994), *Behind Human Error: Cognitive Systems, Computers and Hindsight. CSERIAC SOAR Report 94-01* (Wright-Patterson Air Force Base, Ohio: Crew Systems Ergonomics Information Analysis Center).

Xiao, Y. (1994), 'Interacting with Complex Work Environments: A Field Study and a Planning Model', unpublished dissertation (Department of Industrial Engineering, University of Toronto).

PART 4
Future Trends

Communication as a Sign of Adaptation in Socio-technical Systems: The Case of Robotic Surgery

Anne-Sophie Nyssen and Adélaïde Blavier

Introduction

As investigations of medical accidents have revealed, communication is one of the factors that is most frequently associated with accidents. For instance, in anesthesia 25 per cent of deaths are due to inadequate communication, which represents 39 per cent of reported medical errors (Arbous et al. 2001; Kluger et al. 2000). But, surprisingly, communication has not received much attention from researchers. Better training, better techniques, and better standards of equipment have been recommended in order to improve the patient's safety, but not much effort has been spent on communication training and tools, even though healthcare practitioners designate "improving communication" as an important corrective strategy (Kluger et al. 2000).

During the past decade or so, there have been two important developments in medical care relevant to the study of communication in hospital:

- The increased specialization of medical sciences, which has increased the division and distribution of tasks among experts from different disciplines and, thus, the need for coordination and communication between healthcare providers. Today, a patient will very seldom visit only one hospital department, and furthermore rarely sees only one physician during their stay. Multiple departments and professional skills are brought together in order to provide health services, but also to provide uninterrupted care around the clock. This specialization requires more and more information to be exchanged between departments as well as between individual operators who work cooperatively in hospitals in order to coordinate interventions both in time and space. Hospitals themselves have even become specialized, so that a patient may have to go to several hospitals and institutions to be properly taken care of (Nyssen 2007). This obviously raises the communication challenge at the inter-organization level.
- The development and introduction of new computer-based technology in hospitals, that requires practitioners to communicate with computers, introduces new forms of media and more distance between the operators and

their tasks, as well as between task performers themselves. During the past decade, the healthcare system has seen the introduction of more and more sophisticated technological devices and automated systems. Our fascination for the benefits of such technology has often obscured the fact that technology creates new demands for communication, it changes the way information is exchanged, introduces new media layers into the system, adds complexity, and creates new demands for cooperation. This perverse effect of technology was depicted by Bainbridge (1987) for automated systems as the irony of automation. It is largely due to the fact that the design is still completely cut off from the environment of use as we, and other researchers such as Woods, have shown in various complex systems (Nyssen 2004; Cook and Woods 1996; Woods and Hollnagel 2006).

The aviation industry has attempted to reduce the problems of cooperation between humans and automation by *organizing* both human–machine and human–human communication, using a straightforward and predefined division and distribution of tasks (for example, pilot flying and pilot non-flying), a codification and standardization of the communication language, a principle of systematic verbalization of main intentions, perceptions and actions (call-outs), a principle of systematic cross-checking of actions and understandings, and mandatory training of so-called "non technical skills" (Crew Resource Management). But some problems of communication obviously remain, as we can see with the case of the Sharm-el-Seikh accident (Egypt, January 4, 2004), in which the crew failed to share a proper understanding of the autopilot status. The Flash Airlines flight 604 was an early morning one (take-off at 02:42 am). Unlike required by the standard procedure, no take-off briefing was conducted by the captain. A take-off briefing allows the crew to review and share data about the distinctive details of the intended flight in order to properly anticipate expected events. In this case, there were several such details. For instance, the aircraft, a B737-300, had a few (minor) equipment failures which had not been repaired (in accordance with the Minimum Equipment List tolerance). One of these known anomalies was that the flight director (FD) was not working in take-off/go-around mode, so no FD guidance would be available to the crew just after take-off. Because no briefing had been made, the crew was surprised and a bit confused after lift-off and the captain requested the autopilot engagement in a condition in which by design it could not engage, which further increased his perplexity about the aircraft behavior. The captain then focused his attention on this issue, failed to properly monitor the flight path, and experienced spatial disorientation, progressively banking the aircraft to an inverted flight position. Continued ambiguous communication and cultural shyness prevented the co-pilot from recognizing that the captain was being incapacitated and from taking control early enough to recover. The aircraft dived and crashed into the Red Sea at the speed of 416 KTS, killing all 148 on board.

These difficulties faced in addressing cooperation needs might be grounded in the dominant tendency to use an analytical approach to solve a complex, non-linear problem. The analytical approach attempts to explain a system through division and simplification. For example, an operation is dismantled into a series of tasks to be performed, cooperation is described as a series of mutual constraints (for example, synchronization, input, output) between these tasks, and communication boils down to the information exchange between task performers which is needed to satisfy the constraints. The science of complex systems, however, addresses problems differently. What characterizes a system as complex is not the mere number of its component parts but the heterogeneity of the component parts and their relations among them, leading to a potentially unanticipated and autonomous outcome, namely an emergence. Particularly, the ability of a complex system to adapt itself to its environment and to maintain this adaptation to some extent against internal changes (for example, new equipment, new people), as well as external changes (environmental), can be seen as an emergent property. In this approach, communication flows are seen as a manifestation of the adaptation work (Piaget 1967; Le Moigne 1999; Maturana and Varela 1980 and 1987; constructivism). In most circumstances, the act of communication represents our best attempt to adapt to a specific situation.

The view taken in our research is that analyzing communication will reveal the adaptation strategies and the limits of the adaptation of the "system," taken here as the interaction between the surgeon, the assistant, and the robot. In this sense, our work is in accordance with new approaches to the safety of social-complex systems that have recently been explored under the name of resilience that looks for adaptation capacity instead of breakdowns and accident models. We shall discuss this new approach in the light of the constructivism perspective, in particular, the increasing focus on the emergent adaptive capacity of socio-technical systems through continual interaction with their environment.

This new approach requires analyzing situations where the capacity of adaptation of the system is engaged to face changes in order to capture markers of adaptation in real time. In this chapter, we examine how the introduction of the robotic system in the operating room creates new patterns of communication between surgeons and how the analysis of the communication reveals surgeons' adaptation strategies in addition to the limits of their adaptation to the technology. As a result, we will be able to better assist developers to design ongoing adaptation and, thus, to design communication tools.

Robotic/Laparoscopy Surgery and Communication Environment

Robotic surgery and laparoscopic procedures provide a good system to support a study on communication, adaptation, and new technology. There have been a number of technological advances in surgery, and laparoscopy is certainly one of them. There is little doubt that laparoscopy represents a definite progress in patients' treatment. However, there are a number of important drawbacks. For instance, the fact that long instruments are used through an opening (trocar) in the abdominal wall limits the surgeon's degrees of freedom to four: in and out, rotation around the axis, up and down and from medial to lateral. Robotic surgery has been designed to improve the process of laparoscopy or minimal invasive surgery (MIS). The system allows for: (1) the restoration of the degrees of freedom that were lost, thanks to an intra-abdominal articulation of the surgical tools; (2) three-dimensional visualization of the operative field in the same direction as the working direction; (3) modulation of motion amplitude by stabilizing or by downscaling; and (4) remote control surgery. Because of these improvements, surgical tasks can be performed with greater accuracy (Hubens et al. 2003; Marescaux et al. 2002; Cadière et al. 2000; Pasticier et al. 2001; Carpentier et al. 1999).

Laparoscopy procedures typically involve the simultaneous use of three or more instruments (for example, laparoscope, probe or gripper, and shears or other cutting tools). Because of this, at least one tool must be operated by an assistant. The assistant's task is often limited to static functions of holding the instrument and managing the camera.

In classical laparoscopy, the assistant and the surgeon are face to face, and they use the same 2D representation of the surgical field to tailor the task. In robotic surgery, the surgeon is seated in front of the console at a distant point, looking at an enlarged three-dimensional binocular display on the surgical field while manipulating handles that transmit the electronic signals to the computer that transfer the exact same motions to the robotic arms. Robotic surgery can be performed at distant locations. However, within the actual technological system, the surgeon is still in the same operating room as the patient. The computer-generated electrical impulses are transmitted by a 10-meter long cable that controls the three articulated "robot" arms. Disposable laparoscopic articulated instruments are attached to the distal part of two of these arms. The third arm carries an endoscope with dual optical channels, one for each of the surgeon's eyes, which allows a true binocular depth perception (stereoscopy). The assistant is next to the patient, holding one or two instruments and looking at a 2-D display of the surgical field.

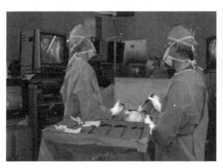 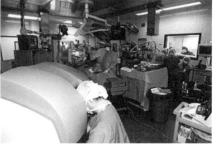

Figure 12.1 Configuration of the operating theater in classical laparoscopy (left) and with the robotic system (right)

Communication as a Sign of Adaptation

Every act of communication, both verbal and non-verbal, can be considered as an adaptive process analogous to biological evolution. Adaptation is the process of adjusting the mental structures and the behavior to cope with the environment.

Because so much of the adaptation processes in real time within the healthcare system are still verbal communication, the analysis of language becomes an important paradigm in order to study the adaptive capacities of a system. It is not the object of this chapter to review the literature concerning whether or not the structure of language determines the structure of thought as several researchers have maintained. However, when activities are distributed across space such as in surgery, the language used by task performers is almost certainly going to serve to organize resources to fit with the environmental constraints. The idea of language as an instrument of development of cognition, and thus serving adaptation, is central to Piaget's theories (1967/1992). Adaptation, in this constructivism framework, is achieved through agent–environment interactions via the conjunction of two processes: (1) the assimilation of new experiences into existing structures, and (2) the accommodation of these structures, that is, adaptation of existing ones and/or the creation of new ones. The latter, learning through accommodation, occurs for the purpose of "conceptual equilibration" and the elimination of perturbations. Some cognitive researches have also examined the relationship between communication, regular interaction and adaptation. When practitioners repeatedly work together, a reduction of verbal information exchanges is observed as practitioners get to know each other. Information taken directly from the work field replaces the verbal exchanges. Indeed, any regular action, parameter or alarm takes on the character of the "initiator" of verbal communication (Savoyant and Leplat 1983; Pavard 1994; Nyssen and Javaux 1996). Other studies (for example, Bressolle et al. 1996) have examined the relationship between communication and non-routine situations in complex systems: the greater the trouble, the greater are the demands for information centered on the task across the members of the team.

Based on the above arguments, three important points can be noted. First, the environment provides feedback, which is the raw material for adaptation. Simple systems tend to have very straightforward feedback, where it is often easy and instantaneous to see the result of an action. Complex systems may have less adequate feedback. The deployment of technology has increased the complexity of communication from non-verbal to verbal, and to complex symbolic patterns. Additionally, introducing media and a distance between the agent and the process to control can delay and/or result in losing feedback information. In laparoscopy surgery, the surgeon loses direct contact with the surgical site. S/he loses tactile feedback and performs operations with only sensory input from the video picture. As the robotic system is introduced in the OR, s/he loses proprioceptive feedback in addition to losing a face-to-face feedback communication channel.

Secondly, communication is a dynamic feedback process which, in turn, affects the communicators. As we shall see, because the assistant and the surgeon have often prior knowledge and experience with the task, the assistant can anticipate the next movement or instrument that the surgeon needs in a routine task and non-verbal communication can be very efficient (for example, when the surgeon makes a hand signal to indicate to stop the movement or when s/he looks at the assistant to verify the receipt of an implicit request).

Third, in this dynamic perspective, short-term adaptation feedback strategies that are exclusively based on verbal communication can be highly resource-consuming for the practitioners over time, and thus may lead to long-term inadequate adaptation.

Each of these points will be dealt with in our working hypotheses:

- In the case of adaptation, it is hypothesized that the environment provides good feedback that supports the system to carry the task. Within our framework that views communication as an adaptive process, the following can be expected with the introduction of a robot system:
  - in the short term, new patterns of communication that reveal adaptation strategies
  - with training and regular interactions, a reduction of communication that reveals the dynamic nature of the adaptation process
- In the case of lack of or inappropriate adaptation, the environment provides inadequate feedback, resulting in increasing and maintaining the verbal communication to compensate for the weakness of feedback from the new environment.

Experimental Study and Verbal Communication Analysis

We carried out three studies to examine our hypotheses:

1. We compared surgical operations that were performed with a robotic system compared with classical laparoscopy. In the two conditions (robotic and classical laparoscopy), the surgical procedures and the team members were identical. They were experts in the use of classical laparoscopy (>100 interventions) and were familiar with the use of a robotic system (> two interventions). We chose two types of surgical procedures (digestive and urology surgery) because it is possible to perform them with either classical laparoscopy or with a robotic system.

   We observed five cholecystectomy (digestive) with the robotic system and four with classical laparoscopy, and seven prostatectomy (urology) with the robotic system and four with classical laparoscopy.

   The robotic system used in our study was the Da Vinci robotic system (Intuitive Surgical, Mountain View, CA, USA) as shown in Figure 12.1.

2. We compared routine and non-routine operations: conversion from robot surgery to classical surgery.

3. We compared teams with different levels of expertise during gynecology surgery with a robotic system. We compared three teams with different levels of expertise who successively performed two tubular re-anastomosis of 36 Fallopian tubes: (1) both the surgeon and the assistant were experts with a robotic system (>50 operations with a robotic system); (2) the surgeon was an expert while the assistant was a novice with a robotic system (<10 operations

with a robotic system); (3) the surgeon and the assistant were novices with a robotic system (<10 operations with a robotic system).

In the three studies, we recorded all the verbal communication between the surgeon and the assistant. We analyzed their content and identified six categories. We also measured the duration of the intervention, as this is an important performance criterion for surgeons.

The six types of communication were:

- Verbal demands concerning the orientation and localization of organs
- Verbal demands concerning the manipulation of instruments and/or organs
- Explicit clarification concerning strategies, plans, and procedures
- Orders referring to tasks such as cutting, changing instruments, and cleaning the camera
- Explicit confirmation of detection or action
- Other communications referring to state of stress or relaxation

For each category, we measured the number of acts of communication, while taking into account the duration of the surgery (ratio = number of acts of communication/time (in seconds) x 100). The Mann-Whitney U test was used to compare the two techniques, classical laparoscopy and robotic surgery, and the Kruskal-Wallis test was used across the board.

Results

Communication as a Feedback Adaptive Process

The average duration of the intervention was significantly longer ($p<0.05$) with the robotic system (cholecystectomy: 82.59±27.37; prostatectomy: 221.39±58.79) than with classical laparoscopic surgery (cholecystectomy: 31.85±9.64; prostatectomy: 95.74±11.53). Figure 12.2 shows that the introduction of the robotic system created a new pattern of communication. Our results show that not only were there more acts of communication with the robotic system, but also that different types of communication between the surgeon and the assistant were used. This pattern of results was similar for the two types of surgery. Following our hypothesis, the increase of communication acts observed in the robotic system suggests that a portion of useful feedback is not provided by the robotic system anymore, and that the surgeon attempts to compensate this weakness of the system via verbal communication acts.

The significant increase in the number of communication acts ($p<0.05$) referring to orientation, manipulation, order, and confirmation within the robotic system suggests that a breakdown occurs in the collaboration between the surgeon and the assistant. The surgeon works alone and continually needs to ask the assistant about the orientation and the placement of the instrument (which is manipulated by the assistant) in order to facilitate the identification of the organs. Explicit demands, order, and confirmation are needed because the system configuration impedes face-to-face communication and prevents the assistant from anticipating the expected course of the surgeon's actions. Additionally, by introducing a distance between the surgeon and the patient, the robot configuration creates a new requirement for collaboration when s/he needs proprioceptive feedback, as illustrated in the following example of communication.

Example of interaction:
Surgeon at the consol: "could you tell me if you are touching something here, because I see a particularity ."
Assistant surgeon near the patient: "yes, I am touching something hard—it is a bone."

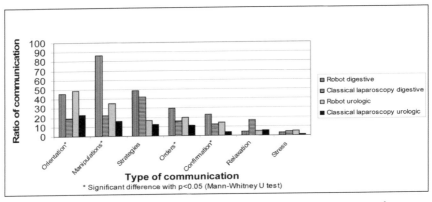

Figure 12.2 Communication during robotic and classical laparoscopy in digestive and urologic surgery

Communication as a Sign of Trouble

We observed two conversions: one in urology from robotic surgery to open surgery, and one in digestive surgery from robotic surgery to classical laparoscopy surgery.

As uncertainty increases during the case due to progression from expected to unexpected variability, initial procedures that are operationalized through preparatory configuration become irrelevant. In this case, conversion becomes imperative and may require the use of procedures that are not practiced by the surgeon anymore, as it was the case for prostatectomy in open surgery.

Each of these conversions is associated with an increased number of verbal communications (see Figure 12.3). These communications concerned explicit clarification of strategies (re-planning) and expectations concerning orientation and manipulations. We also observed less communication that referred to confirmation. During a crisis, the surgeon acts and does not take the time to verify the receipt of his action or request.

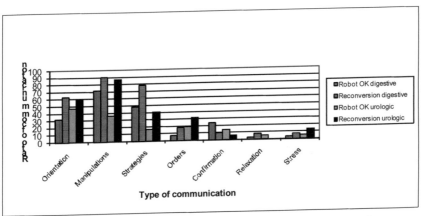

Figure 12.3 Communications during safe operations and reconversion in robotic surgery

Communication as a Dynamic Process

Our results show that the number of acts of communication is reduced with repeated experience: from the first operation to the second operation of Fallopian tube anastomosis, but also with the degree of expertise of the team with the robotic system (see Figure 12.4). The duration of the intervention was significantly different ($p<0.05$) according to the surgeon's expertise level: interventions are longer with novice surgeons (58.37 ± 5.66) than with an expert at the console (32.67 ± 10.46) and with two experts (25.85 ± 8.66).

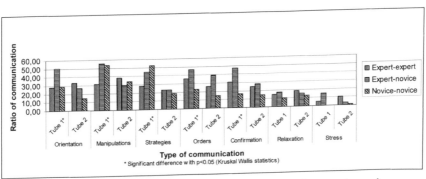

Figure 12.4 Communication during first and second tube anastomosis according to the expertise

Detailed analysis of communication showed that the number of communication acts referring to orientation, manipulation, and strategies was significantly reduced ($p<0.05$) when both surgeons were experts. Not surprisingly, the number of acts of communication referring to order and confirmation was significantly greater when an expert was present. In the contrary, the reduced number of acts of communication referring to orders and confirmation when both surgeons were novices attests to the absence of organization and structure that the surgeons have to compensate through more communication on ongoing action control (manipulation and strategies).

Discussion

Based on our results, it is clear that a robotic environment changes the feedback loop and that verbal communication used by surgeons is a feedback-adaptive process to compensate the feedback information absent in the robotic environment. Verbal demands concerning manipulation, orientation, confirmation, and orders attest to the fact that the surgeons need information in order to carry out their task, identify the organs, and control their action. Indeed, the patterns of communication reveal the need for feedback and, thus, the defeating aspects of feedback from the robotic system.

Our results also show that both the number of communication acts and the type of communication evolves with the agent–robot environment interactions. The fact that there are regular interactions between the surgeon and the assistant creates implicit communication and reduces the need for explicit communication, and furthermore suggests successful adaptation to the environment. However, our results also indicate that the surgeon's emergent adaptive learning response is achieved more readily through interacting with the classical laparoscopy system than with the robotic system. By introducing a distance between the surgeon and the assistant, the robotic system prevents face-to-face communication, which normally serves as a critical feedback for this adaptive process. Instead, the robotic system requires greater attention and continual efforts to communicate during even routine surgical procedures. However, as mentioned earlier, when complications occur, increased verbal communication is required to clarify plans and expectations in order to enable coordinated actions between the surgeon and the assistant.

These results reveal the value of verbal communication as a sign of adaptation or difficulty with adaptation of socio-technical systems. Indeed, our studies suggest that verbal communication can be seen as an adaptive feedback process that allows the agents to maintain an adequate performance level, minimizing the defeating feedback from the technical system. This adaptive response of the system is triggered by the environmental change (the change of the technical system) but emerges and evolves through agent–environment interactions. Thus, it is compatible with Piaget's constructivist view of adaptation: driven by the need to fit environmental constraints and emerging through interaction with the environment.

The concept of adaptation is also central to newer research on resilience engineering that views safety of complex systems as a system property that emerges from agent–environment interactions. In psychology, the term "resilience" is used to designate the human ability to survive after a significant trauma that has destroyed his/her equilibrium (Bowlby 1973; Cyrulnik 2003). We will therefore utilize the term resilience to designate the system's ability to recover from a change that destroys the system's structure.

We have discussed that the conversion cases represent a fundamental breakdown for the system, yet we have also seen how the surgeons, and not the robot, have mechanisms for recovering from the situation before it affects the patient, by replanning the cases into classical surgery. This means that the system's capacity for resilience resides in the human part rather than in the technical part of the system. Indeed, adaptation emerges through the history of different agent–environment coupling over time (open surgery, classical laparoscopic surgery, robotic surgery) that enhances the agent's autonomy towards the variability from the environment. This is similar to Maturana and Varela's work on the biology of cognition and autopoiesis (Maturana and Varela 1980 and 1987). According to Maturana and Varela (1980), living systems are not at all the same as machines made by humans. Machines, including robots, are allopoietic. The organization of an allopoietic machine is given in terms of a concatenation of processes independent of the organization of the machine. Thus, the changes that an allopoietic machine goes through are necessarily subordinated to something different from itself. In contrast, a living system is truly autonomous in the sense that it is an autopoietic machine whose continual interactions between components and environment, their transformations and destruction regenerates and maintains the system to be viable, in an emergent fashion, driven by the need to fit with environmental variability constraints. The result will be what Varela has called "a history of mutual congruent structural changes."

Although recent work from joint cognitive systems engineering discusses issues like autonomy, resilience, variability, and adaptation, much prevention effort is still spent on control mechanisms and how to anticipate breakdown. However, from our point of view, attempting to predict and control the breakdown sterilizes the new approach developed above. The results captured in this chapter support the idea that studying both the behavior of the system and the communication process provides markers of the system's adaptation and inadequate adaptation, and, in turn, will help to develop adaptive technology that enhances coupling between agents and their environment.

References

Amalberti, R. (1996), *La conduite des systèmes à risques* (Paris: Presses Universitaires de France).

Arbous, M.S., Grobbee, D.E., van Kleef, J.W., de Lange, J.J., Spoormans, H.H.A.J.M., Touw, P., Werner, F.M. and Meursing, A.E.E. (2001), 'Mortality Associated with Anaesthesia: A Qualitative Analysis to Identify Risk Factors', *Anaesthesia* 56:12, 1141–53.

Bainbridge, L. (1987), 'The Ironies of Automation', in J. Rasmussen, K. Duncan and J. Leplat (eds), *New Technology and Human Error* (London: Wiley) 271–83.

Bowlby, J. (1973), *Attachment and Loss*, Volume 2: Separation (New-York: Basic Books).

Bressolle, M.C., Decortis, F., Pavard, B. and Salembier, P. (1996), 'Traitement cognitif et organisationnel des micro-incidents dans le domaine du contrôle aérien: analyse des boucles de régulation formelles et informelles', in G. De Terssac and E. Friedberg (eds), *Coopération et conception* (Toulouse: Octares) 267–88.

Cadière, G.B., Himpens, J., Germay, O., Lupinc, N., Degueldre, M., Vandromme, J., Izizaw, R. and Bruyns, J. (2000), 'Chirurgie laparoscopique par robot: Faisabilité. A propos de 78 cas', *Le Journal de Coelio-Chirurgie* 33, 42–8.

Carpentier, A., Loulmet, D., Aupecle, B., Berrebi, A. and Relland, J. (1999), 'Computer-assisted cardiac surgery', *Lancet* 353:9150, 379–80.

Cook, R. and Woods, D.D. (1996), 'Adapting to New Technology in the Operating Room', *Human Factors* 38:4, 593–613.

Cyrulnik, B. (2003), *Le murmure des fantômes* (Paris: Odile Jacobs).

Hatton, F., Tiret, L., Maujol, L., N'Doye, N., Vourc'h, G., Desmonts, J.M., Otteni, J.C. and Scherpereel, P. (1983), 'Enquête épidémiologique sur les accidents d'anesthésie. Premiers résultats', *Annales Françaises d'Anesthésie et de Réanimation* 2, 331–86.

Hollnagel, E., Woods, D. and Leveson, N. (2006), *Resilience Engineering: Concepts and Precepts* (Aldershot, UK: Ashgate Publishing).

Hubens, G., Coveliers, H., Balliu, L., Ruppert, M. and Vaneerdeweg, W. (2003), 'A Performance Study Comparing Manual and Robotically Assisted Laparoscopic Surgery Using the da Vinci System', *Surgical Endoscopy* 17:10, 1595–9.

Hutchins, E. (1995), *Cognition in the Wild* (Cambridge, MA: MIT Press).

Kluger, M.T., Tham, E.J., Coleman, N.A., Runciman, W.B. and Bullock, M.F. (2000), 'Inadequate Pre-operative Evaluation and Preparation: A Review of 197 Reports from the Australian Incident Monitoring Study', *Anaesthesia* 55:12, 1173–8.

Le Moigne, J.L. (1999), *La modélisation des systèmes complexes* (Paris: Dunod).

Marescaux, J., Leroy, J., Rubino, F., Smith, M., Vix, M., Simone, M. and Mutter, D. (2002), 'Transcontinental Robot-assisted Remote Telesurgery: Feasibility and Potential Applications', *Annals of Surgery* 235:4, 487–92.

Maturana, H.R. and Varela, F.J. (1980), *Autopoiesis and Cognition – The Realization of the Living* (Dordrecht, The Netherlands: D. Reidel Publishing).

Maturana, H.R. and Varela, F.J. (1987), *The Tree of Knowledge – The Biological Roots of Human Understanding* (Boston, MA: Shambhala). Nyssen, A.S. (2004), 'Integrating Cognitive and Collective Aspects of Work in Evaluating Technology', *IEEE Transactions on Systems, Man and Cybernetics, Part A: Systems and Humans* 34:6, 743–9.

Nyssen, A.S. (2007), 'Coordination in Hospitals: Organized or Emergent Process?', *Cognition, Technology and Work* 9:3, 149–54.

Nyssen, A.S. and Javaux, D. (1996), 'Analysis of Synchronization Constraints and Associated Errors in Collective Work Environments', *Ergonomics* 39:10, 1249–64.

Pasticier, G., Rietbergen, J.B., Guillonneau, B., Fromont, G., Menon, M. and Vallancien, G. (2001), 'Robotically Assisted Laparoscopic Radical Prostatectomy: Feasibility Study in Men', *European Urology* 40:1, 70–74.

Pavard, B. (1994), *Système coopératifs: de la modélisation à la coopération* (Toulouse: Octares).

Piaget, J. (1967/1992), *Biologie et connaissance* (Lausanne: Delachaux et Niestlé) (1st edition, 1967: Paris: Gallimard).

Samurçay, R. (1995), 'Conceptual Models for Training', in J.-M. Hoc, E. Hollnagel and C. Cacciabue (eds), *Expertise and Technology: Cognition and Human-Computer Cooperation* (Hillsdale, NJ: LEA) 104–24.

Savoyant, A. and Leplat, J. (1983), 'Statut et fonction des communications dans l'activité des équipes de travail (Rule and Communication Function in the Activity of Workteams)', *Psychologie Francaise* 28:3, 247–53.

Woods, D. and Hollnagel, E. (2006), *Joint Cognitive Systems: Patterns in Cognitive Systems Engineering* (New York: Taylor and Francis).

Chapter 13

Telehealth and Healthcare Team Communication

Rod Elford

Introduction

Telehealth can be defined as: "The use of information and communications technology (ICT) to deliver health services and exchange health information when distance separates the participants" (Elford 1998: 207). Telehealth is healthcare at a distance. The aviation and aerospace environment in particular can be considered the ultimate in providing telehealth services as the patients, that is, astronauts, can be extremely far away. Healthcare team communications are impacted by the use of telehealth in a number of ways. Much can be learned from telehealth experiences because telehealth involves not just technology, but health professionals who use, operate, and interact with the technology. When implemented properly, telehealth can enhance communications between healthcare professionals.

Communication between healthcare teams is emerging as one of the most important factors affecting the quality of healthcare. A major US study of almost 3,000 hospitals, conducted from 1995 to 2004, found that communication failures among team members were the primary cause in 60 per cent of sentinel or serious adverse events (Joint Commission 2004). Improvements in team communication were positively correlated with quality of care and higher levels of job satisfaction (Rafferty, Ball and Aiken 2001). Quality communication, interactions, and coordination among health providers resulted in improvements in the quality of care (Higgins and Routhieux 1999; Irvine Doran et al. 2002) and also improved patient outcomes (Irvine Doran et al. 2001; Doran et al. 2002). Because telehealth impacts healthcare communications, it is important for the healthcare professional to be aware of these impacts in order to decrease the limitations of telehealth and increase its potential benefits.

Good Communications are Needed for a Successful Telehealth Consultation

If a patient in a rural community needs to see a specialist in an urban center, one option is to use telehealth for a remote consultation. When using telehealth, there are a number of interactions that need to occur for the consultation to take place. Each interaction requires healthcare professionals to communicate with each other or with the patient. First, someone (usually the patient's doctor) needs to inform the local telehealth booking person that a telehealth consultation is requested. The booking person at the patient's site will need to notify the booking person at the distant site (specialist site) that a telehealth consultation is requested and confirm when it will happen. The patient is then booked into a telehealth clinic and the local and distant information technology (IT) personnel, for example, individuals who look after the telehealth technology, are informed about the consultation. Next, all participants at both sites, for example, patient, nurse, specialist, and so on, are informed when the appointment is. On the day of the consultation, the IT people at each site usually show up prior to the patient and health professionals, and establish a link between the sites. Next, the patient and nurse at the local site and the specialist at the distant site need to arrive at their respective telehealth rooms at the proper time. During the telehealth consultation, the healthcare professionals need to be aware of the technology's limitations and know how to use the technology in order to communicate with it effectively. After the consultation, the specialist will need to send a summary and his/her recommendations to the referring doctor. Finally, appropriate records need to be kept of the encounter at both sites. The above interaction can become increasingly complicated by any of the following: (a) if time zones are crossed; (b) if state or national boundaries are crossed; (c) if the number of participants increases; (d) if more than two sites are linking together at the same time; (e) if translators are required; (f) if there is a technical problem. Obviously, good communication is needed between the healthcare professionals, their support staff, and the patient in order for a telehealth consultation to be a success.

This chapter will introduce telehealth, what it is and how it works. It will then discuss how telehealth impacts communications between healthcare professionals and their patients. Many of these impacts introduce limitations to the communications process; however, telehealth can also provide a number of potential benefits. Examples of how telehealth has been used in the aerospace industry will be described. And then lessons learned from the use of telehealth will be summarized. Finally, the chapter will conclude with a future telehealth scenario.

Telehealth—What Is It?

Telehealth has been around for a number of decades (Gershon-Cohen and Cooley 1950; Wittson and Benschoter 1972). However, it is only in the last few years that it has become a practical way to deliver health services (DeBakey 1995). There are a number of reasons for this, but primarily the cost of clinically acceptable technology has decreased to the point where it is economically sustainable. Today, telehealth is allowing more patients to be diagnosed and cared for at a distance. However, it only makes up a small percentage of interactions in the healthcare system and many people are not fully aware of what it is and what it can do. Telehealth is a general term that includes many different technologies and telecommunications links applied to many different clinical, health education, and health information applications. It is important to understand the different components of telehealth in order to understand how they may impact communications between healthcare professionals.

A telehealth system can be divided into four different components: (1) technology, such as workstation and peripherals; (2) telecommunications link, such as the Internet and satellites; (3) people, including clinicians and patients; and (4) policies and protocols. Each of these components is important and must be properly integrated with the others for telehealth to be successful.

Technology

The technology component of telehealth is the hardware, software, and peripheral devices that are used to perform telehealth activities. It is the component that most people envision when they hear the term telehealth. There are many different technologies used for telehealth including: telephones, store and forward systems (basically personal computers running telehealth software that provide a service similar to sending an email with attachments), videoconferencing systems, and specialized telehealth workstations. Two technologies are shown below.

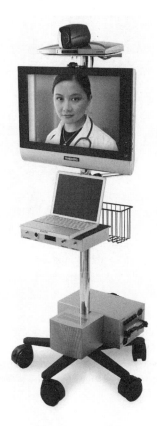

Figure 13.1 Tandberg Intern MXP
Note: Figure 13.1 shows a telehealth workstation developed specifically for conducting medical consultations at a distance, that is, a Tandberg Intern MXP. A number of peripheral devices can be connected to the workstation allowing images, video, text, and sound to be captured and transmitted from one site to another. The Intern can be used for a variety of applications such as teledermatology, telecardiology, and tele-ENT.

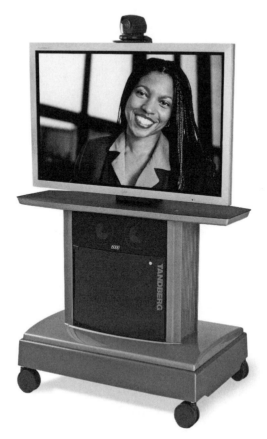

Figure 13.2 Tandberg Educator MXP
Note: Figure 13.2 shows an educational videoconferencing unit, that is, a Tandberg Educator MXP. This technology can be used in the healthcare environment for applications like telepsychiatry, distance medical education, and administrative videoconferencing.

Peripheral Devices Peripheral devices are an important part of many telehealth workstations. Peripherals are devices that can be plugged into or connected to a workstation and allow the local health professional to capture clinical images, video, sounds, and vitals. Some peripheral devices are shown below.

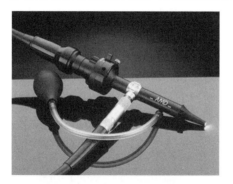

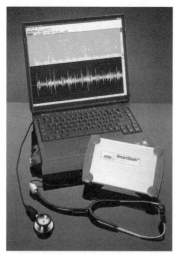

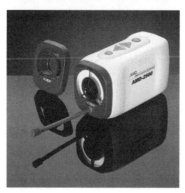

**Figure 13.3 AMD peripheral devices (from top to bottom): (a) otoscope,
(b) electronic stethoscope, (c) general exam camera**

Note: Figure 13.3a shows an otoscope, which allows images from the ear, nose, and throat to be captured and transmitted to a distant site for review. Figure 13.3b shows an electronic stethoscope. This device allows heart, lung, and bowel sounds to be captured and transmitted to a distant site for review. Figure 13.3c shows a general exam camera. This device can be used for multiple purposes such as capturing pictures of the eye, ear, throat, and skin.

Telecommunications Link

The second component of telehealth is the telecommunications link. This is the electronic connection that links the workstations mentioned above. There are many different telecommunications mediums including: telephone lines, coaxial cable, and radio wave/wireless links such as cell phone communications, WiFi (that is, 802.11x), microwave, and satellite. To transmit information over the telecommunications medium, a number of different telecommunications protocols are used including: Internet Protocols (IP), Integrated Service Digital Networks (ISDN), asymmetric digital subscriber line (ADSL), and Asynchronous Transfer Mode (ATM). Most of these protocols can operate over different mediums. For example, you can access the Internet using a dial-up modem over POTS (plain old telephone system), ADSL telephone line, coaxial cable, or cell phone. All these telecommunications modalities can be used to transmit information; however, each one has specific advantages and disadvantages.

An important factor to take into account when choosing a telecommunications link for your telehealth system is the amount of bandwidth required for your application(s). Bandwidth is the amount of information that can be transmitted over a telecommunications medium in a specified period of time. It is often measured in the number of bits of data that can be transmitted per second, for example, kilobits per second (kbps). Different telehealth applications require different bandwidths. For example, real-time medical videoconferencing often requires a minimum bandwidth of 384 kbps. Usually the more bandwidth you require, the higher the cost. The cost of the telecommunications link (installation, ongoing fees, and maintenance) is often a key factor in the sustainability of a telehealth network.

People

The maxim "If you build it, they will come" does not hold true for telehealth. If you set up a telehealth network, healthcare professionals will not automatically come and use it. Many unsuccessful or underutilized telehealth programs testify to this fact. The "people network" is just as important (if not more important) than the technical network. For this reason it is essential that you carefully identify, educate, train, and support your users. Although some people quickly embrace new technologies, the majority of people do not; rather they have neutral or distrustful feelings towards it. As a result, most individuals need to be educated about telehealth, what it is, how it works, and how it is beneficial to them and their patients, before they will consider using it. If they do choose to use telehealth, they then need to be trained how to use it properly. Failure to do so usually leads to users being intimidated by the technology and frustrated when they cannot get it to do what they want. Proper training also increases the probability that the user will be able to take full advantage of what the technology can do. Finally, users need to be supported (ideally 24 x 7) so that when they do have problems, they can quickly interact with a knowledgeable person who can help them solve the problem.

Policies and Protocols

Before telehealth (in particular medical consultations conducted at a distance) can continue as an ongoing service, a number of policy issues must be resolved. Examples of policy issues include reimbursement, licensing, and liability. Questions that need to be answered are: Who pays the clinician to perform a teleconsultation? If the patient and clinician are not in the same province, is the clinician electronically going to the patient or is the patient coming to the clinician? (In most jurisdictions, it has been decided that the physician goes to the patient). If something goes wrong with the patient due to the information exchanged during a teleconsultation, who is liable—the clinician, hospital/clinic, technology vendor, or telecommunications provider?

Protocols are the steps that need to take place for an interaction to occur. Protocols need to be agreed upon by all users and implemented in order for telehealth to happen in an efficient manner. Examples of questions that need to be answered before protocols can be created include: Who initiates the interaction? When is the interaction to be initiated? What documentation is required of the encounter? What happens when there is a technical problem?

Policies and protocols are vital to the long-term operations of a telehealth network. They need to be defined, or users will eventually stop using the network, even if technically it works fine and they know how to use it.

Impact of Telehealth on Communications

Healthcare professionals primarily work with patients and each other in a face-to-face environment. When in a face-to-face environment, healthcare professionals utilize and simultaneously process a number of different sensory stimuli, for example, auditory, visual, smell, tactile. Face-to-face interactions are also conducted in real time with no perceptible delay or degradation of the sensory stimuli. For example, when talking to someone in person, there is no perceptible delay between when their lips move and when you hear their voice. And unless the person has laryngitis, the quality of their voice is usually very good. It is important to note that when using telehealth technology to capture, transmit, and display sensory stimuli, the results are less than perfect.

Telehealth Introduces Limitations to Healthcare Team Communications

Telehealth usually limits healthcare team communications in the following ways (compared to face-to-face communications):

- Less sensory stimuli is communicated
- Decreased quality
- Introduces a delay
- Participants need to consciously think about communicating
- Increases complexity

Each of these limitations will be described and the impact it has on communications will be discussed.

Less Sensory Stimuli is Communicated

Currently, we do not have technology that can perfectly capture, transmit, and reproduce all sensory stimuli. This would require reproducing a virtual 3-D environment, such as the sense of smell and touch at a distance and the background temperature and humidity, and so on. This technology would be similar to the Holodeck on Star Trek. We do, however, have technologies that can capture and reproduce audio and still images very well, and to a lesser extent video. The first major limitation of using telehealth technology for communications is that it decreases the amount of sensory stimuli that can be transmitted. Most telehealth encounters transmit either audio, or audio plus video information. No other senses, such as taste, smell, and touch, are usually transmitted.

> During my Telemedicine Fellowship in the mid-1990s, I remember having discussions with telemedicine practitioners, especially psychiatrists regarding whether using videoconferencing for patient consultations resulted in "missing something". The psychiatrists wondered since only audio and video information was transmitted whether they were missing some form of communication that was neither audio or video; information that would have been communicated if they had been in the same room as the patient. After having used videoconferencing for a number of consultations these clinicians indicated that although they had a preference for face-to-face communications and found them more satisfying, they felt that videoconferencing was an acceptable alternative (Elford 1996).

Impact of Decreased Sensory Stimuli on Communications Transmitting less sensory stimuli during an interaction often results in poorer or more difficult communication between healthcare professionals (Jong et al. 2001; Bischoff 2004; Elford 1997). This makes sense, as studies investigating the effect of sensory loss (specifically as people age) have found that it results in poor communication (Heine and Browning 2004).

Decreasing the amount of sensory stimuli transmitted results in healthcare professionals needing more time to communicate. For example, if a nurse at a remote site has a patient with a skin lesion and is discussing the case with a physician over the phone (auditory only), the nurse will have to take more time explaining what the lesion looks like compared to sending a picture of it. The physician may also ask more questions in order to get an idea of what the lesion looks like.

Telehealth usually results in one healthcare professional having to rely on a remote person to be their sensory surrogate; basically their eyes, ears, nose, and sense of touch at a distance. In the above example, even if the nurse and physician are connected by videoconferencing technology and the physician can see the skin lesion, she still cannot touch the lesion or surrounding area to determine how warm the skin is, see if the skin is indurated or if it is painful to touch. Neither can she smell any odor from the lesion. The nurse at the remote site will have to act as her sense of touch and smell at a distance.

Finally, transmitting decreased sensory stimuli usually results in a decreased level of confidence in the diagnosis and subsequent treatment (Jong et al. 2001; Ball, McLaren and Watson 1996). In a study that involved GPs supporting nurses in a remote community with a store and forward telehealth system, it was found that the physicians had more confidence using the telehealth link compared to the telephone alone (Jong et al. 2001). Basically, having the nurse capture and send images to the physicians to be reviewed, and then having a conversation about it, resulted in physicians being more confident in their diagnosis and in making treatment recommendations. It also made them more confident in deciding whether an evacuation was necessary. This suggests that limiting sensory stimuli to just audio makes communicating about healthcare issues more difficult, and the recipient is not as confident about what is being discussed or in making recommendations about it.

Sometimes It is Not Necessary to Transmit Multiple Sensory Stimuli It is important to note that it is not always necessary to transmit all sensory stimuli in order to have a satisfactory clinical encounter. A landmark Canadian study with 1,015 patients comparing consultations done via audio only, audio plus still images, interactive video, and face-to-face concluded that they were unable to measure any significant differences related to diagnostic accuracy, tests required, patient management practices, efficiency, and referral rates among the four communications modes (Dunn et al. 1977; Dunn and Higgins 1984; Conrath, Dunn and Higgins 1983). This surprised the researchers, who commented, "Surely high-quality color television is a far cry from hands-free audio, and yet the performance of the two is virtually identical" (Dunn et al. 1977: 752). For some types of consultations only one sense is needed. For example, teleradiology involves sending diagnostic images from one site to another to review. As long as the quality of the captured images are high enough and the receiving monitor of high enough resolution, the interpretation of the teleradiology images should be the same as looking at film-based images in person.

Decreased Quality

When telehealth technology is used for communications, it usually results in a decreased quality of the transmitted sensory stimuli compared to face-to-face. For example, the quality of the video seen on a videoconferencing monitor is less than the visual information you would obtain if you were having a face-to-face conversation with someone. There are a number of reasons for this, including: (1) electronics cannot capture the same quality of information as the human senses; (2) usually the sensory stimuli is converted from an analog signal to a digital signal and then back to analog, resulting in some degradation; (3) often compression is used after the signal has been converted to a digital format that results in some loss of quality; (4) the reproduction of the sensory stimuli is of less quality than in person, for example, a computer monitor is two-dimensional versus 3-D, and the resolution is of lower quality than what the eye can sense.

Impact of Decreased Quality of Sensory Stimuli on Communications Decreasing the quality of the sensory stimuli that is transmitted from one site to another impacts communications. If the quality of the transmitted information is too low, it may make communication impossible. For example, if there is too much static on a telephone line, the participants may not be able to understand each other. Similarly, if a chest x-ray image is captured at too low a resolution or compressed too much, the image at the receiving site may not be of sufficient quality to make a diagnosis.

Decreasing the quality of information transmitted can decrease the accuracy of the diagnosis. Studies have shown that lower quality sound, images, and video can decrease the accuracy of, and make it more difficult to make, a diagnosis (Roberge et al. 1982; Zarate et al. 1997). Lower quality can also decrease healthcare professional satisfaction with the consultation (Ball and McLaren 1995; Ball et al. 1995).

Studies have shown that not all sensory stimuli need to be transmitted at the same quality level. For example, mental health consultations that are conducted via a videoconferencing system require a relatively high quality audio and video signal; however, if bandwidth is at a premium, psychiatrists have indicated that it is more important to have high quality audio than high quality video (Elford 1997).

Sometimes the Highest Quality is Not Always Needed What is interesting is that we are now at the point where some of the technology we have is higher definition or more sensory rich than is required for some healthcare applications. For example, an audiophile would consider the audio quality of a standard telephone poor, but it is usually considered adequate for a conversation between healthcare professionals. Interestingly, now that high-definition videoconferencing is available, health professionals are not suddenly jumping on board to use it for medical consultations. The main reason is that most clinicians do not feel that the additional resolution is worth the additional cost. Even when the costs come down, many clinicians may simply feel it is not needed—"Why buy a Ferrari when a Ford will do?"

Introduces a Delay

Using telehealth usually leads to a delay compared to face-to-face communications. Sometimes this delay is imperceptible to the user, at other times it is very obvious and has a negative impact on communication. Some telehealth technologies that are asynchronous, such as store and forward telehealth systems, have a delay built into them. This can be useful at times, as will be discussed later.

Telehealth technology introduces a delay to communications because it takes time to electronically capture, process, transmit, and reproduce an electronic signal. When using simple technology such as the telephone, this delay is usually not perceptible, except when talking across great distances. For example, during the Moon landing of *Apollo 16* on April 21, 1972, a spoken message from the Moon took roughly 1.35 seconds to reach Earth (Keeports 2006). As increasingly large amounts of information are captured, for example, high quality video, more processing is required and delays become evident over smaller distances. In addition, technology can introduce delays when information is compressed and/or encrypted at the sending end and de-compressed and/or de-encrypted at the receiving end. Terrestrially, the longest delays are usually introduced when geosynchronous satellites are used for communications. For example, a telephone signal sent over geosynchronous satellites results in an approximately 0.5 second-delay (Stallings 2005).

Impact of Delays on Communications The impacts of delays on communications depend upon the length of the delay. A delay of 0.5 seconds when using the telephone leads to longer than usual pauses and a stilted conversation. The impact on videoconferencing is even more significant. For example, it may lead to a slight variation between when you see someone's lips move and when the sound is heard. The delay from when you actually say something to when it is heard at the other end results in awkward pauses, with the initial speaker wondering if the other site has heard them.

Sometimes Delays Can Be Beneficial Delayed or asynchronous communication can be useful at times. For example, store and forward telehealth systems allow one person to capture patient information at one site and then send it to another site to be reviewed. If the receiving individual is busy, the information is stored, usually on a server/computer, until the individual has time to review the information. It can also be more efficient as a number of consultations can be sent and stored, then reviewed all at once.

Participants Need to Consciously Think about Communicating

When health professionals communicate with each other in person, they do so without thinking too much about how they do it. When technology is utilized for communication, people need to think more about the communication process. For example, when conducting a videoconference, the participants need to decide who is going to initiate the call so that they can connect. Once connected, each site needs to make sure the other participants can see and hear them. This may require making adjustments such as increasing the volume, zooming in on a person's face or improving the light in the room. Conducting a telehealth consultation requires more forethought and usually is done in a pre-defined order, as it may require switching to different cameras, or require a health professional at the patient's end to perform part of the exam. To facilitate remote consultations, telehealth organizations usually develop telehealth policies and protocols. This means that people have to learn about and adhere to the policies and follow the established protocols.

Impact of Consciously Thinking about Communicating Being more conscious about communicating can make people more self-conscious. During videoconferences, some people are distracted by their out-going video image (the video that is being transmitted to the remote site).

> During a child telepsychiatry project that I was involved in, we had to turn off the out-going monitor. This was because when children saw themselves on TV, they became distracted. They waved their arms and made weird sounds to see what they looked and sounded like (Elford 1997).

When people are new to telehealth, they often focus on the technology and not the conversation, and find communicating awkward. Most participants do seem to adapt quickly.

> During a telemental health consultation, a schizophrenic patient was initially very aware of the technology during a videoconference interview commenting on it a number of times. He also seemed slightly paranoid about it, wondering if the psychiatrists were recording the interview to use against him later and if other people could see him on TV. However, after about 15 minutes he seemed to relax and really got into the interview. At the end of the interview, he got up and extended his arm to shake the psychiatrist's hand forgetting they were not in the same room (Elford 1996).

Having healthcare professionals consciously think about communicating when using telehealth results in them realizing that they need to behave/act in a different manner than in person. For example, when using videoconferencing systems, they learn to look into the camera which is typically just above the monitor, versus looking into the eyes of the person on the monitor. The reason for this is that if they look directly at the person in the monitor, it appears to the patient at the other site that the health professional is looking down at something and not making eye contact. Healthcare professionals also learn that they should try to keep their head and shoulders within the camera's field of view.

Having to Focus More on Communicating Can Have Positive Effects An interesting result of having healthcare professionals focus more on the communication process is that some patients have been more satisfied with videoconferencing interviews than with face-to-face interviews (Zarate et al. 1997; Elford et al. 2000; Elford et al. 2001). Patients have stated that the reason for this is that the specialist appeared to focus more on them than they did in person and seemed more prepared, for example, had read all the information in the chart ahead of time.

Increases Complexity

Telehealth increases complexity and requires an unusually high level of cooperation among participants. Telehealth requires proper communication among people at the local site, at the remote site, and between sites. Increasing complexity occurs when people from different disciplines (specialists, generalists, nurses, allied health professionals, IT, clerks, and so on) need to work together, and when people who do not regularly work together need to do so; this is because they may not understand each other's culture or how things are usually done at the other site. For each telehealth interaction, there are a large number of people involved, who are exchanging information prior to and during the interaction. If any of these exchanges is miscommunicated, then the intended telehealth interaction may not take place.

Impact of Complexity on Healthcare Professional Communications Increasing complexity decreases the probability that healthcare professionals will use telehealth technology for communications. This can result in people not using telehealth because they do not understand it, do not know how to operate it, or are afraid of it, and so on. When people have these feelings, it means that telehealth can lead to decreased communication between healthcare professionals.

Increasing complexity also results in an increased probability that something will go wrong. Whenever there are more variables, even if one of them is out by a bit, it affects the entire equation. In addition, small problems with a number of variables can have a large negative impact.

Mastery of Complexity Can Lead to Other Benefits Healthcare professionals who master using telehealth technology for communications often have an increased sense of self-confidence with ICT in general. Healthcare professionals may then be more open or tolerant of the use of other ICTs in their practice, for example, electronic health records. In addition, healthcare professionals who have had to think about how to communicate using telehealth technology often begin to think about how they communicate with colleagues or patients in person. This leads them to thinking about how they could change/improve their face-to-face communications.

Potential Benefits of Telehealth

The many potential benefits of telehealth can be divided into those for the patient, remote healthcare provider (sender), central healthcare provider (receiver), and the healthcare payer (insurer).

Benefits—Patient

- Improved access to healthcare specialists
- Reduced travel
- Decreased cost (travel, meals, accommodation, lost work)
- Decreased stress
- Quicker, more accurate diagnosis and treatment leading to improved patient outcomes

Benefits—Remote Healthcare Provider

- Improved access to healthcare specialists
- Backed up by specialist leading to increased confidence in management
- Increased opportunities for education (can attend classes/rounds/conferences virtually)
- Decreased professional isolation

Benefits—Central Healthcare Provider

- Decreased need to travel; "see patients, not the road"; can do "electronic house calls")
- Improved screening of patients (can see patients at a distance prior to an in-person consultation)

- Improved follow-up (can see patients at a distance after an in-person consultation or intervention, for example, post-surgery)
- Increased educational opportunities

Benefits—Healthcare Payer

- Decreased overall healthcare costs (per patient) due to:
  - reduced reimbursement of patient travel costs
  - reduced reimbursement of healthcare professional travel costs
  - less admissions to Emergency Department/hospital
  - more patients treated at remote site or at home
- More specialists can visit region, more often, at less expense
- Human resources are used more efficiently, "Do more with less"
- Healthcare professionals are attracted to and kept in the region
- Can back up healthcare professionals at remote sites

Clinical Examples of How Telehealth Can Improve Healthcare Communications

As long as telehealth is set up properly and health professionals are aware of the limitations of telehealth and adapt to them, telehealth has the potential to benefit healthcare professional communications and subsequently improve health services at a distance. Six clinical examples follow, which demonstrate how telehealth has had a positive effect on healthcare communications.

During a telehealth consultation with a pediatric patient with Tourettes, the specialist was able to zoom in on the patient's face and focus on the patient's subtle facial tics and other movement disorders. The physician indicated that if he had wanted to do the same thing in person, he would have had to stand right in front of the patient and stare into his face, which he believed would have made the patient very uncomfortable.

A Norwegian psychiatrist mentioned that it was much easier for him to conduct a consultation with a very anxious, agoraphobic patient using telepsychiatry versus in-person. The reason was because the patient usually needed to sit a long distance from the psychiatrist in order to feel comfortable during an interview. During the telepsychiatry interview, both the patient and psychiatrist sat a few feet in front of their respective videoconferencing systems, but the camera focusing on the psychiatrist was zoomed out so that it looked to the patient like the psychiatrist was really far away. In addition, when the patient became very anxious, he would sometimes back up his chair away from the psychiatrist. During the videoconference, the psychiatrist could control the camera at the patient's end, and simply zoomed in a bit on the patient and increased the volume. This allowed the interview to proceed with fewer interruptions than usual and with less anxiety for the patient.

Teleradiology has facilitated faster turnaround times for the interpretation of diagnostic images. This has been particularly beneficial for sites where there is no local radiologist or sporadic coverage or limited coverage at night. Teleradiology facilitates the electronic transfer of digital diagnostic images to a radiologist located at a distant site versus having to physically courier film images or a DVD/hard disk containing the images. This can speed up turnaround time for reporting and allow for urgent review of a case if necessary. A controversial practice that is becoming increasingly popular in developed countries is using teleradiology to transmit diagnostic images to radiologists in foreign countries for review. In the United States, hundreds of hospitals are sending their diagnostic images to foreign radiologists, in particular India, to review (Wachter 2006). The two major benefits of this service are: (1) fast turnaround time, and (2) decreased cost. Turnaround times are fast because images are sent during the evening/night in the USA, which is daytime in India, allowing Indian radiologists to review diagnostic images during regular office hours. A report is transmitted back to the USA and available the next morning. This service can also be less expensive, since radiologists in India are reimbursed at a lower rate than their American counterparts.

Some child telepsychiatry studies have found that children preferred the TV doctor to the real one (Elford et al. 2000; Elford et al. 2001). Informal discussions with parents indicated that they thought that their children may not have felt as intimidated by seeing a psychiatrist over the videoconferencing system compared to being in the same room with a strange adult. They also surmised that their children were comfortable with the TV doctor because they were so used to watching TV and playing videogames.

Videoconferencing technology was used in a large city to facilitate bringing together healthcare professionals from different hospitals for meetings and grand rounds. Participating clinicians indicated that they would not have been able to physically travel to one hospital for these activities (or would not have been able to attend as often). Benefits included increased educational opportunities and increased connection with their colleagues.

It is not convenient on some occasions to communicate in real time, that is, telephone or face-to-face. This is particularly relevant to surgeons who are operating or physicians with extremely busy clinics, as they would have to interrupt their activities to answer a call or talk to someone. Sometimes it is more efficient and easier to communicate asynchronously, for example, store and forward telehealth. Studies have shown that some store and forward telehealth systems have increased clinician satisfaction with their communications compared to using the telephone or telephone/pager. This is partly because more information such as images or video can be sent using store and forward systems compared to the phone, but also because it can be more convenient. It allows the healthcare professional to review the transmitted information on his or her own schedule.

Examples of Telehealth in Aerospace

Aerospace agencies have been pioneers in the use of telehealth. Some of the National Aeronautics and Space Administration's and the Canadian Department of Communication's early telehealth activities are summarized below.

NASA Telemetry

The National Aeronautics and Space Administration (NASA) has utilized telecommunications to support space exploration as a means of coordinating, monitoring, and commanding remotely located facilities to conduct science and operations at a distance. When NASA began preparing for human space flight, they began to develop telehealth capabilities (telecommunications support for the delivery of medical care). In the early 1960s, NASA used telemetry of basic physiological data from astronauts to understand the effects of launch, space flight, and re-entry on the human body (Doarn, Ferguson and Nicogossian 1996; Nicogossian, Huntoon and Pool 1994). Specifically, telemetry was used for acquiring biomedical and physiological parameters (for example, EKG, blood pressure, heart rate, and respiration) and environmental parameters from the space vehicles (for example, radiation, CO_2, O_2, H_2O). Medical telemetry has been utilized on all subsequent human space flights, including monitoring of astronauts during extra-vehicular activities.

STARPAHC

Space Technology Applied to Rural Papago Advanced Health Care (STARPAHC), was a large-scale telehealth project, sponsored jointly by the Indian Health Service (IHS), NASA, and the Papago Indian Reservation (NASA 1974; Bashshur 1980). Beginning in 1973, STARPAHC provided healthcare to Papago Indians using a mobile health unit (MHU). This mobile unit was staffed by non-MD providers and linked by two-way television, radio, and remote telemetry to physicians at an IHS hospital approximately 100 miles away. The rationale for NASA's involvement was to obtain data on how to provide medical care at a distance. Outcomes from the project indicated that the technology was considered costly (for terrestrial purposes), in some cases inconvenient to physicians, and was not always considered essential for making a diagnosis and for treatment. The major benefit was improved access to healthcare for a population who were not previously receiving care near their homes. Non-physicians considered the link to remote physicians via television and voice communications to be a major benefit.

Communications Technology Satellite

The Communications Technology Satellite (CTS), also called Hermes, was a joint project by NASA and the Canadian Department of Communications (DOC), and was the world's most powerful satellite at the time of its launch in 1976. The satellite was used for a number of different experiments, including three Canadian telehealth projects: the Moose Factory Telemedicine Programme (Carey and Russell 1978; Carey et al. 1979); Memorial University Telemedicine Project (House and Roberts 1977; House, McNamara and Roberts 1977); and the Baffin Zone Telemedicine Study (Roberts and Picot 1981). All three projects utilized two-way audio and one-way video, and linked urban tertiary care centers to extremely remote northern hospitals and clinics. The projects demonstrated remote consultations in a variety of specialties, as well as conducting continuing medical education and community health education activities.

Anik-B Satellite

The Anik-B satellite was used for two telehealth projects, specifically the Offshore Telemedicine Project (House 1980) and the Telemedicine in Quebec Project (Roberge et al. 1982). Phase 1 of the offshore project began in 1979 and evaluated the ability to provide a telephone channel from the sick bay of a drill ship operating in the Labrador Sea to the Emergency Department at Memorial University of Newfoundland's (MUN) Health Science Center. Although successful audio and slow-scan images could be transmitted in calm waters, the terminal did not work well in choppy seas. Phase 2 evaluated a gyroscopically stabilized terminal that could automatically position itself towards the satellite. This project linked the semi-submersible drilling rig to MUN's Emergency Department. Slow-scan images (mainly patient skin lesions) were routinely transmitted to supplement the audio link. EKGs were also successfully sent. The Telemedicine in Quebec Project compared using two-way, black and white television (340 horizontal lines) transmission of x-rays to slow-scan transmission (275 horizontal lines) to in-person review. The overall conclusion was that "real-time bi-directional television was well suited to all types of telemedicine applications. However, its costs become prohibitive over long distances and the technical complexity is forbidding for routine use in isolated areas" (Roberge et al. 1982).

Spacebridge Activities

In the late 1980s and early 1990s, NASA was involved in a number of activities that involved using satellite communications systems (a spacebridge) to provide medical consultations (Doarn, Ferguson and Nicogossian 1996; Ferguson, Doarn and Scott 1995). In December 1988, a massive earthquake devastated the Soviet Republic of Armenia, leaving much of the country's medical care capability in ruins. Under the US/USSR Joint Working Group on Space Biology and Medicine, NASA offered assistance to the medical care workers in Armenia, linking them via satellite (DOMSAT and INTELSAT) to medical facilities in the US. The link provided one-way full-motion color video and two-way audio to support the clinical consultations. Telephone and facsimile were used for regular communications and to transmit information and medical records for case preparation. Consultations across the spacebridge resulted in 25 per cent of the cases having the treatment plans altered. During this project, there was a train accident in Ufa, Russia, injuring hundreds. The spacebridge was extended to Ufa to support medical consultation for the burn victims. This program was the first use of telemedicine for a large-scale international disaster response (Llewellyn 1995). A major outcome of this program was that interactive remote consultations by specialists could provide valuable assistance to on-site physicians and positively influence clinical decisions in the aftermath of major disasters.

Based on the success of the spacebridge to Armenia, NASA conducted a second international telemedicine demonstration, Spacebridge to Moscow, beginning in 1993 (Doarn, Ferguson and Nicogossian 1996; Willis et al. 1995). Under the sponsorship of the US/Russian Joint Working Group on Biomedical and Life Support Systems, NASA and the Russian Medical Information Agency operated the spacebridge. The communications network was established using a US satellite and a former Russian military satellite. Spacebridge to Moscow linked two diverse medical cultures for medical interactions including 14 formal clinical sessions. These clinical sessions provided expert consultation in diverse areas such as space medicine, internal and preventive medicine, disaster and trauma management, cardiology, surgery, and cancer treatment.

These collaborative spacebridge activities led to NASA Johnson Space Center (JSC) developing an operational telemedicine capability at the Gargarin Cosmonaut Training Facility in Star City, Russia, to support NASA flight surgeons and astronauts training in Moscow for Phase I of the International Space Station Program (ISS).

NASA and Internet-based Telehealth

Spacebridge to Moscow highlighted the need for reliable, inexpensive, regular medical communications. Consequently, in the late 1990s NASA began developing an Internet-based link to Russia (Angood et al. 1998). Clinical consultations were developed using a variety of electronic media, packaged as digital files, and transmitted using Internet and World Wide Web tools. These systems also offered the capability of real-time video teleconferencing.

IIU Telehealth Network

The IIU Telehealth Network was initiated in 1999 and used videoconferencing technology linked via satellite to connect all healthcare facilities in Nunavut (Nunavut Government 2004). Nunavut is Canada's largest Territory (three times the size of Texas), most northern (it includes the magnetic North Pole) and least populated (28,000 people). The only access to Nunavut's 25 communities is by plane or boat (in the summer). The IIU Telehealth Network links all communities to each other and to a number of tertiary healthcare centers in southern Canada. Most sites have peripheral devices attached to their workstations to allow remote clinicians to look into the patient's mouth, ears, and eyes at a distance. The network is used for multiple types of consultations, health education and rounds, and for health-related meetings. Previous to the implementation of the network, all patients had to be flown at great expense from their remote communities to a regional health center, or to a hospital in southern Canada. A unique use of the network is to link patients that are being treated in southern hospitals to family members that are back home in their local Nunavut community.

Current Space Telehealth Activities

Currently, astronauts that travel on space flights to the International Space Station have biomedical parameters telemetered to the ground during extra-vehicular activities and while performing biomedical research. Private medical conferences are conducted between the flight surgeons and each individual crew member on a regular basis.

Lessons Learned

The aerospace industry was one of the pioneers in telehealth and has been involved in a number of terrestrially based telehealth projects. Because telehealth requires an unusually high level of cooperation in order to function successfully, there are eight lessons to be learned from it in regards to healthcare communications.

It is extremely important to define your need. This means not only defining what type of consultation or healthcare activity you will be conducting, but specifically what type of sensory stimuli/information will need to be transmitted between sites in order for that consultation to occur. Once you have defined your need, you can then select telehealth technology that will meet your need, that is, what you will need to capture, transmit, and reproduce the sensory stimuli/information required during the interaction.

Telehealth technology limits the amount of sensory stimuli that can be captured, transmitted, and reproduced, and often decreases the quality of the information that has been transmitted to the distant site (compared to face-to-face). Clinicians have determined that when using telehealth technology, one needs to transmit a minimum number of sensory stimuli (audio, visual, and so on) and a minimum quality of information in order for health professionals to feel that the consultation is acceptable compared to face-to-face. The number of sensory stimuli and the quality of each varies depending upon the application. Many clinical specialties have developed minimum standards for the type of consultations they perform.

When setting up a telehealth network, it is best to connect individuals at sites/ organizations that already have a good working relationship. Telehealth can enhance communications between groups that already communicate well.

Technology that facilitates synchronous (real-time) interaction such as videoconferencing can introduce delays that make communication more challenging. Participants need to adapt to these delays, that is, it is best to let one person talk at a time, decrease interruptions, and prepare for longer pauses.

Synchronous (real-time) communication is not always needed for a consultation to occur. Asynchronous communication is often all that is needed. At times, asynchronous communication, such as store and forward telehealth, is more convenient.

Users have to be properly trained and supported in order to fully take advantage of telehealth technology. They also need to learn about how to communicate most effectively using the technology, in order to minimize the limitations of the technology and take advantage of its potential benefits.

Telehealth can act as a catalyst, causing healthcare professionals to think about how to communicate with others, not only at a distance but in person as well.

Telehealth can change the way healthcare is practiced. It can facilitate the provision of care in ways and locations where it was not possible in the past.

Looking to the Future

Telehealth has been practiced for a number of decades and currently there are many successful telehealth programs that see thousands of patients annually. However, telehealth activities make up only a small percentage of the total number of healthcare interactions. What will telehealth look like in the future?

The author believes that telehealth activities will increase significantly in the future and they will become much more commonplace. This expansion of telehealth activities will mirror the increased use and capabilities of computers and the Internet. This is because an increasing number of telehealth networks are using computer-based workstations and linking using the Internet. At the present time, dedicated videoconferencing systems are usually used to conduct real-time telehealth consultations; however, as computing power and Internet bandwidth increase, more and more telehealth will be conducted on high-end desktops or wireless mobile computers. In addition, store and forward telehealth (similar to sending an email with an attachment) will make up the majority of telehealth consultations. Most people will also have telehealth capabilities in their homes, and some will regularly use mobile telehealth devices.

Future Telehealth Scenario

The year is 2015. Joe Smith is 68 and recently retired to an adult community. He and his wife chose the community because they both have chronic diseases and the builder informed them that the community has state-of-the-art health monitoring built into the homes, plus the ability to link to a nurse or physician as needed via telehealth technology. Joe gets up at 7:00. He steps on a scale in the bathroom, which informs him that his weight has increased almost 5 lbs overnight. It also senses the temperature of his feet and notes that one area is two degrees higher than it should be. He then goes to the bathroom and the toilet automatically performs a urinalysis, finding some WBC, nitrates, and glucose in the urine. The scale and toilet wirelessly transmit the collected data to a computer/server in the house, which compares the data to parameters that have been pre-defined by his physician. The values fall outside normal, so Joe is informed that there is an abnormality. At the same time, a message is transmitted from the server to a nursing call center. The nurse at the call center receives the message and pulls up the patient's electronic chart, then calls the patient over a videophone. While the patient talks to the nurse, a sensor on the videophone records his vitals, including heart rate, blood pressure, temperature, and oxygen saturation. This is also transmitted automatically to the nurse to review, who notes an elevated temperature and heart rate. The nurse asks him to focus the phone on his lower legs and push on the skin near his ankles. The video shows pitting edema. He is also asked to take a few high-resolution pictures with the videophone of his left foot, which had the higher temperature. The nurse notes some swelling and redness near the big toe plus some streaking up the lower leg. The nurse informs Joe that she is concerned that his congestive heart failure might be worsening, that his blood sugar is elevated, that he may have a bladder and foot infection. She recommends that he go down the block to the telehealth room at the community center and have a formal teleconsultation with his physician. The nurse emails the video clips, still images, sound clips plus data over a secure link to the patient's physician. The patient arrives at the community center and uses a videoconferencing system to link to his physician. The physician conducts a remote consultation with the help of the telehealth nurse. This includes listening to the patient's heart and lungs using a wireless, electronic stethoscope. The physician hears decreased air entry and fine crackle breath sounds at both lung bases. It is recommended that the patient get a digital x-ray, EKG, and blood tests (using a single drop of blood), which are all done at the telehealth room. The images, EKG tracing, and test results are all autoanalyzed by an expert system and then sent to the doctor. The physician confirms an acute exacerbation of CHF and hyperglycemia (out of control diabetes), likely secondary to a left-foot cellulitis and bladder infection. In addition, a bacterial infection has also been found in the blood. The physician has a discussion with the nurse and they decide that the patient has too many issues to be monitored from home. Instead the patient is told he should probably go to a hospital. Joe is surprised as he has not had to see a doctor in person for years (his health problems have always been caught soon enough).

Summary

Telehealth is the use of information and communications technology to deliver health services and exchange health information when distance separates the participants. Although telehealth has been around for a number of decades, it is only in the last few years that it has become a practical alternative to traditional in-person consultations. Healthcare professionals primarily work with patients and each other in a face-to-face environment. Telehealth introduces a new way to communicate. Telehealth usually limits healthcare professional communications in a number of ways, such as decreasing the amount of sensory stimuli transmitted and decreasing the quality of the information. All these limitations impact healthcare professional communications. As long as telehealth is set up properly and health professionals are aware of the limitations of telehealth and adapt to them, telehealth has the potential to benefit healthcare communications and subsequently improve health services at a distance. The aerospace industry was one of the pioneers in telehealth and has been involved in a number of terrestrially based telehealth projects. There are many lessons to be learned from these activities in regards to healthcare communications. Currently, telehealth is used in only a small percentage of healthcare interactions. In the future, it is expected that telehealth will become much more commonplace, with telehealth workstations located in every healthcare facility, and many people having telehealth capabilities in their homes.

References

Angood, P.B., Doarn, C.R., Holaday, L., Nicogossian, A.E. and Merrell, R.C. (1998), 'The Spacebridge to Russia Project: Internet-based Telemedicine', *Telemedicine Journal* 4:4, 305–11.

Ball, C.J. and McLaren, P.M. (1995), 'Comparability of Face-to-face and Videolink Administration of the Brief Psychiatric Rating Scale', *American Journal of Psychiatry* 152:6, 958–9.

Ball, C.J., McLaren, P.M., Summerfield, A.B., Lipsedge, M.S. and Watson, J.P. (1995), 'A Comparison of Communication Modes in Adult Psychiatry', *Journal of Telemedicine and Telecare* 1:1, 22–6.

Ball, C.J., McLaren, P.M. and Watson, J.P. (1996), 'Psychiatry: Communications Technology and Education in Mental Health', *Journal of Telemedicine and Telecare* 2:2, 62–4.

Bashshur, R. (1980), 'Technology Serves the People: The Story of a Co-operative Telemedicine Project by NASA, the Indian Health Service and the Papago People. STARPAHC', Superintendent of Documents, US Government Printing Office, Washington, DC, 20402 (Stock No. 017-028-00009-0).

Bischoff, R. (2004), 'Considerations in the Use of Telecommunications as a Primary Treatment Medium: The Application of Behavioral Telehealth to Marriage and Family Therapy', *American Journal of Family Therapy* 32:3, 173–87.

Carey, L.S. and Russell, E.S. (1978), Canadian Telemedicine Experiment U-6. Final Report of a Telemedicine Experiment in Canada Using Satellite, Hermes: A Telecommunications Experiment between a Remote Nursing Station (Kashechewan), a Base Hospital (Moose Factory General) and a Health Science Center (University of Western Ontario). January.

Carey, L.S., Russell, E.S., Johnston, E.E. and Wilkins, W.W. (1979), 'Radiologic Consultation to a Remote Canadian Hospital Using Hermes Spacecraft', *Journal of the Canadian Association of Radiologists* 30:1, 12–20.

Conrath, D.W., Dunn, E.V. and Higgins, C.A. (1983), *Evaluating Telecommunications Technology in Medicine* (Washington, DC: Artech House).

DeBakey, M.E. (1995), 'Telemedicine Has Now Come of Age', *Telemedicine Journal* 1:1, 3–4.

Doarn, C.R., Ferguson, E.W. and Nicogossian, A.E. (1996), 'Telemedicine and Telescience in the US Space Program', paper presented at the 20th ISTS, Gifu, Japan, May 19–25, 1996, available at: <http://www.quasar.org/21698/nasa/gifu.html>.

Doran, D.I., Sidani, S., Keatings, M. and Doidge, D. (2002), 'An Empirical Test of the Nursing Role Effectiveness Model', *Journal of Advanced Nursing 38:1*, 29–39.

Dunn, E.V., Conrath, D.W., Bloor, W.G. and Tranquada, B. (1977), 'An Evaluation of Four Telemedicine Systems for Primary Care', *Health Services Research* 77:5, 748–54.

Dunn, E.V. and Higgins, C.A. (1984), 'Telemedicine in Canada: An Overview', *Dimensions in Health Services* 61:7, 16–18.

Elford, D.R. (1996), personal experience while completing Telemedicine Fellowship at the Telemedicine Centre in Tromso, Norway.

Elford, D.R. (1997), 'The Child Telepsychiatry Project – A Randomized Controlled Trial. Community Medicine', Master's thesis, Memorial University of Newfoundland.

Elford, D.R. (1998), 'Telemedicine Activities at Memorial University of Newfoundland: A Historical Review, 1975–1997', *Telemedicine Journal* 4:3, 207–24.

Elford, D.R., White, H., Bowering, R., Ghandi, A., Maddigan, B., St. John, K., House, M., Harnett, J., West, R. and Battcock, A. (2000), 'A Randomized, Controlled Trial of Child Psychiatric Assessments Conducted Using Videoconferencing', *Journal of Telemedicine and Telecare* 6:2, 73–82.

Elford, D.R., White, H., St. John, K., Maddigan, B., Ghandi, M. and Bowering, R. (2001), 'A Prospective Satisfaction Study and Cost Analysis of a Pilot Child Telepsychiatry Service in Newfoundland', *Journal of Telemedicine and Telecare* 7:2, 73–81.

Ferguson, E.W., Doarn, C.R. and Scott, J.C. (1995), 'Survey of Global Telemedicine', *The Electronic Library* 13:4, 35–46.

Gershon-Cohen, J. and Cooley, A.G. (1950), 'Telediagnosis', Radiology 55:4, 582–7.

Heine, C. and Browning, C. (2004), 'The Communication and Psychosocial Perceptions of Older Adults with Sensory Loss: A Qualitative Study', *Aging and Society* 24:1, 113–30.

Higgins, S.E. and Routhieux, R.L. (1999), 'A Multiple-level Analysis of Hospital Team Effectiveness', *Health Care Supervisor 17:4,* 1–13.

House, A.M. (1980), 'Application of Anik B Telephony Channels to Meet Health and Education Needs in Remote Areas', Telemedicine Center document.

House, A.M., McNamara, W.C. and Roberts, J.M. (1977), Report on Memorial University's Experimental Use of the Communications Satellite 'Hermes' in Telemedicine. Final report submitted to the Department of Communications. January.

House, A.M. and Roberts, J. (1977), 'Telemedicine in Canada', *Canadian Medical Association Journal* 117:4, 386–8.

Irvine Doran, D., Baker, G.R., Murray, M., Bohnen, J., Zahn, C., Sidani, S. and Carryer, J. (2002), 'Achieving Clinical Improvement: An Interdisciplinary Intervention', *Health Care Management Review 27:4,* 42–56.

Irvine Doran, D., McGillis Hall, L., Sidani, S., O'Brien-Pallas, L., Donner, G., Baker, G. and Pink, G.H. (2001), 'Nursing Staff Mix and Patient Outcome Achievement: The Mediating Role of Nurse Communication', *International Nursing Perspective 1:2–3,* 74–83.

Joint Commission on Accreditation of Healthcare Organizations (2004), 'Root Causes of Sentinel Events: All Categories, 1995–2004', available at: <www.jointcommission. org/NR/rdonlyres/FA465646-5F5F-4543-AC8F-E8AF6571E372/0/root_cause_se.jpg>.

Jong, M.K.K., Horwood, K., Robbins, C.W. and Elford, D.R. (2001), 'A Model for Remote Communities using Store and Forward Telemedicine to Reduce Health Care Cost', *Canadian Journal of Rural Medicine* 6:1, 15–20.

Keeports, D. (2006), 'Estimating the Speed of Light from Earth–Moon Communication', *The Physics Teacher* 44:7, 414–15.

Llewellyn, C.H. (1995), 'The Role of Telemedicine in Disaster Medicine', *Journal of Medical Systems* 19:1, 29–34.

NASA (1974), Space Technology in Remote Health Care, NASA publication JSC-09161 (Houston, TX, August, 1974),

Nicogossian, A.E., Huntoon, C.L. and Pool, S.L. (1994), *Space Physiology and Medicine*, 3rd edition (Philadelphia: Lea and Febiger).

Nunavut Government (2004), <http://www.telehealth.ca/downloads/cipa.pdf> or <http://cipa.com/award_winners/winners_04/NunavutGov.html> or <http://www.rnantnu.ca/biennial/bridging_gap.ppt>.

Rafferty, A.M., Ball, J. and Aiken, L.H. (2001), 'Are Teamwork and Professional Autonomy Compatible, and Do They Result in Improved Hospital Care?', *Quality in Health Care 10:II*, ii32–7.

Roberge, F.A., Page, G., Sylvestre, J. and Chahlaoui, J. (1982), 'Telemedicine in Northern Quebec', *Canadian Medical Association Journal* 127:8, 707–9.

Roberts, J. and Picot, J. (1981), A Telehealth – Telemedicine Bibliography (Ottawa: Council on Medical Education, Canadian Medical Association).

Stallings, W. (2005), *Wireless Communications and Networks*, 2nd edition (New Jersey: Prentice Hall).

Wachter, R.M. (2006), 'International Teleradiology', *New England Journal of Medicine* 354:7, 662–3.

Willis, C.E., Leckie, R.G., Brink, L. and Goeringer, F. (1995), 'Integrated Telemedicine Workstation for Intercontinental Grand Rounds', in Y. Kim (ed.), *Proceedings of SPIE- Medical Imaging 1995: Image Display* 2431, 374–81.

Wittson, C.L. and Benschoter, R.A. (1972), 'Two-way Television: Helping the Medical Center Reach Out', *American Journal of Psychiatry* 129:5, 136–9.

Zarate, C.A., Weinstock, L., Cukor, P., Mroabito, C., Leahy, L., Burns, C. and Baer, L. (1997), 'Applicability of Telemedicine for Assessing Patients with Schizophrenia: Acceptance and Reliability', *Clinical Psychiatry* 58:1, 22–5.

Chapter 14

A Healthcare Team Communication Research Agenda

Christopher P. Nemeth and Robert L. Wears

There is always an easy solution to every human problem—neat, plausible, and wrong.
H.L. Mencken

Research into clinical work reveals the day-to-day difficulties that healthcare workers confront, as well as the means they conceive to surmount them. These are the *messy details* (Nemeth, Cook and Woods 2004a) that comprise the actual clinical experience in which communication plays such a vital role. This approach contrasts with the popular rush to provide solutions for reported patient safety problems without the benefit of understanding the problem. The notion that a "silver bullet" can solve patient safety problems is neat, plausible … and wrong. David Musson provided an example of such a solution in Chapter 4: crew resource management (CRM). While interest continues in the use of CRM to improve healthcare communication, the data do not support such enthusiasm. Rigorous reviews such as Salas et al. (2001) have surveyed the literature on crew resource management and found that, while CRM seems to have a positive effect on behavior, its effect on safety is unproven. CRM is not the only popular trend. Surveys such as Sexton et al. (2006) have applied the aviation model to healthcare by assessing *perceptions* of clinical teamwork. Surveys of perceptions, though, do not reveal what actually happens in the clinical setting. Improvements to healthcare team communications are intended to ultimately improve healthcare for clinicians and patients alike.

Improving Healthcare Team Communication grounds the understanding of issues related to healthcare team communications in well-considered, methodical, valid research. The chapters have drawn the connection between original research into aviation and aerospace team communication and current work that is underway in healthcare. Each of the chapters reflects original research of actual work as it is performed. This is in marked contrast to the way that work is imagined by those who have not done it, or by practitioners trying to reconstruct what they have done. The chapters provide part of the foundation of understanding technical work, which is the planning and management of care.

A select number of researchers featured in Nemeth, Cook and Woods (2004b) currently use *systems engineering* (Samaras and Horst 2005) and *cognitive engineering* (Woods and Roth 1988) to reveal and support sharp end (operator) cognition. Emily Patterson analyzed an adverse event involving communication of an order for an oncology medication, using a case-based analysis to shed light on how communication mechanisms and breakdowns contribute to undesired outcomes. Anne-Sophie Nyssen assessed the effect of adding new technology such as an infusion device and robotic surgical system on healthcare team collaboration. Yan Xiao discovered care providers are predisposed to respond in certain ways to acoustic alarms, due to the large numbers of alarms, confusion among alarms, temporary episodes of high workload, and external economic pressures. He also uncovered a number of proactive interventions at unit and organizational levels that sometimes had unanticipated effects. Meghan Dierks demonstrated how the implementation of a "count" protocol during surgical procedures to reduce the likelihood of leaving a tool in a body cavity actually had negative consequences. Stephanie Guerlain determined that viewing video clips of procedures improved medical student perception and procedural knowledge about laparoscopic surgery. Helen Klein and Amy Meininger found that as Type II diabetics try to manage their own care, they typically do not understand the dynamics of controlling their disease, which often renders their efforts ineffective.

Other similar contributions to understanding group cognition can be found in two special issues of the journal *Cognition, Technology and Work* on the large scale coordination of cognitive work (Nemeth 2007a and 2007b). In the first special issue, authors explore the use of naturalistic decision making (NDM) methods to reveal how groups of operators have developed ways to perform inter-group work in real world settings. The first two papers examine theoretical issues in coordination at large scale. Björn Johansson and Erik Hollnagel's paper discusses how control at large scale emerges as a product of human interaction. Jill Ritter et al. propose a framework to assist the development of widely distributed systems and teams to support military logistics coordination. The second two papers describe the results of efforts to simulate large scale coordination. Laura Militello et al. account for the successes and shortcomings among ad hoc teams that sought to manage emergency response to natural disasters. Colin Mackenzie et al. explored large scale coordination at international scale, experimenting with complex communications technologies to support expert decision making during an emergency. The final paper by Phil Smith et al. discusses improvements to managing the complex, dynamic US national air transportation system. Larry Hirshhorn's reflections offer insights into what such work may reveal.

In the second special issue, authors focus on large scale coordination in healthcare. Yan Xiao and colleagues found the goal of operating room (OR) team stability is nested within longer term goals of equity in the assignment of work and allocation of resources. Nemeth et al. explained how clearing space to accommodate sicker patients in a patient care unit is nested within the longer term goal of accommodating the demand for care. Sara Albolino and Richard Cook revealed how making sense of diagnostic and therapeutic needs "on the fly" in a hospital intensive care unit (ICU) is nested within a plan for a course of treatment that serves as a defense against future days, weeks, or months to come. Anne-Sophie Nyssen discovered how local action by workers outstrips the ability of centralized ICT (for example, medical records) to share information, which resulted in a failure to integrate crucial healthcare information among medical units. Emily Patterson et al. found that cross-checking methods such as hand-offs can make processes more evident, and detect and correct erroneous assessments and actions, although poor versions can create gaps in care continuity.

These contributions have added new insight to the conventional view of healthcare and its management. We believe the above authors would agree that this is just the start of understanding a complex and little explored domain. Where do we go from here? The next section lays out an agenda for how to conduct substantive work in this area.

A Research Agenda

The ability to truly improve healthcare requires a well-grounded understanding of the nature of actual work. This understanding requires insight that comes from thoughtful, repeated, deep looks into the way work is performed. Judith Orasanu and Ute Fischer's thorough understanding of aircrew communications described in Chapter 3 has taken years to cultivate. Healthcare, which is an even more complex and variable work domain than aviation, will take even longer to understand. The process requires time because the complexities of the daily work setting are too entangled to gain insight by asking for opinions or making quick, superficial observations. It is necessary to visit and revisit actual work settings. Such rigorous scrutiny makes it possible to discover the driving forces that underlie work; forces that are apparently simple, but are in reality quite complex.

This approach has a direct bearing on the communication of information within and among teams. As in other high hazard settings, expertise (Feltovich, Ford and Hoffman 1997) in healthcare is the ability to know what is, and what is not, important. Healthcare activities rely on the acquisition, portrayal, and analysis of therapeutic and diagnostic information as an integral part of individual patient care. The need for accurate, timely information exists not only at the individual patient level but also at the unit level—that is, the OR, ICU, and emergency department (ED). Unit-level planning and management directs who will get care, what type of care will be provided, and when it will be provided. As a result, the daily work of the clinician requires representations that serve as a map of the ever-changing territory of work that must be successfully navigated (Rasmussen and Pejtersen 1995: 132). What information is presented, and how it is presented, depends on the individual and group cognitive work that it is intended to support. Individual elements of information vary enormously in the length of time that they remain reliable, and their weight depends a great deal on their context and other elements that are present in the same moment. Language provides us with a useful analogy. Linguistic signs have little intrinsic meaning, but derive it instead from their relationship to other signs (Cilliers 1998). All well and good, but what can we do to proceed?

As two of their strategies to improve patient safety, the Institute of Medicine (Kohn, Corrigan and Donaldson 2000) advocated improving access to accurate, timely information, and making relevant information available at point of patient care. Soon thereafter, the IOM (Aspden et al. 2004: 6, 8, 17, 20) recommended developing a national health information infrastructure, facilitating the use of decision support in clinical information systems. The recent National Academy of Engineering/IOM report (Reid et al. 2005) encourages federal research and mission agencies to significantly increase their support for research to advance the application and utility of systems engineering in healthcare, including research on new systems tools and the adaptation, implementation, and improvement of existing tools at all levels. The NAE/IOM report recommends the creation of 30 to 50 multidisciplinary research centers that include both human factors and healthcare professionals. The report also recommends three initiatives for these research centers: (1) demonstrate and disseminate the use of tools that support communication and coordination—this includes, but is not limited to, information and telecommunications systems; (2) conduct basic and applied research on the systems challenges to healthcare; and (3) educate current and future healthcare researchers in the science, practice, and challenges of systems engineering for healthcare. Woods and Cook (2002) outline nine steps that would make it possible to realize these goals:

1. Pursue second stories beneath the surface to discover multiple contributors
2. Escape the hindsight bias
3. Understand work as performed at the sharp end of the system
4. Search for systemic vulnerabilities
5. Study how practice creates safety
6. Search for underlying patterns
7. Examine how change will produce new vulnerabilities and paths to failure
8. Use new technology to support and enhance human expertise
9. Tame complexity through new forms of feedback

Translating these steps into action requires a few essential initiatives:

1. *Develop a coherent program of study* using healthcare institutions as living laboratories. Academic medical centers are in a position to coordinate efforts to study technical work, including communication. However, they may not be in a position to successfully lead it (Wears, Perry and Sutcliffe 2005). These programs will need an infrastructure to coordinate research scope, methods, and initiatives in a substantive, long-term collaboration with research professionals from other fields such as human factors.
2. *Develop a program of study to build a base of understanding and improve practice*. Individual studies performed on a shoestring are necessarily limited in scope and offer only limited "keyhole" views of a complex world. Support for ongoing research in healthcare technical work will make it possible to understand healthcare as a whole, not just as individual parts such as communication. Ongoing studies that build on the work of others will develop reliable, useful results.
3. *Cultivate a cadre of human factors and healthcare professionals* who are adept at this kind of research. Produce a continuing stream of well-qualified and trained researchers with a clear career path who will be able to carry this work forward through decades, not a project at a time. This research cadre will be well qualified to engage crucial issues that are related to information and

clinical care, but are not currently grounded in science. Such issues include: "How do clinicians make decisions with regard to changes in their approach to a particular patient?" and "How do clinician working groups recognize, identify, and re-prioritize problems in their work?"

Funding, attitude, and organizational support need to change in order to pursue such changes. Above all, a constancy of purpose will be crucial to success. At the moment, studies in technical work are done occasionally when grant funding permits, or as unfunded initiatives. This fragments and blunts the progress that could be made. An ongoing program of activities, rather than occasional studies, would develop the intellectual capital and data that is essential for such a body of knowledge.

Summary

Human factors skills and knowledge can be successfully teamed with healthcare expertise to inform the work of healthcare, including team communications. It is difficult at this stage, though, to see a career for the study of technical work in healthcare until academic, professional, and funding organizations provide a path to follow. Manager and senior clinician support for joint research initiatives by human factors professionals and clinicians can open the way.

References

Aspden, P., Corrigan, J., Wolcott, J. and Erikson, S. (2004), Patient Safety: Achieving a New Standard of Care (Washington, DC: The National Academies Press).

Cilliers, P. (1998), *Complexity and Postmodernism: Understanding Complex Systems* (London: Routledge).

Cook, R., Woods, D. and Miller, C. (1998), *A Tale of Two Stories: Contrasting Views of Patient Safety* (Chicago: National Health Care Safety Council of the National Patient Safety Foundation, American Medical Association), available at: <http://www.npsf.org>, accessed June 8, 2002.

Feltovich, P.J., Ford, K.M. and Hoffman, R.R. (eds) (1997), *Expertise in Context: Human and Machine* (Cambridge, MA: MIT Press).

Kohn, L., Corrigan, J. and Donaldson, M. (eds) (2000), *To Err is Human. Building a Safer Health System* (Washington, DC: National Academies Press).

Mencken, H.L. (1949), 'The Divine Afflatus', Chapter 25, *A Mencken Chrestomathy*, 443. Cited in S. Platt (ed.), *Respectfully Quoted: A Dictionary of Quotations* (New York: Barnes and Noble Books) 325.

Nemeth, C. (2007a), 'Groups at Work: Lessons from Research into Large Scale Coordination', in C. Nemeth (ed.), Special Issue on Large Scale Coordination, *Cognition, Technology and Work* 9:1, 1–4.

Nemeth, C. (2007b), 'Healthcare Groups at Work: Further Lessons from Research into Large Scale Coordination', in C. Nemeth (ed.), Second Special Issue on Large Scale Coordination, *Cognition, Technology and Work* 9:3, 127–76.

Nemeth, C., Cook, R. and Woods, D. (2004a), 'The Messy Details: Insights from Technical Work in Healthcare', in C. Nemeth, R. Cook and D. Woods (eds), Special Issue on Studies in Healthcare Technical Work, *IEEE Transactions on Systems, Man and Cybernetics-Part A* 34:6, 689–92.

Nemeth, C., Cook, R. and Woods, D. (eds) (2004b), Special Issue on Studies in Healthcare Technical Work, *IEEE Transactions on Systems, Man and Cybernetics-Part A* 34:6.

Rasmussen, J. and Pejtersen, A. (1995), 'Virtual Ecology of Work', in J. Flasch, P. Hancock, J. Caird and K. Vincente (eds), *Global Perspectives on the Ecology of Human-Machine Systems* (Hillsdale, NJ: Lawrence Erlbaum Associates) 121–56.

Reid, P.R., Compton, W.D., Grossman, J.H. and Fanjiang, G. (eds) (2005), *Building a Better Delivery System: A New Engineering/Health Care Partnership* (Washington, DC: The National Academies Press).

Salas, E., Burke, C.S., Bowers, C.A. and Wilson, K.A. (2001), 'Team Training in the Skies: Does Crew Resource Management (CRM) Training Work?', *Human Factors* 43:4, 641–74.

Samaras, G.M. and Horst, R.L. (2005), 'A Systems Engineering Perspective on the Human-centered Design of Health Information Systems', *Journal of Biomedical Informatics* 38:1, 61–74.

Sexton, J.B., Makary, M.A., Tersigni, A.R., Pryor, D., Hendrich, A., Thomas, E.J., Holzmueller, C.G., Knight, A.P., Wu, Y. and Pronovost, P.J. (2006), 'Teamwork in the Operating Room: Frontline Perspectives among Hospitals and Operating Room Personnel', *Anesthesiology* 105:5, 877–84.

Wears, R., Perry, S.J. and Sutcliffe, K.M. (2005), 'The Medicalization of Patient Safety', *Journal of Patient Safety* 1:1, 4–6.

Woods, D.D. and Cook, R.I. (2002), 'Nine Steps to Move Forward from Error', *Cognition, Technology and Work* 4:2, 137–44.

Woods, D. and Roth, E. (1998), 'Cognitive Systems Engineering', in M. Helander (ed.), *Handbook of Human-Computer Interaction* (New York: North Holland) 3–43.

Index